American Medical Association
Physicians dedicated to the health of America

Council on Ethical and Judicial Affairs

Code of Medical Ethics

Current Opinions with Annotations

W9-AHA-563

1998–1999 Edition

Annotations prepared by the
Southern Illinois University Schools of Medicine and Law

Additional copies (product number OP632398) may be ordered from:
Order Department
American Medical Association
515 N State Street
Chicago, IL 60610
800 621-8335

Also available in an unannotated version.

ISBN 0-89970-960-5

BP25:98-500:2M:6/98

Contents

1.00 Introduction

2.00 Opinions on Social Policy Issues

3.00   Opinions on Interprofessional Relations

4.00   Opinions on Hospital Relations

5.00   Opinions on Confidentiality, Advertising, and Communications Media Relations

6.00   Opinions on Fees and Charges

7.00   Opinions on Physician Records

8.00   Opinions on Practice Matters

9.00   Opinions on Professional Rights and Responsibilities

Appendix

Preface

This edition of *Current Opinions with Annotations* of the Council on Ethical and Judicial Affairs replaces all previous editions of *Current Opinions* and includes opinions based on reports adopted through June 1997. It is one component of the American Medical Association's Code of Ethics; the other components are the Principles of Medical Ethics, Fundamental Elements of the Patient-Physician Relationship, and the Reports of the Council on Ethical and Judicial Affairs. The Principles and Fundamental Elements precede the opinions in this volume.

The Principles of Medical Ethics are the primary component of the Code. They establish the core ethical principles from which the other components of the Code are derived. The Principles were most recently revised in 1980.

Fundamental Elements of the Patient-Physician Relationship enunciates the basic rights to which patients are entitled from their physicians.

Current Opinions with Annotations reflects the application of the Principles of Medical Ethics to 140 specific ethical issues in medicine, including health care rationing, genetic testing, withdrawal of life-sustaining treatment, and family violence. Much as courts of law elaborate on constitutional principles in their holdings, the Council develops the meaning of the Principles of Medical Ethics in its opinions. Accordingly, each opinion is followed by one or more roman numerals that identify the Principle(s) from which the opinion is derived.

Each opinion is also followed by a list of annotations reflecting citations to the opinion in judicial rulings and the medical, ethical, and legal literature.

The Reports—from which many of the opinions are derived—discuss the rationale behind the Council's opinions, providing a detailed analysis of the relevant ethical considerations.

All four components of the AMA's Code of Ethics need to be consulted to determine the Association's positions on ethical issues. In addition, the AMA's House of Delegates at times issues statements on ethical issues. These statements are contained in a separate publication, the AMA *Policy Compendium*. Because the Council on Ethical and Judicial Affairs is responsible for determining the AMA's positions on ethical issues, statements by the House of Delegates should be construed as the view of the House of Delegates but not as the ethics policy of the Association.

Medical ethics involve the professional responsibilities and obligations of physicians. Behavior relating to medical etiquette or custom is not addressed in *Current Opinions with Annotations*. The opinions which follow are intended as guides to responsible professional behavior.

No one Principle of Medical Ethics can stand alone or be individually applied to a situation. In all instances, it is the overall intent and influence of the Principles of Medical Ethics which shall measure ethical behavior for the physician. Council opinions are issued under its authority to interpret the Principles of Medical Ethics and to investigate general ethical conditions and all matters pertaining to the relations of physicians to one another and to the public.

The Council on Ethical and Judicial Affairs encourages comments and suggestions for future editions of this publication.

Council on Ethical and Judicial Affairs

1996–1997
Charles W. Plows, MD, Chair

Robert M. Tenery, Jr., MD, Vice Chair

Alan Hartford, MD, PhD

Dwight Miller

Leonard J. Morse, MD

Herbert Rakatanksy, MD

Frank A. Riddick, Jr., MD

Victoria N. Ruff, MD

George T. Wilkins, Jr., MD

1997–1998
Robert M. Tenery, Jr., MD, Chair

Herbert Rakatanksy, MD, Vice Chair

Alan Hartford, MD, PhD

John C. Madden, III

Leonard J. Morse, MD

John M. O'Bannon, III, MD

Frank A. Riddick, Jr., MD

Victoria N. Ruff, MD

George T. Wilkins, Jr., MD

Linda L. Emanuel, MD, PhD, Vice President, Ethics Standards

Michael Ile, JD, Council Secretary

Stephen R. Latham, JD, PhD, Council Secretary

Jeffrey C. Munson, Staff Associate

Jessica W. Berg, JD, Staff Consultant

H. Nina Kim, Staff Associate

Blaire S. Osgood, Staff Associate

P. John Seward, MD, AMA Executive Vice President

Lynn E. Jensen, PhD, AMA Executive Vice President

Daniel Seckinger, MD, AMA Group Vice President, Professional Standards

Reed V. Tuckson, MD, AMA Senior Vice President, Professional Standards

History

The Oath of Hippocrates, a brief statement of principles, has come down through history as a living statement of ideals to be cherished by the physician. This Oath was conceived some time during the period of Grecian greatness, probably in the fifth century B.C. It protected rights of the patient and appealed to the inner and finer instincts of the physician without imposing sanctions or penalties on him or her. Other civilizations subsequently developed written principles, but the Oath of Hippocrates (Christianized in the tenth or eleventh century A.D. to eliminate reference to pagan gods) has remained in Western Civilization as an expression of ideal conduct for the physician.

The most significant contribution to Western medical ethical history subsequent to Hippocrates was made by Thomas Percival, an English physician, philosopher, and writer. In 1803, he published his Code of Medical Ethics. His personality, his interest in sociological matters, and his close association with the Manchester Infirmary led to the preparation of a "scheme of professional conduct relative to hospitals and other charities" from which he drafted the code that bears his name.

At the first official meeting of the American Medical Association at Philadelphia in 1847, the two principal items of business were the establishment of a code of ethics and the creation of minimum requirements for medical education and training. Although the Medical Society of the State of New York and the Medico-Chirurgical Society of Baltimore had formal written codes of medical ethics prior to this time, it is clear the AMA's first adopted Code of Ethics was based on Percival's Code.

In general, the language and concepts of the original Code adopted by the Association in 1847 remained the same throughout the years. There were revisions, of course, which reflected the temper of the times and the eternal quest to express basic concepts with clarity. Major revisions did occur in 1903, 1912, 1947, and 1994.

In December 1955, an attempt was made to distinguish medical ethics from matters of etiquette. A draft of a two-part code seeking to accomplish this was submitted to the House of Delegates at that time but was not accepted. This proposal was, in effect, a separation of then existing statements found in the Principles into two categories. Little or no change was made in the language of the 48 sections of the Principles.

Subsequently, in June 1956, a seemingly radical proposal was submitted to the House of Delegates for consideration. This proposal, a short version of the Principles, was discussed at the December 1956 session of the House after wide publication and broad consideration among members of the medical profession. It was postponed for final consideration until the June 1957 meeting of the House of Delegates, when the short version was adopted.

The format of the Principles adopted in June 1957 is a change from the format of the Principles promulgated by Percival in 1803 and accepted by the Association in 1847. Ten short sections, preceded by a preamble, "succinctly express the fundamental concepts embodied in the present (1955) Principles," according to the report of the Council on Constitution and Bylaws. That Council assured the House of Delegates in its June 1957 report that "every basic principle has been preserved; on the other hand, as much as possible of the prolixity and ambiguity which in the past obstructed ready explanation, practical codification and particular selection of basic concepts has been eliminated."

In 1977, the Judicial Council recommended to the House of Delegates that the AMA Principles of Medical Ethics be revised to clarify and update the language, to eliminate reference to gender, and to seek a proper and reasonable balance between professional standards and contemporary legal standards in our changing society. Given the desire of the Judicial Council for a new version of the Principles to be widely accepted and accurately understood, in 1978 the Judicial Council recommended that a special committee of the House be appointed to consider such a revision. This was done in 1980, and the House of Delegates adopted the revision of the AMA Principles of Medical Ethics at its Annual Meeting in June 1980.

In June 1985, the Judicial Council became the Council on Ethical and Judicial Affairs.

Guide to Use of Annotations

Over the years, the AMA Principles of Medical Ethics and the Current Opinions of the Council on Ethical and Judicial Affairs have emerged as an important source of guidance for responsible professional medical behavior, as well as the primary compendium of medical professional value statements in the United States.

The Opinions included in this volume are derived from two sources. The Council may issue Opinions directly at any time, usually during the Annual and Interim meetings of the AMA House of Delegates. Other Opinions are derived from the conclusions or recommendations of longer reports of the Council that are available from the AMA. Many of the reports from which Opinions are derived are also published in peer-reviewed medical journals.

In this volume, an Opinion that is derived from a longer report is followed by a citation to that report and, if applicable, in a peer-reviewed medical journal. Opinions that are issued directly rather than derived from reports are followed by information giving the date of issuance or most recent revision. For some of the older Opinions, however, this information is not available.

The impact of the Principles and Opinions has been significant. In this regard, attorneys and judges have shown an increasing willingness to look to the Principles and Opinions as a predicate for legal advocacy and decision making in matters of health care law and litigation.

Against this backdrop of increasing reliance on the Principles and Opinions, these annotations have been prepared. They are designed to provide a research and reference tool for practitioners, scholars, jurists, and others who seek ready access to the Principles and Opinions in their work.

The annotations include summaries of all reported court decisions and selected state attorney general opinions, which make substantive reference to the Principles or Opinions. Additionally, the annotations summarize selected articles from the medical, legal, and ethical literature.

These materials were gathered on the basis of carefully structured searches of a variety of computerized research services including WESTLAW, LEXIS, and MEDLINE. Further, more generalized review of various medical and legal journals resulted in evaluation of approximately 2,000 articles. The annotations are inclusive through December, 1997.

The annotations have been prepared to maximize their usefulness as reference and research tools. After a brief synopsis of the facts and legal issues, each case annotation focuses on the court's reference to the Principle(s) or Opinion(s) and the role it played in the decision. In addition to the particular source referred to by the court, case annotations include, where necessary, a cross reference to the relevant provision(s) of the present version of the Principles and Opinions.

Journal annotations provide a general summary of the subject article, along with an indication of the specific Principle(s) or Opinion(s) referenced therein. Again, a cross-reference feature is included. For convenience, consistent terminology is used in the journal annotations. When an author generally refers to the Principle or Opinion, the term "references" is used. When a Principle or Opinion is "cited," this term is used. Finally, if an author directly quotes from a Principle or a Current Opinion, then the annotation so indicates.

With respect to both case and journal annotations, specific page references are provided to identify where the Principle(s) or Current Opinion(s) are discussed. This feature is intended to facilitate efficient use of these annotations. A Table of Cases and a Table of Articles also have been compiled to further enhance the usefulness of this compendium.

It is important to recognize that the Principle(s) and Opinion(s) have a long and evolving history. Many of the cases included herein refer to older versions of the Principles and Opinions, some of which have been eliminated or have changed considerably over the years. Nonetheless, these cases may be valuable to the user. Efforts were made to identify the most appropriate provisions of the present Principles and Opinions to which to assign these cases. However, in some instances the correspondence is not exact and the user will need to review carefully the particular case under consideration with respect to the user's specific interests.

As a final observation, it should be noted that the majority of annotations included herein relate to Principle(s) and Opinion(s). Nevertheless, references to the sections on Fundamental Elements of the Patient-Physician Relationship and Patient Responsibilities have been noted in the literature. Accordingly, annotations have been prepared which relate to these sections. This will further enhance the usefulness of this publication.

The annotators would like to express appreciation to Keleigh Biggins, Frank Choi, Michelle Dillon, Charles Ellington, Elizabeth Foster, Jean Kirchner, Elizabeth Lingle, Thomas Morrow, Holly Noyes, Susan Tedrick, and Christopher White, who provided valuable research, editing, and other assistance on this project. Finally, we owe a special debt of thanks to Pamela Graham of the School of Law who handled the difficult task of entry of annotations into the database and preparation of the final manuscript with skill, enthusiasm, and infinite patience.

This project was supported by a grant from the American Medical Association.

Annotators

Theodore R. LeBlang, J.D.
Southern Illinois University
School of Medicine
Department of Medical Humanities

Frank G. Houdek, J.D., M.L.S.
Southern Illinois University
School of Law

W. Eugene Basanta, J.D., LL.M.
Southern Illinois University
School of Law

Connie Poole, A.M.L.S.
Southern Illinois University
School of Medicine
Department of Information and
Communication Sciences

March 1998

American Medical Association
Principles of Medical Ethics

Preamble

The medical profession has long subscribed to a body of ethical statements developed primarily for the benefit of the patient. As a member of this profession, a physician must recognize responsibility not only to patients, but also to society, to other health professionals, and to self. The following Principles adopted by the American Medical Association are not laws, but standards of conduct which define the essentials of honorable behavior for the physician.

I.   A physician shall be dedicated to providing competent medical service with compassion and respect for human dignity.

II. A physician shall deal honestly with patients and colleagues, and strive to expose those physicians deficient in character or competence, or who engage in fraud or deception.

III. A physician shall respect the law and also recognize a responsibility to seek changes in those requirements which are contrary to the best interests of the patient.

IV. A physician shall respect the rights of patients, of colleagues, and of other health professionals, and shall safeguard patient confidences within the constraints of the law.

V.   A physician shall continue to study, apply and advance scientific knowledge, make relevant information available to patients, colleagues, and the public, obtain consultation, and use the talents of other health professionals when indicated.

VI. A physician shall, in the provision of appropriate patient care, except in emergencies, be free to choose whom to serve, with whom to associate, and the environment in which to provide medical services.

VII. A physician shall recognize a responsibility to participate in activities contributing to an improved community.

Fundamental Elements of the Patient-Physician Relationship

From ancient times, physicians have recognized that the health and well-being of patients depends upon a collaborative effort between physician and patient. Patients share with physicians the responsibility for their own health care. The patient-physician relationship is of greatest benefit to patients when they bring medical problems to the attention of their physicians in a timely fashion, provide information about their medical condition to the best of their ability, and work with their physicians in a mutually respectful alliance. Physicians can best contribute to this alliance by serving as their patients' advocate and by fostering these rights:

1. The patient has the right to receive information from physicians and to discuss the benefits, risks, and costs of appropriate treatment alternatives. Patients should receive guidance from their physicians as to the optimal course of action. Patients are also entitled to obtain copies or summaries of their medical records, to have their questions answered, to be advised of potential conflicts of interest that their physicians might have, and to receive independent professional opinions.

2. The patient has the right to make decisions regarding the health care that is recommended by his or her physician. Accordingly, patients may accept or refuse any recommended medical treatment.

3. The patient has the right to courtesy, respect, dignity, responsiveness, and timely attention to his or her needs.

4. The patient has the right to confidentiality. The physician should not reveal confidential communications or information without the consent of the patient, unless provided for by law or by the need to protect the welfare of the individual or the public interest.

5. The patient has the right to continuity of health care. The physician has an obligation to cooperate in the coordination of medically indicated care with other health care providers treating the patient. The physician may not discontinue treatment of a patient as long as further treatment is medically indicated, without giving the patient reasonable assistance and sufficient opportunity to make alternative arrangements for care.

6. The patient has a basic right to have available adequate health care. Physicians, along with the rest of society, should continue to work toward this goal. Fulfillment of this right is dependent on society providing resources so that no patient is deprived of necessary care because of an inability to pay for the care. Physicians should continue their traditional assumption of a part of the responsibility for the medical care of those who cannot afford essential health care. Physicians should advocate for patients in dealing with third parties when appropriate.

Report of the Council on Ethical and Judicial Affairs of the American Medical Association, adopted June 1990.

Updated 1993.

American Medical Association

Principles of Medical Ethics

Preamble

The medical profession has long subscribed to a body of ethical statements developed primarily for the benefit of the patient. As a member of this profession, a physician must recognize responsibility not only to patients, but also to society, to other health professionals, and to self. The following Principles adopted by the American Medical Association are not laws, but standards of conduct which define the essentials of honorable behavior for the physician.

Haw. 1995 After physician was convicted of attempted first degree sexual abuse and kidnapping, the civil court affirmed the Board of Medical Examiner's decision to suspend him from practicing medicine for one year. In challenging Board's action, physician argued, among other things, that convictions were not related to his qualifications, functions, or duties as a physician. The court disagreed with all of physician's points of error on appeal. In considering physician's claim that convictions were not related to his duties as a physician, the court referred to the Preamble as reflecting a duty to the public generally. *Loui v. Board of Medical Examiners*, 78 Haw. 21, 889 P.2d 705, 714.

Ind. 1991 Plaintiff sued physician for injuries caused by physician's patient as the result of medication administered by the physician. Weighing (1) the relationship between the parties, (2) the reasonable foreseeability of harm to the injured party, and (3) public policy, the court held that a physician generally owes no duty to unknown third parties who may be injured by the physician's treatment of a patient. Concurring opinion quoted the Preamble which mandates that a physician "recognize responsibility...to society" arguing that there is no absolute immunity to third-party suits. *Webb v. Jarvis*, 575 N.E.2d 992, 998.

N.J. 1979 In wrongful death action against a psychiatrist whose patient murdered plaintiff's decedent, the court concluded, in accord with Principle 9 (1957) [now Principle IV], that a psychiatrist may owe a duty to warn potential victims of possible danger from psychiatrist's patient despite the general emphasis on confidentiality. The court also noted the Preamble and Principles 1 and 3 (1957) [now revised Preamble, Principle I and Opinion 5.05] in discussing the psychiatrist-patient relationship. *McIntosh v. Milano*, 168 N.J. Super. 466, 403 A.2d 500, 510, 512-13.

Journal 1997 Examines noncompetition clauses in the medical field. Reviews policy concerns and historical and common-law analyses of agreements not to compete. Posits that, the more commercialized the medical profession becomes, the more noncompetition clauses infringe upon the physician-patient relationship and patients' rights. Quotes Opinions 9.02 and 9.06. Cites Preamble and Opinion 6.11. Comment, *Noncompetition Clauses in Physician Employment Contracts in Oregon*, 76 Or. L. Rev. 195, 204-06 (1997).

Journal 1997 Considers principles of confidentiality in the physician-patient relationship. Notes the current trend emphasizing public reporting obligations of physicians to protect members of society. Emphasizes need for balance between patient rights and societal interests. Quotes Principle IV and Opinion 5.05. References Preamble. Jozefowicz, *The Case Against Having "Professional Privilege" in the Physician-Patient Relationship*, 16 Med. & L. 385, 386-87, 391 (1997).

Journal 1997 Discusses the need for balance between business ethics and medical ethics in the context of managed care. Explores two models for integrating ethics and managed care. Proposes the adoption of a collective responsibility model to improve quality of care. Quotes Principles I, II, III, IV, and V. Cites Preamble. References Opinion 8.13. Regan, *Regulating the Business of Medicine: Models for Integrating Ethics and Managed Care*, 30 Colum. J.L. & Soc. Probs. 635, 651, 656, 657 (1997).

Journal 1996 Considers the impact of gag clauses on the physician-patient relationship. Undertakes an extensive legal, ethical, and policy analysis. Concludes that gag clauses are violative of legal and ethical principles. Quotes Principles II, V, and VI, and Fundamental Elements (1). Cites Preamble. Martin & Bjerknes, *The Legal and Ethical Implications of Gag Clauses in Physician Contracts*, XXII Am. J. Law & Med. 433, 465-66 (1996).

Journal 1996 Considers prearraignment forensic evaluations. Notes the prohibition against use of such evaluations. Examines underlying ethical precepts. Observes that principles of beneficence are misapplied to forensic psychiatry in this context. Advocates a new ethical framework. Quotes Preamble. References Principle IV and Opinion 5.05. Ornish, Mills, & Ornish, *Prearraignment Forensic Evaluations: Toward a New Policy*, 24 Bull. Am. Acad. Psychiatry Law 453, 454, 469 (1996).

Journal 1995 Examines the metaphor of physicians as fiduciaries. Considers how the law holds physicians accountable in this regard. Discusses limits to this way of perceiving the physician-patient relationship in a changing health care environment. Quotes Preamble. Cites Opinion 8.03 (1986) [now Opinion 8.032]. Rodwin, *Strains in the Fiduciary Metaphor: Divided Physician Loyalties and Obligations in a Changing Health Care System*, XXI Am. J. Law & Med. 241, 246, 250 (1995).

Journal 1994 Reviews the evolution of the physician-patient relationship. Describes legal responses to increasing awareness of the importance of ensuring patient autonomy. Examines the changing health care delivery environment. Concludes with a discussion of the impact of these changes on patient participation in medical decision-making. Quotes Preamble, Principles I, II, III, IV, V, and VI, Fundamental Elements (1) and (2), and Opinions 1.02 and 8.07 (1981) [now Opinion 8.08]. Cites Opinion 1.01. Szczygiel, *Beyond Informed Consent*, 21 Ohio N.U.L. Rev. 171, 217, 218, 220, 225, 226, 256 (1994).

Journal 1993 Discusses ethical issues that may arise in the context of caring for the critically ill. Emphasizes the need for organization of patient care when multiple providers are involved. Proposes solutions to ethical dilemmas that confront providers in these types of situations. Quotes Preamble. Bruening, Andrew, & Smith, *Concurrent Care: An Ethical Issue for Family Physicians*, 36 J. Fam. Practice 606, 607 (1993).

Journal 1991 Examines the informed consent doctrine and how it was broadened in *Moore v. Regents of the University of California*. Concludes that, in California, under *Moore*, a physician must disclose to patients any economic or research interest he or she might have in the patient's medical treatment. Quotes Preamble to Principles. Guise, *Expansion of the Scope of Disclosure Required Under the Informed Consent Doctrine: Moore v. The Regents of the University of California*, 28 San Diego L. Rev. 455, 462 (1991).

Journal 1990 Discusses the moral dilemma in deciding whether to withdraw artificial nutrition and hydration from a patient and the appropriate role of the judiciary. States that part of the reason for judicial activism in this private area is because legislatures have not adequately expressed public policy. Concludes that judicial decisions do not represent the moral viewpoint of society and that moral pronouncements should not be made in the courtroom. Quotes Preamble, Principles I, II, III, IV, V, VI, and VII, and Opinion 2.20. Peccarelli, *A Moral Dilemma: The Role of Judicial Intervention in Withholding or Withdrawing Nutrition and Hydration*, 23 John Marshall L. Rev. 537, 539, 540, 541 (1990).

I. A physician shall be dedicated to providing competent medical service with compassion and respect for human dignity.

D. Kan. 1995 Plaintiff, an occupational medicine physician, alleged that defendant-medical group wrongfully discharged him in violation of public policy and in breach of the implied covenant of good faith and fair dealing. Defendant complained that plaintiff consistently granted excess time off to patients. Even though defendant warned plaintiff that he would be terminated if he continued this practice, plaintiff refused to comply stating that he was ethically obligated to serve the best interests of his patients. Plaintiff claimed that to place the defendant's interests above his legal and ethical duties to his patients would violate public policy as set out by statute and the Principles of Medical Ethics, with apparent reference to Principle I. Since plaintiff failed to show that defendant's practice caused harm to patients or deviated from accepted standards, the court disregarded plaintiff's public policy exception to the employment at-will doctrine and granted defendant's motion for summary judgment. *Aiken v. Business & Indus. Health Group*, 886 F. Supp. 1565, 1571.

N.J. 1979 In wrongful death action against a psychiatrist whose patient murdered plaintiff's decedent, the court concluded, in accord with Principle 9 (1957) [now Principle IV], that a psychiatrist may owe a duty to warn potential victims of possible danger from psychiatrist's patient despite the general emphasis on confidentiality. The court also noted the Preamble and Principles 1 and 3 (1957) [now revised Preamble, Principle I and Opinion 5.05] in discussing the psychiatrist-patient relationship. *McIntosh v. Milano*, 168 N.J. Super. 466, 403 A.2d 500, 510, 512-13.

Ohio 1991 State medical board revoked license of physician who had consensual sexual relations with his patient. The court upheld the board's ruling that this violated Principles I, II and IV. Dissenting judge, citing AMA Council on Ethical and Judicial Affairs, Sexual Misconduct in the Practice of Medicine, 266 JAMA 2741 [now Opinion 8.14], argued that until 1991, the AMA did not clearly deem sexual contact with a patient unethical. *Pons v. Ohio State Medical Bd.*, 66 Ohio St. 3d 619, 623, 625, 614 N.E.2d 748, 752, 753.

Journal 1997 Discusses the need for balance between business ethics and medical ethics in the context of managed care. Explores two models for integrating ethics and managed care. Proposes the adoption of a collective responsibility model to improve quality of care. Quotes Principles I, II, III, IV, and V. Cites Preamble. References Opinion 8.13. Regan, *Regulating the Business of Medicine: Models for Integrating Ethics and Managed Care*, 30 Colum. J.L. & Soc. Probs. 635, 651, 656, 657 (1997).

Journal 1996 Discusses the trend toward conserving resources expended on health care by withholding services absent a showing of necessity. Claims that the high standard of care physicians owe patients is jeopardized by medical treatment decisions based on coverage concerns. Concludes that the legal structure regarding health care plans should be changed. Quotes Preamble, Principles I, II, III, IV, V, VI, and VII and Opinion 2.03. Hirshfeld & Thomason, *Medical Necessity Determinations: The Need for a New Legal Structure*, 6 Health Matrix 3, 8-9 (1996).

Journal 1995 Examines the rights of health care professionals to refuse to participate in patient care on the basis of conscientious objection. Discusses rights and duties of health care facilities in this context. Suggests steps that facilities may take when dealing with health care professionals who object to participating in patient care. Quotes Principles I and VI and Opinions 1.02, 2.035, and 9.055. Dellinger & Vickery, *When Staff Object to Participating In Care*, 28 J. Health & Hospital Law 269, 272, 276 (1995).

Journal 1994 Considers whether an exception should be made to physician-patient confidentiality that would allow a physician to reveal parental medical history to a child. Discusses whether parents should be required to divulge their medical history to their children. Concludes that such an exception would not completely erode physician-patient confidentiality. Quotes Principles IV, Fundamental Elements (4), and Opinion 5.05. Cites Principle I and Fundamental Elements (1). Friedland, *Physician-Patient Confidentiality: Time to Re-Examine a Venerable Concept in Light of Contemporary Society and Advances in Medicine*, 15 J. Legal Med. 249, 257, 264, 276 (1994).

Journal 1994 Argues that physician aid-in-dying should be protected by the United States Constitution and that patients should have a federal cause of action to challenge prohibitive state statutes. Considers how such a cause of action might affect public policy. Quotes Principles I and III. References Opinion 2.06. Note, *Toward a More Perfect Union: A Federal Cause of Action for Physician Aid-In-Dying*, 27 U. Mich. J.L. Ref. 521, 538 (1994).

Journal 1994 Reviews the evolution of the physician-patient relationship. Describes legal responses to increasing awareness of the importance of ensuring patient autonomy. Examines the changing health care delivery environment. Concludes with a discussion of the impact of these changes on patient participation in medical decision-making. Quotes Preamble, Principles I, II, III, IV, V, and VI, Fundamental Elements (1) and (2), and Opinions 1.02 and 8.07 (1981) [now Opinion 8.08]. Cites Opinion 1.01. Szczygiel, *Beyond Informed Consent*, 21 Ohio N.U.L. Rev. 171, 217, 218, 220, 225, 226, 256 (1994).

Journal 1993 Discusses physicians' duty to disclose medical treatment alternatives to patients that are not readily available. Proposes that based on the historical development and legal requirements of the informed consent doctrine, physicians should be required to inform patients of nonreadily available alternatives or face liability for breach of such obligation. Quotes Principles I, II, III, IV, and V and Opinion 8.08. Note, *Informed Choice: Physicians' Duty to Disclose Nonreadily Available Alternatives*, 43 Case W. Res. L. Rev. 491, 491, 498-499, 508, 509 (1993).

Journal 1990 Discusses the moral dilemma in deciding whether to withdraw artificial nutrition and hydration from a patient and the appropriate role of the judiciary. States that part of the reason for judicial activism in this private area is because legislatures have not adequately expressed public policy. Concludes that judicial decisions do not represent the moral viewpoint of society and that moral pronouncements should not be made in the courtroom. Quotes Preamble, Principles I, II, III, IV, V, VI, and VII, and Opinion 2.20. Peccarelli, *A Moral Dilemma: The Role of Judicial Intervention in Withholding or Withdrawing Nutrition and Hydration*, 23 John Marshall L. Rev. 537, 539, 540, 541 (1990).

Journal 1986 Observes that the AMA policy on capital punishment expressly forbids psychiatrists from making determinations of competency for execution. Such a practice places the psychiatrist in the position of a "double agent," employed by the state, yet required to serve the patient. Compares the psychiatrist's determination of competency for execution to the behavior of Nazi physicians, and condemns as inherently dishonest any therapy not grounded in the patient's best interests. References Principle I and Opinion 2.06. Sargent, *Treating the Condemned to Death*, 16 Hastings Center Rep. 5, 5 (Dec. 1986).

II. A physician shall deal honestly with patients and colleagues, and strive to expose those physicians deficient in character or competence, or who engage in fraud or deception.

Cal. App. 1956 Physician-petitioner sought mandamus against local medical association whose bylaws provided for the expulsion of any member who violated the Principles. Petitioner had been expelled under the provision for alleged violation of Principles Ch. III, Art IV, Sec.4 (1947) [now Opinions 9.04 and 9.07] for making disparaging statements regarding another physician in a report used in judicial proceedings. In holding that application of the provision to petitioner was contrary to public policy, the court noted that the physician's statements had been made at the request of a civil litigant and enjoyed a statutory testimonial privilege. Further, the court found that the American Medical Association's right to formulate ethical principles did not extend to defining the duties of witnesses. Expulsion was also based on petitioner's critical comments about other physicians overheard by their patients in violation of Principles Ch. III, Art. IV, Sec.1 (1947) [now Principle II and Opinion 9.04]. The court found application of this Principle under the circumstances reasonable and not contrary to public policy. *Bernstein v. Alameda-Contra Costa Medical Ass'n*, 139 Cal. App. 2d 241, 293 P.2d 862, 863, 863 nn.1, 2, 865 nn.4, 6, 866, 866 n.8, 867.

Fla. App. 1995 The court considered the issue of the effect of § 455.241(2) of the Florida Statutes on right of defense in a medical malpractice action to engage in ex parte communications with plaintiff's non-party treating physician. The court held that a 1988 amendment to § 455.241(2) negated the applicability of the statute to medical malpractice cases. The dissent, citing Petrillo v. Syntex Laboratories, Inc., 148 Ill. App. 3d 581, 499 N.E.2d 952 (1986), quoted Principles II and IV and Opinions 5.05, 5.06, and 5.08 as strong public policy support for its position that ex parte communications should be barred altogether. *Castillo-Plaza v. Green*, 655 So. 2d 197, 206 n.4.

Ill. App. 1986 Defense attorney in product liability suit was held in contempt of court for conducting ex parte discussions with plaintiff-patient's treating physician without patient's consent and contrary to authorized methods of discovery. The court held that the strong public policy favoring physician-patient confidentiality articulated in Principles II and IV and Opinions 5.05, 5.06, 5.07, and 5.08 justified a rule against such ex parte discussions. Further, the court held that the public has the right to rely on physicians to faithfully execute their ethical obligations. *Petrillo v. Syntex Laboratories, Inc.*, 148 Ill. App. 3d 581, 499 N.E.2d 952, 957, 958, 959.

Ky. App. 1978 Plaintiff-physician attempted to enjoin defendant medical society from expelling him for actions contrary to a variety of Principles, the most relevant to his alleged unethical behavior being Principle 4 (1957) [now Principles II and III]. After reviewing the procedures followed by the medical society in considering the evidence pertaining to the charges, the court affirmed judgment dismissing the action, concluding that plaintiff was not deprived of due process. *Kirk v. Jefferson County Medical Soc'y*, 577 S.W.2d 419, 421.

Md. App. 1993 State Board of Physician Quality Assurance received a complaint that psychiatrist was having a romantic relationship with a former patient. When, as part of its investigation, the Board subpoenaed psychiatrist's records, patient raised the constitutional right to privacy. The court held that the state's interest in investigating possible disciplinary action against psychiatrist outweighed patient's constitutional right to privacy. The court cited Principle II as a potential basis to justify the Board's investigation of possible unprofessional conduct by physician. *Dr. K. v. State Board of Physician Quality Assur.*, 98 Md. App. 103, 632 A.2d 453, 456, *cert. denied*, 334 Md. 18, 637 A.2d 1191 (1994), *and cert. denied*, 115 S. Ct. 75, 130 L. Ed. 29 (1994).

Mass. 1955 Plaintiff-physician was charged under state licensing statute by defendant-board with conspiracy and fee-splitting. Both parties sought a declaratory judgment as to whether the defendant-board had jurisdiction to determine plaintiff's guilt or innocence. In holding that the board was qualified to determine if plaintiff's actions constituted "gross misconduct" under the statute, the court referred to Principles Ch.I, Secs.1 and 6 (1947) [now Principle II and Opinion 6.02] delineating, in part, limitations on payment for medical services. These provisions, the court said, reflected the medical profession's understanding of its "peculiar obligations." *Forziati v. Board of Registration in Medicine*, 333 Mass. 125, 128 N.E.2d 789, 791.

Mich. App. 1968 Physician was properly dismissed from hospital staff for violating Principle 4 (1957) [now Principle II and Opinion 9.11] when on numerous occasions physician "vilified" other physicians, swore and screamed in the hospital, and quarreled with staff and hospital visitors. *Anderson v. Board of Trustees of Caro Community Hosp.*, 10 Mich. App. 348, 159 N.W.2d 347, 348-50.

Minn. 1970 Defendant-physician appealed order to answer interrogatories, claiming that a medical malpractice plaintiff is prohibited from compelling expert testimony from a defendant to prove a charge of malpractice without calling other medical witnesses. In holding that a defendant could be compelled to provide expert medical opinion in response to interrogatories, the court quoted Principle 1 (1957) [now Principle II and Opinion 8.12] for the proposition that physicians owe a duty of disclosure to their patients. *Anderson v. Florence*, 288 Minn. 351, 181 N.W.2d 873, 880, 880 n.7.

N.Y. Sup. 1965 Physician sued publishing company to bar insertion of advertisement for baby and child care products in physician's book, seeking declaration that book contract was void to the extent that it allowed inclusion of such an advertisement. Physician asserted that the advertisement was contrary to public policy, citing Opinions and Reports of the Judicial Council Sec. 5, Para. 29 (1965) [now Opinion 5.02] which stated that a doctor should not lend his name to any product. In rejecting the physician's claim, the court was willing to give careful consideration to the Association's view but concluded that it did not, in itself, constitute an expression of public policy. *Spock v. Pocket Books, Inc.*, 48 Misc. 2d 812, 266 N.Y.S.2d 77, 79.

Ohio 1991 State medical board revoked license of physician who had consensual sexual relations with his patient. The court upheld the board's ruling that this violated Principles I, II and IV. Dissenting judge, citing AMA Council on Ethical and Judicial Affairs, Sexual Misconduct in the Practice of Medicine, 266 JAMA 2741 [now Opinion 8.14], argued that until 1991, the AMA did not clearly deem sexual contact with a patient unethical. *Pons v. Ohio State Medical Bd.*, 66 Ohio St. 3d 619, 623, 625, 614 N.E.2d 748, 752, 753.

Ohio 1980 A physician, charged with violating the state medical licensing statute by distributing controlled substances without a proper license and writing prescriptions for narcotics in the name of one person when they were intended for another, challenged the state medical board's decision to suspend his license and place him on two years probation. Under the statute, a physician could be disciplined for various activities including "violation of any provision of a code of ethics of a national professional organization" such as the American Medical Association. The board found in part that the physician's actions violated Principles 4 and 7 (1957) [now Principles II and III and Opinions 6.04 and 9.04]. The trial court reversed, holding that the board had insufficient evidence for its decision, and the court of appeals affirmed. On appeal, the supreme court held that expert testimony was not required at a hearing before a medical licensing board because they were experts and could determine for themselves whether the Principles had been violated. *Arlen v. State*, 61 Ohio St. 2d 168, 399 N.E.2d 1251, 1252, 1253-54.

Journal 1997 Reports on a study of physician attitudes regarding expert witnesses. Notes that a majority of physicians believe that medical expert testimony should be subject to peer review and, when appropriate, medical licensing board discipline. Quotes Principles II and VI, and Opinion 9.07. Eitel, Hegeman, & Evans, *Medicine on Trial: Physicians' Attitudes about Expert Medical Witnesses*, 18 J. Legal Med. 345, 355, 358 (1997).

Journal 1997 Discusses physician frustration with managed care plans caused by gag clauses and cost-containment mechanisms. Reviews the development of managed care organizations and federal attempts at limiting the use of gag clauses. Concludes that gag clauses are "inherently flawed" and compromise quality health care. Quotes Principles II and V, Fundamental Elements (1), and Opinion 8.13. Note, *Physicians, Bound and Gagged: Federal Attempts to Combat Managed Care's Use of Gag Clauses*, 21 Seton Hall Legis. J. 567, 601-02 (1997).

Journal 1997 Discusses the need for balance between business ethics and medical ethics in the context of managed care. Explores two models for integrating ethics and managed care. Proposes the adoption of a collective responsibility model to improve quality of care. Quotes Principles I, II, III, IV, and V. Cites Preamble. References Opinion 8.13. Regan, *Regulating the Business of Medicine: Models for Integrating Ethics and Managed Care*, 30 Colum. J.L. & Soc. Probs. 635, 651, 656, 657 (1997).

Journal 1996 Discusses the trend toward conserving resources expended on health care by withholding services absent a showing of necessity. Claims that the high standard of care physicians owe patients is jeopardized by medical treatment decisions based on coverage concerns. Concludes that the legal structure regarding health care plans should be changed. Quotes Preamble, Principles I, II, III, IV, V, VI, and VII and Opinion 2.03. Hirshfeld & Thomason, *Medical Necessity Determinations: The Need for a New Legal Structure*, 6 Health Matrix 3, 8-9 (1996).

Journal 1996 Considers the impact of gag clauses on the physician-patient relationship. Undertakes an extensive legal, ethical, and policy analysis. Concludes that gag clauses are violative of legal and ethical principles. Quotes Principles II, V, and VI, and Fundamental Elements (1). Cites Preamble. Martin & Bjerknes, *The Legal and Ethical Implications of Gag Clauses in Physician Contracts*, XXII Am. J. Law & Med. 433, 465-66 (1996).

Journal 1996 Examines the issue of attorney-client sexual relationships and the ethical problems inherent in such conduct. Recommends promulgation of a rule regulating such relationships. Quotes Principle II. Myers, Sonenshein, & Hofstein, *To Regulate or Not To Regulate Attorney-Client Sex? The Ethical Question in Pennsylvania*, 69 Temp. L. Rev. 741, 780 (1996).

Journal 1996 Discusses the ethical implications of sexual misconduct in the medical field. Examines the current civil and criminal tools used to curb physician-patient misconduct. Notes the inadequacy of physician reporting. Proposes a statutory approach to discipline physicians who abuse their fiduciary duties. Quotes Principle II. References Opinion 8.14. Note, *Sexual Conduct Within the Physician-Patient Relationship: A Statutory Framework for Disciplining this Breach of Fiduciary Duty*, 1 Widener L. Symp. J. 501, 507 (1996).

Journal 1994 Compares Texas law with Illinois law on the issue of ex parte communications between defense counsel and the patient/plaintiff's physician in civil litigation. Argues that preservation of the physician-patient relationship requires prohibition of such contact. Quotes Principles II and IV and Opinion 5.05. Comment, *From the Land of Lincoln a Healing Rule: Proposed Texas Rule of Civil Procedure Prohibiting Ex Parte Contact Between Defense Counsel and a Plaintiff's Treating Physician*, 25 Tex. Tech L. Rev. 1081, 1081, 1082 (1994).

Journal 1994 Reviews the evolution of the physician-patient relationship. Describes legal responses to increasing awareness of the importance of ensuring patient autonomy. Examines the changing health care delivery environment. Concludes with a discussion of the impact of these changes on patient participation in medical decision-making. Quotes Preamble, Principles I, II, III, IV, V, and VI, Fundamental Elements (1) and (2), and Opinions 1.02 and 8.07 (1981) [now Opinion 8.08]. Cites Opinion 1.01. Szczygiel, *Beyond Informed Consent*, 21 Ohio N.U.L. Rev. 171, 217, 218, 220, 225, 226, 256 (1994).

Journal 1993 Discusses physicians' duty to disclose medical treatment alternatives to patients that are not readily available. Proposes that based on the historical development and legal requirements of the informed consent doctrine, physicians should be required to inform patients of nonreadily available alternatives or face liability for breach of such obligation. Quotes Principles I, II, III, IV, and V and Opinion 8.08. Note, *Informed Choice: Physicians' Duty to Disclose Nonreadily Available Alternatives*, 43 Case W. Res. L. Rev. 491, 491, 498-499, 508, 509 (1993).

Journal 1993 Evaluates self-policing mechanisms for addressing incompetent and unethical behavior in the medical profession. Discusses the problems physicians may encounter by exposing the errant colleague, such as harm to the reporting physician's reputation and the fear of litigation. States that problems involving physician competency and unethical behavior should be investigated, and that physicians should take personal responsibility for reporting problems they observe. References Principle II and Opinions 8.14 and 9.031. Morreim, *Am I My Brother's Warden? Responding to the Unethical or Incompetent Colleague*, 23 Hastings Center Rep. 19, 23 (May/June 1993).

Journal 1993 Explores problems associated with parental requests to withhold diagnoses from children. Discusses the physician's conflict between a duty to respect parents' wishes and a duty to tell children the truth. Examines clinical factors that may be considered when dealing with this dilemma. Quotes Principle II. Sigman, Kraut, & La Puma, *Disclosure of a Diagnosis to Children and Adolescents When Parents Object*, 147 Am. J. Diseases Children 764, 766 (1993).

Journal 1991 Examines the issues surrounding judicial use of professional ethics codes in private litigation. Explores the history and major characteristics of the "professions." Explains how courts currently apply codes of ethics. Concludes that judges should more extensively use professional ethics codes to define public policy, standards of care, and legal causes of action. Quotes Principle II and Opinion 2.19. Note, *Professional Ethics Codes in Court: Redefining the Social Contract Between the Public and the Professions*, 25 Georgia L. Rev. 1327, 1335, 1351 (1991).

Journal 1990 Examines the extent to which forensic psychiatrists are consulted in medical malpractice cases. Considers the appropriate standard of care, particularly for psychiatric malpractice cases, and the problems associated with its determination. In cases where a practitioner was negligent, criteria for establishing damages are considered. References Principles II and IV. Modlin, *Forensic Psychiatry and Malpractice*, 18 Bull. Am. Acad. Psychiatry Law 153, 161 (1990).

Journal 1990 Discusses the moral dilemma in deciding whether to withdraw artificial nutrition and hydration from a patient and the appropriate role of the judiciary. States that part of the reason for judicial activism in this private area is because legislatures have not adequately expressed public policy. Concludes that judicial decisions do not represent the moral viewpoint of society and that moral pronouncements should not be made in the courtroom. Quotes Preamble, Principles I, II, III, IV, V, VI, and VII, and Opinion 2.20. Peccarelli, *A Moral Dilemma: The Role of Judicial Intervention in Withholding or Withdrawing Nutrition and Hydration*, 23 John Marshall L. Rev. 537, 539, 540, 541 (1990).

Journal 1989 Discusses the history of the physician-patient privilege up through changes implemented under the Ohio Tort Reform Act of 1987. Aspects of the physician-patient privilege that are most significantly affected by this Tort Reform Act are highlighted, with recommendations for further refinement of the privilege in Ohio. Quotes Principles II, IV and Opinion 5.05. Note, *The Ohio Physician-Patient Privilege: Modified, Revised, and Defined*, 49 Ohio St. L. J. 1147, 1167 (1989).

Journal 1985 Focuses on the importance of patient autonomy in medical decision making. Initially describes how existing doctrines protect the value of autonomy in the context of the physician-patient relationship, then examines various problems in the current protective scheme. Case law is evaluated wherein enhanced protection is afforded to patient autonomy. Concludes by recommending the creation of an independent articulable protected interest in patient autonomy. Quotes Principles II and IV. Cites Opinions 4.04 (1984) [now Opinion 8.08] and 6.03 (1984) [now Opinion 6.02]. Shultz, *From Informed Consent to Patient Choice: A New Protected Interest*, 95 Yale L. J. 219, 275 (1985).

III. A physician shall respect the law and also recognize a responsibility to seek changes in those requirements which are contrary to the best interests of the patient.

Ariz. 1965 Physician appealed denial of medical license which was based on alleged violations of local medical society rules and Principles 3, 5, and 10 (1957) [now Principles III and VII, and Opinions 3.01, 8.11, and 9.06]. Alleged violations included treating a patient without first obtaining a prior treating physician's permission, inadequate patient care, performing operations without hospital privileges, and signing the medical record of a deceased patient who had been treated by interns. The court held that the evidence failed to show any clear violation of the Principles and that a local medical society had no right to prescribe a code of ethics for state licensing purposes. *Arizona State Bd. of Medical Examiners v. Clark*, 97 Ariz. 205, 398 P.2d 908, 914-15, 915 n.3.

Ky. App. 1978 Plaintiff-physician attempted to enjoin defendant medical society from expelling him for actions contrary to a variety of Principles, the most relevant to his alleged unethical behavior being Principle 4 (1957) [now Principles II and III]. After reviewing the procedures followed by the medical society in considering the evidence pertaining to the charges, the court affirmed judgment dismissing the action, concluding that plaintiff was not deprived of due process. *Kirk v. Jefferson County Medical Soc'y*, 577 S.W.2d 419, 421.

Ohio 1980 A physician, charged with violating the state medical licensing statute by distributing controlled substances without a proper license and writing prescriptions for narcotics in the name of one person when they were intended for another, challenged the state medical board's decision to suspend his license and place him on two years probation. Under the statute, a physician could be disciplined for various activities including "violation of any provision of a code of ethics of a national professional organization" such as the American Medical Association. The board found in part that the physician's actions violated Principles 4 and 7 (1957) [now Principles II and III and Opinions 6.04 and 9.04]. The trial court reversed, holding that the board had insufficient evidence for its decision, and the court of appeals affirmed. On appeal, the supreme court held that expert testimony was not required at a hearing before a medical licensing board because they were experts and could determine for themselves whether the Principles had been violated. *Arlen v. State*, 61 Ohio St. 2d 168, 399 N.E.2d 1251, 1252, 1253-54.

Journal 1997 Discusses the need for balance between business ethics and medical ethics in the context of managed care. Explores two models for integrating ethics and managed care. Proposes the adoption of a collective responsibility model to improve quality of care. Quotes Principles I, II, III, IV, and V. Cites Preamble. References Opinion 8.13. Regan, *Regulating the Business of Medicine: Models for Integrating Ethics and Managed Care*, 30 Colum. J.L. & Soc. Probs. 635, 651, 656, 657 (1997).

Journal 1996 Discusses the trend toward conserving resources expended on health care by withholding services absent a showing of necessity. Claims that the high standard of care physicians owe patients is jeopardized by medical treatment decisions based on coverage concerns. Concludes that the legal structure regarding health care plans should be changed. Quotes Preamble, Principles I, II, III, IV, V, VI, and VII and Opinion 2.03. Hirshfeld & Thomason, *Medical Necessity Determinations: The Need for a New Legal Structure*, 6 Health Matrix 3, 8-9 (1996).

Journal 1995 Provides legal and medical definitions of physician-assisted suicide and euthanasia. Offers relevant historical perspectives and provides comprehensive ethical and legal discussion of these compelling social issues. Highlights important legislative developments, including the Oregon Death with Dignity Act, and analyzes significant judicial opinions. Advocates legal tolerance of physician-assisted suicide and euthanasia. Quotes Principles III, IV, and VI and Opinions 2.21 and 9.12. Cites Opinions 2.20 and 8.11. Stone & Winslade, *Physician-Assisted Suicide and Euthanasia in the United States: Legal and Ethical Observations*, 16 J. Legal Med. 481, 483, 490, 497, 498, 499 (1995).

Journal 1994 Explores the ethical issues involved in a multidisciplinary team working with children in legal proceedings. Focuses on the relationships between professionals and the conflicts that arise regarding disclosure of confidential information and forced disclosure of non-privileged information. Examines theories supporting protection of client information. Quotes Principles III, IV, Fundamental Elements (4) and Opinions 1.02 (1992) and 5.07 (1992) [now Opinion 5.05]. Cites Opinions 2.02. Glynn, *Multidisciplinary Representation of Children: Conflicts Over Disclosures of Client Communications*, 27 J. Marshall L. Rev. 617, 625, 626, 630-32, 637, 639, 643 (1994).

Journal 1994 Argues that physician aid-in-dying should be protected by the United States Constitution and that patients should have a federal cause of action to challenge prohibitive state statutes. Considers how such a cause of action might affect public policy. Quotes Principles I and III. References Opinion 2.06. Note, *Toward a More Perfect Union: A Federal Cause of Action for Physician Aid-In-Dying*, 27 U. Mich. J.L. Ref. 521, 538 (1994).

Journal 1994 Reviews the evolution of the physician-patient relationship. Describes legal responses to increasing awareness of the importance of ensuring patient autonomy. Examines the changing health care delivery environment. Concludes with a discussion of the impact of these changes on patient participation in medical decision-making. Quotes Preamble, Principles I, II, III, IV, V, and VI, Fundamental Elements (1) and (2), and Opinions 1.02 and 8.07 (1981) [now Opinion 8.08]. Cites Opinion 1.01. Szczygiel, *Beyond Informed Consent*, 21 Ohio N.U.L. Rev. 171, 217, 218, 220, 225, 226, 256 (1994).

Journal 1993 Discusses physicians' duty to disclose medical treatment alternatives to patients that are not readily available. Proposes that based on the historical development and legal requirements of the informed consent doctrine, physicians should be required to inform patients of nonreadily available alternatives or face liability for breach of such obligation. Quotes Principles I, II, III, IV, and V and Opinion 8.08. Note, *Informed Choice: Physicians' Duty to Disclose Nonreadily Available Alternatives, 43 Case W. Res. L. Rev. 491, 491, 498-499, 508, 509 (1993)*.

Journal 1991 Examines the wisdom and likely results of medicalizing psychoactive drugs of abuse. Notes that claimed advantages of medicalizing recreational drugs could be more efficiently achieved through legalization. Concludes that although many physicians would consider prescribing psychoactive drugs of abuse for drug abusers in order to end dependence, few would be willing to prescribe such drugs for recreational purposes. Quotes Principle III. Levine, *Medicalization of Psychoactive Substance Use and the Doctor-Patient Relationship, 69 Milbank Quarterly 623, 624 (1991)*.

Journal 1990 Discusses the moral dilemma in deciding whether to withdraw artificial nutrition and hydration from a patient and the appropriate role of the judiciary. States that part of the reason for judicial activism in this private area is because legislatures have not adequately expressed public policy. Concludes that judicial decisions do not represent the moral viewpoint of society and that moral pronouncements should not be made in the courtroom. Quotes Preamble, Principles I, II, III, IV, V, VI, and VII, and Opinion 2.20. Peccarelli, *A Moral Dilemma: The Role of Judicial Intervention in Withholding or Withdrawing Nutrition and Hydration, 23 John Marshall L. Rev. 537, 539, 540, 541 (1990)*.

IV.   A physician shall respect the rights of patients, of colleagues, and of other health professionals, and shall safeguard patient confidences within the constraints of the law.

D. Kan. 1991 With apparent reliance on Principle IV and Opinion 5.05, plaintiff claimed that other than in discovery or judicial proceedings, the physician-patient privilege is absolute and precludes ex parte communications with defense counsel. While recognizing the confidential nature of the physician-patient relationship, the court held that the ethical standards promulgated by the AMA are not binding law and that, where a litigant-patient has placed his or her medical status in issue, the physician is released from the constraints imposed by the physician-patient relationship for the purposes of the litigation. *Bryant v. Hilst, 136 F.R.D. 487, 490*.

N.D. Ohio 1965 Plaintiff-patient alleged that the defendant-malpractice insurer induced physician to reveal confidential information about plaintiff on pretext that plaintiff filed a malpractice suit. In denying defendant's motion for reconsideration of the court's earlier opinion, the court confirmed its holding that actions of a third party inducing a physician to divulge confidential information may result in liability to the patient. In so holding, the court quoted (with incorrect citation to Ch. II, Sec.1) Principles Ch. I, Sec.2 (1912), [now Principle IV and Opinion 5.08], to emphasize the medical profession's established views regarding confidentiality. *Hammonds v. Aetna Casualty & Sur. Co., 243 F. Supp. 793, 803*.

M.D. Pa. 1987 Plaintiff in a medical malpractice action sought to preclude his treating physicians from serving as defendant's expert witnesses at trial. The court held that defense counsel's failure to provide prior notice of ex parte communication with plaintiff's treating physicians barred their use as defense experts. Referring to Petrillo v. Syntex Laboratories, Inc., 148 Ill. App. 3d 581, 499 N.E.2d 952 (1986), the court noted that the court there favorably cited Principle IV and Opinions 5.05, 5.06, and 5.07 (1984) in support of a public policy protecting confidentiality between physician and patient and against ex parte discussion. *Manion v. N.P.W. Medical Ctr. of N.E. Pa., Inc., 676 F.Supp. 585, 591*.

Ala. 1973 Physician revealed patient information to the patient's employer, contrary to instructions of patient. Patient sued for breach of fiduciary duty. Citing Principle 9 (1957) [now Principle IV and Opinion 5.05] as well as cases from other states, the court held that even in the absence of a testimonial privilege statute, as a matter of public policy, a physician has a fiduciary duty not to make extrajudicial disclosures of patient information acquired in the course of treatment unless the public interest or the private interest of the patient demands otherwise. In holding that the physician had breached his contract with patient, the court found the Principles together with state licensing requirements sufficient to establish the public policy of confidentiality. *Horne v. Patton,* 291 Ala. 701, 287 So. 2d 824, 829, 832.

Alaska 1977 Physician-school board member failed to fully comply with state's conflict of interest law by refusing to reveal the names of patients from whom he had received over $100 in income. The physician claimed a legal privilege or ethical duty not to disclose the information under Principle 9 (1957) [now Principle IV and Opinion 5.05] and, alternatively, that the conflict of interest law unconstitutionally invaded a patient's right to privacy. The court held that disclosure was not barred by a legal privilege or ethical mandate, but that the conflict of interest law unconstitutionally invaded patient privacy due to the absence of protective regulations. In ruling on the ethical duty issue, the court noted that under Alaska law, a physician's license may be revoked for violating the Principles. However, the court found this licensing provision irrelevant to the privileged relationship exception in the conflict of interest law. The court found that otherwise the privilege exception in the statute could be changed by the American Medical Association, a private organization, simply by amending the Principles. *Falcon v. Alaska Pub. Offices Comm'n,* 570 P.2d 469, 474 n.13.

Ariz. App. 1992 Employer argued that workers' compensation statute abrogated the physician-patient privilege statute, permitting ex parte communications with employee's treating physician. Recognizing that a physician is ethically bound to protect the confidentiality of privileged information pursuant to Principle IV, yet lacks the legal training to distinguish between privileged and unprivileged information, the court held that a claimant has the right to insist that his attorney be present when his employer interviews the employee's physician. *Salt River Project v. Industrial Comm'n,* 1992 Ariz. App. LEXIS 323, 129 Ariz. Adv. Rep. 39.

Ariz. App. 1989 In a medical malpractice action, defense counsel interviewed several of plaintiff's treating physicians ex parte and notified plaintiff of this in preparation for a medical liability review panel hearing. Plaintiff moved to bar all testimony by those physicians and to disqualify defense counsel from representing defendants. The appellate court noted a physician's obligation of confidentiality pursuant to Principle IV and Opinion 5.05 and held that "defense counsel in a medical malpractice action may not engage in non-consensual ex parte communications with plaintiff's treating physicians." *Duquette v. Superior Court,* 161 Ariz. 269, 778 P.2d 634, 641.

Cal. 1976 Parents sued psychotherapists to recover for murder of daughter by psychiatric patient, alleging that failure to warn victim of patient's violent threat was a proximate cause of her death. In considering whether such a revelation would have been a violation of professional ethics, the Court noted that Principle 9 (1957) [now Principle IV and Opinion 5.05] recognized that the confidential nature of a physician-patient communication must yield when disclosure is necessary to protect an individual or community as a whole. The court concluded that, in the circumstances of this case, disclosure would not have violated medical ethics and held that psychotherapists are under a duty to warn when they determine or should determine that a patient poses a serious danger of violence to someone else. *Tarasoff v. Regents of Univ. of Cal.,* 17 Cal.3d 425, 551 P.2d 334, 347, 131 Cal. Rptr. 14, 27.

Cal. 1970 Psychiatrist-witness in civil assault case applied for writ of habeas corpus after being held in contempt of court for refusing to produce patient's psychiatric records. Patient, plaintiff in the assault action, neither expressly claimed nor waived the statutory psychotherapist-patient privilege. The court held that the litigant-patient exception to the statutory psychotherapist-patient privilege does not unconstitutionally infringe rights of privacy of either psychotherapists or their patients. The court noted that in such a context a psychiatrist does not violate Principle 9 (1957) [now Principle IV and Opinion 5.05] since the Principle allows for legally compelled disclosure. *In re Lifschutz,* 2 Cal. 3d 415, 467 P.2d 557, 565-66 n.9, 85 Cal. Rptr. 829, 837-38 n.9.

Cal. App. 1982 Defendant was convicted of lewd act with a child and child molestation or annoyance, after licensed clinical psychologist reported defendant's admission of sexual conduct to authorities. The court held that the psychologist's testimony was properly admitted since a statute requiring the reporting of actual or suspected child abuse expressly made the psychotherapist-patient privilege inapplicable. The court quoted Principle 9 (1957) [now Principle IV and Opinions 2.02 and 5.05] in concluding the disclosure was not a breach of professional ethics. *People v. Stritzinger,* 137 Cal. App. 3d 126, 186 Cal. Rptr. 750, 752 rev'd, 34 Cal.3d 505, 668 P.2d 738, 194 Cal. Rptr. 431 (1983).

Colo. 1989 Spouse of police officer killed by released psychiatric patient sued state mental hospital and psychiatrist for negligence. Patient had blamed police for his misfortunes during repeated involuntary commitments for paranoid schizophrenia, and psychiatrist knew that patient would have access to a gun after release. The court held that a psychiatrist owed a duty of care in determining whether patient had propensity for violence and posed unreasonable risk of serious bodily harm to others. In so holding, the court cited Principle 9 (1957) [now Principle IV and Opinion 5.05], in support of the view that there are situations in which the need to protect an individual or the community from the threat of harm from a patient may outweigh the strong policy in favor of non-disclosure of patient confidences. *Perreira v. State, 768 P.2d 1198, 1210 n.7.*

Del. Super. 1993 Plaintiff-patient brought action for invasion of privacy, breach of confidentiality, and breach of implied contract against defendants, a physician and nurse. Plaintiff alleged that defendant-nurse, without plaintiff's consent, informed plaintiff's mother and grandmother that she was pregnant. Plaintiff also alleged that defendant-physician was liable for the nurse's conduct based on respondeat superior. The defendants questioned whether plaintiff had stated a cause of action and if so, whether the cause should be treated as a medical malpractice action. Quoting Principle IV and noting that the legislature and the courts had recognized the duty of confidentiality, the court held that plaintiff had a cause of action for breach of confidentiality. *Martin v. Baehler, 1993 Del. Super. LEXIS 199.*

D.C. App. 1985 Patient sued plastic surgeon for breach of confidential physician-patient relationship following surgeon's use of before and after photographs of her plastic surgery in a department store presentation. In considering whether such a breach was an actionable tort, the court made reference to an earlier case quoting Principles Ch. II, Sec. 2 (1947) [erroneously cited in the earlier case as Ch. II, Sec. 1 (1943) [now Principle IV and Opinion 5.05], as evidence of the strong public policy which exists in favor of maintaining a patient's confidences. *Vassiliades v. Garfinckel's, Brooks Bros., 492 A.2d 580, 590, 591.*

Fla. App. 1995 The court considered the issue of the effect of § 455.241(2) of the Florida Statutes on right of defense in a medical malpractice action to engage in ex parte communications with plaintiff's non-party treating physician. The court held that a 1988 amendment to § 455.241(2) negated the applicability of the statute to medical malpractice cases. The dissent, citing Petrillo v. Syntex Laboratories, Inc., 148 Ill. App. 3d 581, 499 N.E.2d 952 (1986), quoted Principles II and IV and Opinions 5.05, 5.06, and 5.08 as strong public policy support for its position that ex parte communications should be barred altogether. *Castillo-Plaza v. Green, 655 So. 2d 197, 206 n.4.*

Ill. 1997 Trial court held various statutory sections, including those permitting unlimited disclosure of a patient's medical records, unconstitutional. On appeal, state supreme court affirmed. Regarding provisions mandating consent to the disclosure of medical records, the court noted, with reference to Principle IV and Opinion 5.05, the crucial importance of confidentiality in the physician-patient relationship. *Best v. Taylor Machine Works, 179 Ill. 2d 367, 689 N.E. 2d 1057, 1099.*

Ill. 1997 Plaintiffs brought action for medical malpractice and loss of consortium against physicians. Defendants sought the release of medical information according to a statute providing for unlimited access to a plaintiff's medical records. The trial court found this provision unconstitutional as a violation of separation of powers and of patients' privacy rights. On appeal, the court agreed that the statute violated separation of powers. Further, with apparent reference to Principle IV, the court noted the ethical duty of physicians to maintain patient confidentiality. The court, in turn, held that the statute violated the right to privacy, as patients hold confidentiality of personal medical information to be an integral part of privacy interests. *Kunkel v. Walton, 179 Ill. 2d 519, 689 N.E. 2d 1047, 1055.*

Ill. App. 1987 In appeal of malpractice action, an issue was whether expert testimony of plaintiff's treating physician, based upon discussions with the defense counsel without patient's consent, was admissible. The court held that ex parte communications between a plaintiff's treating physician and legal adversary violated public policy. In determining the existence of such a policy favoring the sanctity of the doctor-patient relationship, the court noted Petrillo v. Syntex Laboratories Inc., 148 Ill. App. 3d 581, 499 N.E.2d 952 (1st Dist. 1986) and its reference to the Principles and Opinions, namely Principle IV and Opinion 5.05 (1984), which establish an ethical obligation to keep physician-patient communications confidential, generally requiring a patient's consent before information is released. *Yates v. El-Deiry, 160 Ill. App. 3d 198, 513 N.E.2d 519, 522.*

Ill. App. 1986 Defense attorney in product liability suit was held in contempt of court for conducting ex parte discussions with plaintiff-patient's treating physician without patient's consent and contrary to authorized methods of discovery. The court held that the strong public policy favoring physician-patient confidentiality articulated in Principles II and IV and Opinions 5.05, 5.06, 5.07, and 5.08 (1984) justified a rule against such ex parte discussions. Further, the court held that the public has the right to rely on physicians to faithfully execute their ethical obligations. *Petrillo v.*

Syntex Laboratories, Inc., 148 Ill. App. 3d 581, 499 N.E.2d 952, 957, 958, 959 cert. denied, 483 U.S. 1007 (1987).

Ill. App. 1979 Patient filed suit against physician for breach of contract and breach of confidential relationship after physician's employee disclosed patient's name to police. Patient alleged that implied contract arose out of a statutory physician-patient privilege, and provisions of the "Canons of Medical Ethics," with apparent reference to Principle 9 (1957) [now Principle IV and Opinion 5.05]. The court held that disclosure of patient's name alone by a physician or the physician's agents is insufficient to state a cause of action in contract and does not violate the physician-patient privilege. *Geisberger v. Willuhn*, 72 Ill. App. 3d 435, 390 N.E.2d 945, 946, 948.

Ind. App. 1996 A patient filed suit against a mental health counseling center for disclosing to a third party death threats made by the patient during therapy. The patient claimed this was a breach of the standard of care owed to her. The trial court found that the counseling center was not statutorily prohibited from disclosing death threats the patient made. On appeal, the court affirmed the decision. It noted, with apparent reference to Principle IV and Opinion 5.05, that physicians may disclose confidential information to ensure the safety of the public or of individuals. In clarifying its holding, the court observed that while free and frank communication should be promoted to aid proper diagnosis and treatment, public policy supports disclosure of confidential information when appropriate. *Rocca v. Southern Hills Counseling Center, Inc.*, 671 N.E. 2d 913, 916.

Md. Att'y Gen. 1989 Except as required by statute, physicians are not legally obligated to report that an adult has been sexually assaulted. Quoting Principle IV regarding the safeguarding of patient confidences within the constraints of the law, the opinion concludes that a physician must consider the confidential nature of the physician-patient relationship when deciding whether to report that a patient has been sexually assaulted. *Maryland Att'y Gen. Op. No. 89-022.*

Md. Att'y Gen. 1986 State attorney general opined that statute authorized physicians to report to the Motor Vehicle Administration patients with certain disorders that would impair their ability to drive. The opinion cites Principle IV in support of the conclusion that, where required by law, a physician's disclosure of patient information is proper. *Maryland Att'y Gen. Op. No. 86-030 71 Op. Att'y. Gen. 407, 410.*

Md. Att'y Gen. 1977 Opinion addresses the obligation of a psychiatrist to report child abuse information obtained from a parent-patient. Referring to state statutes and to Principle 9 (1957) [now Principle IV and Opinions 2.02 and 5.05] the opinion concludes that the question of whether to disclose suspected child abuse is a matter left to the individual psychiatrist's professional and moral judgment. *Maryland Att'y. Gen. Opinion, 62 Op. Att'y Gen. 157, 160.*

Mass. 1989 Physician appealed after being disciplined for discussing anticipated deposition testimony with malpractice defendant's attorney one day prior to scheduled deposition. The court, referring to Principle IV noted that the American Medical Association's ethical standards did not specifically address situation presented. After weighing the fact that physician had specifically asked attorney whether discussion was appropriate, the court held that the physician's behavior did not constitute "gross misconduct" and thus he could not be disciplined under licensing statute. *Hellman v. Board of Registration in Medicine*, 404 Mass. 800, 537 N.E.2d 150, 153 n.4.

Mass. 1984 Employee sued employer for libel and invasion of privacy following disclosure of medical facts about employee to other employees. In part, claim involved disclosure of opinion about employee's mental state to his supervisor by physician retained by employer. Citing Principle 9 (1957) [now Principle IV and Opinions 5.05 and 5.09], the court held that a physician retained by an employer may disclose to the employer information concerning an employee if receipt of the information is reasonably necessary to serve a substantial and valid business interest of the employer. *Bratt v. Intn'l Business Mach. Corp.*, 392 Mass. 508, 467 N.E.2d 126, 137 n.23.

Minn. 1976 Plaintiff-patient in malpractice action appealed trial court's order to provide authorization for private, informal interview between defense counsel and patient's treating physician. In holding that formal pretrial discovery provided the exclusive procedure by which defendant could obtain medical testimony, the court noted, without deciding the issue, that a physician who discloses confidential patient information in a private interview may be subject to tort liability for breach of patient's right to privacy or professional discipline for unprofessional conduct, citing Principle 9 (1957) [now Principle IV and Opinion 5.05]. *Wenninger v. Muesing*, 240 N.W.2d 333, 337 n.3.

Mo. 1993 Patient sued physicians alleging a breach of fiduciary duty of confidentiality for participating in an unauthorized ex parte discussion with defendant's attorney. While recognizing this duty, the court held that, where the plaintiff's medical condition is in issue, this constitutes a waiver of both the testimonial privilege and the physician's fiduciary duty in so far as the information is related to the medical issues. Quoting Opinion 5.05 and citing Principle IV, the court stated that courts may apply ethical principles to frame the specific limits of the legal duty of confidentiality. *Brandt v. Medical Defense Assoc.*, 856 S.W.2d 667, 671 n.1.

Mo. 1989 In a personal injury suit, plaintiff challenged trial court's authority to compel plaintiff to authorize ex parte meetings between defendant insurance company and plaintiff's treating physician. Applying a balancing test between preserving the physician-patient confidential and fiduciary relationship, the physician-patient testimonal privilege, and the quest for truth in civil litigation, the court held that such information could be obtained through the methods of formal discovery. The court quoted Principle IV and Opinion 5.05 (1984) as statements of the policy underlying medical confidentiality and a basis for a patient's affirmative right to rely on the confidential nature of disclosures to a treating physician. *State ex. rel. Woytus v. Ryan*, 776 S.W.2d 389, 392-93.

Mo. App. 1985 In a prohibition proceeding arising from a medical malpractice action, defense attorneys sought order compelling plaintiff to authorize a private interview between defense attorneys and physician who treated plaintiff for injuries allegedly caused by defendant-physician. The appellate court, after discussing Principle IV and Opinion 5.05 (1984), held that the defense attorneys had the right to seek an ex parte interview with the treating physician, subject to the willingness of the physician to grant the interview. Furthermore, the court noted that Opinion 5.05 prevents a physician from revealing a patient's confidences only where there is a lack of consent from the patient and found that consent did exist here in the form of a medical authorization executed by plaintiff during pendency of the malpractice action. *State ex rel. Stufflebam v. Appelquist*, 694 S.W.2d 882, 886, 888 n.7, *overruled by State ex. rel. Woytus v. Ryan*, 776 S.W.2d 389 (Mo. 1989).

N.J. 1985 Plaintiff provided authorization for release of decedent's medical records from former treating physicians but refused to consent to depositions or interviews between defense counsel and physicians. The court noted physicians' ethical duty to avoid unauthorized disclosure, as stated in Principle 9 (1957) [now Principle IV and Opinion 5.05], but recognized that a patient's right to confidentiality was not absolute. After balancing the competing interests involved, the court held that defense counsel had a right to seek ex parte interviews of decedent's other treating physicians regarding litigation matters, provided procedural safeguards were met including clear statements that participation in such an interview is voluntary on the part of a physician. *Stempler v. Speidell*, 100 N.J. 368, 495 A.2d 857, 860, *cert. denied*, 483 U.S. 1007 (1987).

N.J. 1979 In wrongful death action against a psychiatrist whose patient murdered plaintiff's decedent, the court concluded, in accord with Principle 9 (1957) [now Principle IV], that a psychiatrist may owe a duty to warn potential victims of possible danger from psychiatrist's patient despite the general emphasis on confidentiality. The court also noted the Preamble and Principles 1 and 3 (1957) [now revised Preamble, Principle I and Opinion 5.05] in discussing the psychiatrist-patient relationship. *McIntosh v. Milano*, 168 N.J. Super. 466, 403 A.2d 500, 510, 512-13.

N.J. 1962 Parents sued pediatrician for unauthorized disclosure to life insurer of deceased infant's congenital heart defect. The court quoted Principle 9 (1957) [now Principle IV and Opinion 5.05] as an articulation of a physician's legal duty to his or her patient subject to exceptions of compelling social or patient interests. The court held that the parents had lost their limited right to nondisclosure by filing an insurance claim. *Hague v. Williams*, 37 N.J. 328, 181 A.2d 345, 347.

N.J. Super. 1991 Physician's estate sued hospital alleging that it violated state law against discrimination by restricting the physician's surgery privileges and requiring him to inform patients of his HIV-infected status before performing invasive procedures. The defendant hospital was also alleged to have breached its duty to maintain confidentiality of his seropositive diagnosis. The court held that the hospital had not discriminated against the physician since the hospital had relied on ethical and professional standards, including a report of the Council on Ethical and Judicial Affairs of the AMA dealing with the issue of AIDS [now Opinions 9.13 and 9.131]. However, the hospital was held to have breached its fiduciary duty to maintain the confidentiality of the physician's medical records. Referring to McIntosh v. Milano, 168 N.J. Super. 466, 403 A.2d 500 (1979) which had quoted AMA Principles of Medical Ethics sec. 9 (1957) [now Principle IV and Opinion 5.05] in applying the "duty to warn" exception, the court noted that the disclosure in this case went far beyond the medical personnel directly involved in the treatment of the physician and those patients entitled to informed consent. *Estate of Behringer v. Medical Ctr.*, 249 N.J. Super. 597, 614, 633, 592 A.2d 1251, 1259, 1268.

N.J. Super. 1988 Several portions of state Department of Corrections regulations concerning exceptions to privileged communications between psychologist and inmates were invalidated by appellate court because they permitted disclosure of confidences that did not present clear and imminent danger to the inmate or others, or failed to identify any intended victim. Court made general reference (with erroneous quotation) to Principle 9 (1957) [now Principle IV and Opinion 5.05]. *In re Rules Adoption, 224 N.J. Super. 252, 540 A.2d 212, 215.*

N.J. Super. 1987 Defendant in a personal injury suit sought to offer testimony from plaintiff's treating physician regarding plaintiff's prognosis. The court denied plaintiff's motion to exclude that evidence, despite the ethical obligation of physicians to uphold patients' communications as confidential under Principle 9 (1957) [now Principle IV and Opinion 5.05]. The court's decision was based on New Jersey case law permitting disclosure of a patient's medical condition to someone having a legitimate interest "where the physical condition of the patient is made an element of a claim." *Kurdek v. West Orange Bd. of Educ., 222 N.J. Super. 218, 536 A.2d 332, 335.*

N.J. Super. 1967 In a suit for separate maintenance, communications between plaintiff-wife and her psychiatrist were not protected from disclosure during depositions, despite Principle 9 (1957) [now Principle IV and Opinion 5.05] which prohibited physicians from disclosing patient confidences except where "necessary to protect the welfare of the individual or of the community." The court concluded that the patient had only a limited right of nondisclosure, subject to exceptions created by "supervening interest of society" and that the institution of litigation by the patient constituted a vitiation of that right. *Ritt v. Ritt, 98 N.J. Super. 590, 238 A.2d 196, 199 rev'd, 52 N.J. 177, 244 A.2d 497 (1968).*

N.Y. Sup. 1977 Plaintiff, a psychiatric patient, sued her psychiatrist and the psychiatrist's spouse for violating several state statutes and her privacy rights by publishing a book about the intimate details of plaintiff's psychotherapy. The court found for plaintiff, basing its decision in part upon Principle 9 (1957) [now Principle IV and Opinion 5.05] which requires a physician to uphold the confidences of a patient. *Doe v. Roe, 93 Misc. 2d 201, 400 N.Y.S.2d 668, 674.*

N.Y. Surr. 1977 In a discovery proceeding, respondent-psychiatrist, who had treated some patients of deceased psychiatrist subsequent to his death, allegedly misappropriated decedent's patient records. Estate petitioned court for return of records and damages for injury to value of decedent's practice. Respondent sought dismissal of claim arguing that estate could not sell patient records. The court rejected respondent's request. In so ruling, the court noted that under Principle 9 (1957) [now Principle IV and Opinion 5.05] prohibiting physicians from revealing patient confidences, various guidelines had been issued regarding sale of a medical practice [now Opinion 7.04]. Whether respondent's actions had interfered with the estate's efforts to dispose of decedent's practice in keeping with these guidelines presented the court with factual issues for later resolution. *Estate of Finkle, 90 Misc. 2d 550, 395 N.Y.S.2d 343, 346.*

N.C. 1990 Plaintiff in a malpractice case was granted an order prohibiting ex parte conferences between defendant's attorney and non-party treating physicians. The court noted that both the Principles of Medical Ethics and Current Opinions affirm the physician's duty to protect patient confidentiality, in apparent reference to Principle IV and Opinion 5.05. In consideration of (1) the patient's right to privacy, (2) physician-patient confidentiality, (3) the adequacy of formal discovery procedures, and (4) the dilemma in which non-party treating physicians are placed by ex parte conferences, the court held that an attorney may not interview a patient's non-party treating physicians privately without express authorization. *Crist v. Moffatt, 326 N.C. 326, 333, 389 S.E.2d 41, 46.*

Ohio 1997 Estates of victims who were killed by their mentally ill son brought suit against son's psychotherapist for failing to disclose potential for violence. Son had been institutionalized and treated for schizophrenia. After release, he continued to take medication and see a psychotherapist. Despite parents' objections and attempts to have him involuntarily recommitted, psychotherapist reduced his medication and continued to recommend outpatient treatment. The court held that the psychotherapist had a duty to exercise reasonable care to control the son so as to prevent him from causing harm to his family. The court expressed concern for safeguarding the confidentiality of psychotherapeutic communications but noted that Principle 9 (1957) [now Principle IV and Opinion 5.05] has long allowed breaches of confidence when it becomes necessary to protect the welfare of the individual or the community. *Estates of Morgan v. Fairfield Family Counseling Center, 77 Ohio St. 3d 284, 303, 673 N.E.2d 1311, 1326.*

Ohio 1991 State medical board revoked license of physician who had consensual sexual relations with his patient. The court upheld the board's ruling that this violated Principles I, II and IV. Dissenting judge, citing AMA Council on Ethical and Judicial Affairs, Sexual Misconduct in the

Practice of Medicine, 266 JAMA 2741 [now Opinion 8.14], argued that until 1991, the AMA did not clearly deem sexual contact with a patient unethical. *Pons v. Ohio State Medical Bd.*, 66 Ohio St. 3d 619, 623, 625, 614 N.E.2d 748, 752, 753.

Ohio 1988 Administrator sued psychiatrist for wrongful death after recently discharged patient killed her infant daughter. In determining whether a professional judgment rule should be adopted in the malpractice standard of care where the prediction of violent behavior is involved, the court referred favorably to Principle 9 (1957) [now Principle IV and Opinion 5.05] which allows breaches of patient confidences when necessary to protect potential victims. *Littleton v. Good Samaritan Hosp.*, 39 Ohio St. 3d 86, 529 N.E.2d 449, 459 n.19.

Okla. 1988 In response to a police request, physician reported patient treated for a penile bite. Patient sued physician for negligence after information furnished by physician led to patient's arrest and conviction for rape. Patient alleged a tortious breach of the physician-patient confidential relationship, breach of contract, violation of licensing statute and breach of Principle 9 (1957) [now Principle IV and Opinion 5.05]. The court reasoned that the benefit of the divulgence inured to the public at large and thus fell within the public policy exception to the testimonial privilege, created no liability in tort or contract, and was not a breach of medical ethics under the licensing statute or the Principles. *Bryson v. Tillinghast*, 749 P.2d 110, 113, 114.

Pa. 1973 Plaintiff in personal injury suit resulting from auto accident claimed that trial court should have allowed showing on cross-examination that defendant's expert medical witness, who had treated plaintiff, violated Principle 9 (1957) [now Principle IV and Opinion 5.05] by ex parte communications with defense counsel, in order to impeach his medical testimony. The court held that any connection between an alleged breach of medical ethics and the credibility of a physician on the witness stand was tenuous. Therefore, the trial court's decision barring further inquiry in this regard was proper. *Downey v. Weston*, 451 Pa. 259, 301 A.2d 635, 638.

Pa. Super. 1988 Plaintiff-patient sued her physician for breach of confidentiality when physician conferred with defense counsel in plaintiff's malpractice suit against the hospital (physician's employer). In its majority opinion, the court cited Principle IV, commenting that it gave very little guidance to physicians but nonetheless was not violated by the physician. The court also noted Opinion 5.07 (1986) finding that the plaintiff's suit minimized her expectations of confidentiality. The dissent, however, interpreted these same provisions, along with Opinion 5.05 (1986), as protecting plaintiff's expectations of confidentiality. *Moses v. McWilliams*, 379 Pa. Super. 150, 549 A.2d 950, 956, 962 (dissent), appeal denied, 521 Pa. 630, 558 A.2d 532 (1989).

S.C. App. 1997 Patient sued physician for breaching duty of confidentiality after physician divulged patient's emotional health status in a letter which was introduced during patient's divorce proceeding. The trial court dismissed the action for failure to state a cause of action, finding state law did not support a duty of confidentiality. The appeals court reversed. In part, it found a basis for such an action in medical and ethical principles, with apparent reference to Principle IV. Absent a compelling public interest in disclosure, confidences must be preserved. The court remanded to consider whether the disclosure was essential to the best interests of the patient or others. *McCormick v. England*, 328 S.C. 627, 494 S.E. 2d 431, 435.

Tenn. App. 1994 Plaintiff sought damages for wrongful death from defendant-surgeon. Defendant requested that the court require plaintiff to sign a form authorizing release of medical records and information to defense counsel. Trial court denied defendant's motion noting, with apparent reference to Principle IV and Opinion 5.05, that confidential relationship exists between physician and patient. Appellate court affirmed although it did not reach the ethical issue of the propriety of disclosures by a physician. *Wright v. Wasudev*, 1994 Tenn. App. LEXIS 657.

Utah Att'y Gen. 1978 A physician who, acting in good faith, discloses confidential information to proper authorities concerning a patient's unfitness to drive is not liable for doing so. Reference is made to Principle 9 (1957) [now Principle IV and Opinion 5.05] to support propriety of such disclosure where the public interest is involved. *Utah Att'y Gen. Op. No. 77-294.*

Wash. 1988 Personal representative brought wrongful death action against decedent's physicians. At issue was whether defense counsel in a personal injury action may communicate ex parte with plaintiff's treating physician where plaintiff has waived the physician-patient relationship. In holding that defense counsel may not engage in ex parte communication, and is limited to formal discovery methods, the court cited Principle IV and Opinion 5.05 (1986) with approval, reasoning that the mere threat of disclosure of private conversations between a physician and defense counsel would chill the physician-patient relationship and hinder further treatment. *Loudon v. Mhyre*, 110 Wash. 2d 675, 756 P.2d 138, 141, 141 n.3.

W. Va. 1993 Plaintiff, in a malpractice action, sought a writ of prohibition to prevent the enforcement of a trial court order allowing ex parte interviews. The court, in granting the writ, held that any benefit from ex parte interviews that occurs is minimal compared to the danger that they will undermine the confidential nature of the physician-patient relationship. Quoting Principles of Medical Ethics Ch. II, sec. 1 (1943) [now Principle IV and Opinion 5.05], the court noted that the medical profession is well aware of the importance of patient confidentiality. *State ex. rel. Kitzmiller v. Henning, 437 S.E.2d 452, 454.*

W. Va. 1988 Patient-wife sued psychiatrist who disclosed subpoenaed confidential information to her husband's attorney in divorce proceedings. The court held that a tort action lies when confidential communications regarding mental health patients are released, except under limited circumstances such as a binding court order. The court however declined to recognize an enforceable contractual right to confidentiality, although it noted that some states have recognized such a right based upon Principle IV. *Allen v. Smith, 368 S.E.2d 924, 928.*

Wis. 1995 In medical malpractice suit, the court held that (1) subject to restrictions, defense counsel may engage in ex parte communications with plaintiff's treating physician if the communications do not involve disclosure of confidential information; (2) outside a judicial proceeding, defendant-physician may communicate ex parte with plaintiff's treating physician subject to a physician's duty of confidentiality; and (3) if defense counsel elicits confidential information from a treating physician during ex parte communications, the appropriate sanction is within the discretion of the court. The court expressly overruled State ex rel. Klieger v. Alby, 125 Wis. 2d 468, 373 N.W.2d 57 (Ct. App. 1985) and the cases applying it. The majority and concurring opinions referred to Principle IV and Opinion 5.05. *Steinberg v. Jensen, 194 Wis. 2d 440, 534 N.W.2d 361, 370, 377.*

Wis. App. 1994 In medical malpractice suit, defense counsel engaged in ex parte communications with plaintiff's consulting physicians. Plaintiff amended her complaint seeking punitive damages for breach of confidentiality. The court concluded that the rule of State ex rel. Klieger v. Alby, 125 Wis. 2d 468, 373 N.W.2d 57 (Ct. App. 1985), which prohibits ex parte communications that have the potential to breach physician-patient confidentiality, was violated and sanctions were required. The court referred to Petrillo v. Syntax Labs., Inc., 148 Ill. App. 3d 581, 499 N.E.2d 952 (1986) and its use of Principle IV and Opinion 5.05. *Steinberg v. Jensen, 186 Wis. 2d 237, 519 N.W.2d 753, 761 n.9, rev'd, 194 Wis. 2d 440, 534 N.W.2d 361 (1995).*

Wis. Att'y Gen. 1987 Physicians may report cases of suspected child abuse or neglect when a patient discloses that he or she has abused a child in some manner. Where report is made in good faith, physicians are immune from any civil or criminal liability. Passing reference is made to Principle 9 (1957) [now Principle IV and Opinions 2.02 and 5.05] in support of this position. *Wisconsin Att'y Gen. Op. 10-87 (Mar. 16, 1987) (LEXIS, States library, Wis. file).*

Journal 1997 Discusses the need for health care providers to have accurate medical information to treat patients effectively. Explains the benefits of computerized patient medical records and the privacy and confidentiality concerns raised. Concludes that patient privacy needs to be assured to improve service. Quotes Principle IV. Cuzmanes & Orlando, *Automation of Medical Records: The Electronic Superhighway and Its Ramifications for Health Care Providers, 6 J. Pharmacy & L. 19, 27 (1997).*

Journal 1997 Discusses principles of autonomy in the physician-patient relationship. Notes that rights to privacy and confidentiality are grounded in patient autonomy. Concludes that patients may be harmed when privacy rights are breached. Quotes Principle IV. Doyal, *Human Need and the Right of Patients to Privacy, 14 J. Contemp. Health L. & Pol'y 1, 3 (1997).*

Journal 1997 Considers principles of confidentiality in the physician-patient relationship. Notes the current trend emphasizing public reporting obligations of physicians to protect members of society. Emphasizes need for balance between patient rights and societal interests. Quotes Principle IV and Opinion 5.05. References Preamble. Jozefowicz, *The Case Against Having "Professional Privilege" in the Physician-Patient Relationship, 16 Med. & L. 385, 386-87, 391 (1997).*

Journal 1997 Suggests that ex parte conferences between treating physicians and opposing counsel undermine the physician-patient relationship. Notes that there are no significant benefits within the fact-finding process that justify the conflicts of interest created. Concludes that ex parte conferences are unnecessary. Quotes Principle IV and Opinion 5.05. Kassel, *Counterpoint . . . Defense Counsel's Ex Parte Communication with Plaintiff's Doctors: A Bad One-Sided Deal, 9 S.C. Law. 42, 43 (Sept./Oct. 1997).*

Journal 1997 Discusses the need for balance between business ethics and medical ethics in the context of managed care. Explores two models for integrating ethics and managed care. Proposes the adoption of a collective responsibility model to improve quality of care. Quotes Principles I, II, III, IV, and V. Cites Preamble. References Opinion 8.13. Regan, *Regulating the Business of Medicine: Models for Integrating Ethics and Managed Care*, 30 Colum. J.L. & Soc. Probs. 635, 651, 656, 657 (1997).

Journal 1997 Explores confidentiality problems that arise as a result of new health information systems. Examines legal aspects of medical records confidentiality. Advocates legislation at the national level to protect privacy of personal health information. Cites Principles of Medical Ethics § 9 (1957) [now Principle IV]. Turkington, *Medical Record Confidentiality Law, Scientific Research, and Data Collection in the Information Age*, 25 J. Law, Med. & Ethics 113, 126 (1997).

Journal 1996 Explores whether patients have a duty to disclose their HIV status to treating physicians. Suggests that recognizing such a duty may subject patients to a lower standard of care and provide a disincentive to be tested. Concludes that courts should not impose a duty to disclose on patients. Quotes Principle 9 (1957) [now Principle IV] and Opinion 9.131. DeNatale & Parrish, *Health Care Workers' Ability to Recover in Tort for Transmission or Fear of Transmission of HIV from a Patient*, 36 Santa Clara L. Rev. 751, 782-83, 787 (1996).

Journal 1996 Discusses the trend toward conserving resources expended on health care by withholding services absent a showing of necessity. Claims that the high standard of care physicians owe patients is jeopardized by medical treatment decisions based on coverage concerns. Concludes that the legal structure regarding health care plans should be changed. Quotes Preamble, Principles I, II, III, IV, V, VI, and VII and Opinion 2.03. Hirshfeld & Thomason, *Medical Necessity Determinations: The Need for a New Legal Structure*, 6 Health Matrix 3, 8-9 (1996).

Journal 1996 Discusses sexual abuse litigation in which accusers have recovered memories of molestation in psychotherapy sessions. Observes that, to successfully defend against such claims, it is necessary for the accused to have access to the clinical record. Posits that confidentiality problems can be eliminated with *in camera* record inspections. References Principle IV and Opinion 5.05. Loftus, Paddock, & Guernsey, *Patient-Psychotherapist Privilege: Access to Clinical Records in the Tangled Web of Repressed Memory Litigation*, 30 U. Rich L. Rev. 109, 127 (1996).

Journal 1996 Reviews two Washington state supreme court decisions in which subsequent treating physicians testified against their patients and on behalf of defendant physicians in malpractice litigation. Observes that these decisions erode the physician-patient privilege. Posits that the decisions are inconsistent with current medical ethics and proposes a statutory enactment as a solution. Quotes Opinion 5.05. Cites Principle 9 (1957) [now Principle IV]. Oppenheim, *Physicians as Experts Against Their Own Patients? What Happened to the Privilege?*, 63 Def. Couns. J. 254, 257, 261 (1996).

Journal 1996 Considers prearraignment forensic evaluations. Notes the prohibition against use of such evaluations. Examines underlying ethical precepts. Observes that principles of beneficence are misapplied to forensic psychiatry in this context. Advocates a new ethical framework. Quotes Preamble. References Principle IV and Opinion 5.05. Ornish, Mills, & Ornish, *Prearraignment Forensic Evaluations: Toward a New Policy*, 24 Bull. Am. Acad. Psychiatry Law 453, 454, 469 (1996).

Journal 1996 Examines the psychiatrist-patient duty of confidentiality. Notes that Principles of Medical Ethics prohibit the disclosure of patient confidences and medical records. Observes that exceptions to this prohibition exist when required by law or to protect the community. Quotes Principle 9 (1957) [now Principle IV and Opinion 5.05]. Sadoff, *Ethical Obligations for the Psychiatrist: Confidentiality, Privilege, and Privacy in Psychiatric Treatment*, 29 Loy. L.A. L. Rev. 1709, 1710, 1711 (1996).

Journal 1996 Examines the theories courts have used when evaluating claims for emotional distress damages arising from HIV misdiagnosis. Observes that the physical injury requirement is outdated but notes that alternatives may give rise to potentially unlimited liability. Concludes that physicians should be afforded good faith immunity from suits. Quotes Principle 9 (1957) [now Principle IV]. Schmid, *Protecting the Physician in HIV Misdiagnosis Cases*, 46 Duke L. J. 431, 458 (1996).

Journal 1995 Discusses the belief of health care providers that they have an ethical obligation to warn the partners of HIV-positive patients. Provides an overview of the ethical and legal principles concerning confidentiality and the duty to warn. Examines both the scope of a Massachusetts statute that prevents providers from releasing HIV test results of patients and possible defenses that providers may assert. Quotes Principle IV and Opinion 5.05. Friedland, *HIV Confidentiality and the Right to Warn—The Health Care Provider's Dilemma*, 80 Mass. L. Rev. 3, 4 (March 1995).

Journal 1995 Examines federal legislative proposals intended to protect confidentiality of computerized medical records. Notes flaws in these proposals. Concludes that proposed legislation will significantly undermine confidentiality. Cites Opinion 5.07. References Principle IV. Hoge, *Proposed Federal Legislation Jeopardizes Patient Privacy*, 23 Bull. Am. Acad. Psychiatry Law 495, 498, 500 (1995).

Journal 1995 Provides legal and medical definitions of physician-assisted suicide and euthanasia. Offers relevant historical perspectives and provides comprehensive ethical and legal discussion of these compelling social issues. Highlights important legislative developments, including the Oregon Death with Dignity Act, and analyzes significant judicial opinions. Advocates legal tolerance of physician-assisted suicide and euthanasia. Quotes Principles III, IV, and VI and Opinions 2.21 and 9.12. Cites Opinions 2.20 and 8.11. Stone & Winslade, *Physician-Assisted Suicide and Euthanasia in the United States: Legal and Ethical Observations*, 16 J. Legal Med. 481, 483, 490, 497, 498, 499 (1995).

Journal 1994 Compares Texas law with Illinois law on the issue of ex parte communications between defense counsel and the patient/plaintiff's physician in civil litigation. Argues that preservation of the physician-patient relationship requires prohibition of such contact. Quotes Principles II and IV and Opinion 5.05. Comment, *From the Land of Lincoln a Healing Rule: Proposed Texas Rule of Civil Procedure Prohibiting Ex Parte Contact Between Defense Counsel and a Plaintiff's Treating Physician*, 25 Tex. Tech L. Rev. 1081, 1081, 1082 (1994).

Journal 1994 Considers whether an exception should be made to physician-patient confidentiality that would allow a physician to reveal parental medical history to a child. Discusses whether parents should be required to divulge their medical history to their children. Concludes that such an exception would not completely erode physician-patient confidentiality. Quotes Principles IV, Fundamental Elements (4), and Opinion 5.05. Cites Principle I and Fundamental Elements (1). Friedland, *Physician-Patient Confidentiality: Time to Re-Examine a Venerable Concept in Light of Contemporary Society and Advances in Medicine*, 15 J. Legal Med. 249, 257, 264, 276 (1994).

Journal 1994 Explores the ethical issues involved in a multidisciplinary team working with children in legal proceedings. Focuses on the relationships between professionals and the conflicts that arise regarding disclosure of confidential information and forced disclosure of non-privileged information. Examines theories supporting protection of client information. Quotes Principles III, IV, Fundamental Elements (4) and Opinions 1.02 (1992) and 5.07 (1992) [now Opinion 5.05]. Cites Opinions 2.02. Glynn, *Multidisciplinary Representation of Children: Conflicts Over Disclosures of Client Communications*, 27 J. Marshall L. Rev. 617, 625, 626, 630-32, 637, 639, 643 (1994).

Journal 1994 Discusses physician-patient confidentiality and the exception that permits breach of a patient's confidence if required by law. Argues that this is always a legitimate exception to the confidentiality rule. Quotes Principle IV and Fundamental Elements (4). McConnell, *Confidentiality and the Law*, 20 J. Med. Ethics 47, 47 (1994).

Journal 1994 Discusses the importance of confidentiality in the physician-patient relationship and under what circumstances patient information may be released. Examines unique considerations that apply when a physician provides medical care to a minor or an HIV-infected individual. Addresses medical record retention. Discusses threats to medical record privacy caused by new advances in communications technology. Quotes Principle IV and Fundamental Elements (4). Weiner & Wettstein, *Confidentiality of Patient-Related Information*, 112 Arch. Ophthalmology 1032, 1033 (1994).

Journal 1993 Discusses family privacy rights and a physician's ethical responsibility to report violence. Considers the meaning of justice, self respect, and the fundamental principles of physician ethics. Concludes that physicians have an ethical duty to intervene in domestic violence so long as such intervention does not breach confidentiality or violate patient autonomy. Quotes Principle IV and Opinion 5.05. References Opinions 8.14 and 9.131. Jecker, *Privacy Beliefs and the Violent Family: Extending the Ethical Argument for Physician Intervention*, 269 J.A.M.A. 776, 778, 779 (1993).

Journal 1993 Discusses physicians' duty to disclose medical treatment alternatives to patients that are not readily available. Proposes that based on the historical development and legal requirements of the informed consent doctrine, physicians should be required to inform patients of nonreadily available alternatives or face liability for breach of such obligation. Quotes Principles I, II, III, IV, and V and Opinion 8.08. Note, *Informed Choice: Physicians' Duty to Disclose Nonreadily Available Alternatives*, 43 Case W. Res. L. Rev. 491, 491, 498-499, 508, 509 (1993).

Journal 1993 Explores the idea of reverse informed consent, which would impose a duty on patients to inform health care professionals of their infectious status. Concludes that such a duty is justified. Quotes Principles IV and VI and Opinions 8.11 and 9.131. Oddi, *Reverse Informed Consent: The Unreasonably Dangerous Patient*, 46 Vand. L. Rev. 1417, 1449, 1463, 1465, 1479 (1993).

Journal 1993 Discusses the issues surrounding the confidentiality of electronic and computerized medical records. Examines the factors that conflict with desirable security measures, such as cost and accessibility. Concludes that any legal standard addressing this problem should balance the need to protect patient confidentiality with the practical constraints limiting ideal security. References Principle IV and Opinion 5.07. Waller & Fulton, *The Electronic Chart; Keeping it Confidential and Secure*, 26 J. Health & Hosp. L. 104, 105 (April 1993).

Journal 1992 Discusses legal issues in the context of disclosing health information in adoptions. Presents the arguments for and against disclosure, including the traditional view favoring nondisclosure. Analyzes current disclosure statutes and argues that many of them do not go far enough in protecting the interests of the various parties involved. References Principle IV. Blair, *Lifting the Genealogical Veil: The Blueprint for Legislative Reform of the Disclosure of Health-Related Information in Adoption*, 70 No. Carolina L. Rev. 681, 692 (1992).

Journal 1991 Discusses the case of *Crist v. Moffat*, which prohibits ex parte communications with a plaintiff's treating physician in North Carolina. Examines the physician-patient privilege and looks at various jurisdictions that permit and forbid ex parte communications. Concludes that *Crist* is a reaffirmation of North Carolina's commitment to protecting the physician-patient relationship. Quotes Principle IV and Opinion 5.06. Comment, *Shielding the Plaintiff and Physician: The Prohibition of Ex Parte Contacts With a Plaintiff's Treating Physician*, 13 Campbell L. Rev. 233, 243, 248 (1991).

Journal 1990 Focuses on the concept of health care rationing. Examines the relationship between professional ethics and professional autonomy, perceived problems of rationing under a prospective payment versus a fee-for-service system, and the relationship between professional ethics and the problem of rationing. Concludes that rationing is inevitable, forcing important ethical questions to be addressed. Quotes Principles IV and VI. Agich, *Rationing and Professional Autonomy*, 18 Law, Med. & Health Care 77, 79, 82 (1990).

Journal 1990 Examines the extent to which forensic psychiatrists are consulted in medical malpractice cases. Considers the appropriate standard of care, particularly for psychiatric malpractice cases, and the problems associated with its determination. In cases where a practitioner was negligent, criteria for establishing damages are considered. References Principles II and IV. Modlin, *Forensic Psychiatry and Malpractice*, 18 Bull. Am. Acad. Psychiatry Law 153, 161 (1990).

Journal 1990 Discusses the moral dilemma in deciding whether to withdraw artificial nutrition and hydration from a patient and the appropriate role of the judiciary. States that part of the reason for judicial activism in this private area is because legislatures have not adequately expressed public policy. Concludes that judicial decisions do not represent the moral viewpoint of society and that moral pronouncements should not be made in the courtroom. Quotes Preamble, Principles I, II, III, IV, V, VI, and VII, and Opinion 2.20. Peccarelli, *A Moral Dilemma: The Role of Judicial Intervention in Withholding or Withdrawing Nutrition and Hydration*, 23 John Marshall L. Rev. 537, 539, 540, 541 (1990).

Journal 1990 Presents current issues, policies, legislation, and judicial decisions regarding impaired physicians. Considers confidentiality problems that arise in the disciplinary process. Concludes by proposing enhanced confidentiality requirements in disciplinary proceedings and nationwide adoption of a uniform law in this area. Quotes Opinion 4.07. References Principle IV. Walzer, *Impaired Physicians: An Overview and Update of the Legal Issues*, 11 J. Legal Med. 131, 174, 192 (1990).

Journal 1989 Discusses the history of the physician-patient privilege up through changes implemented under the Ohio Tort Reform Act of 1987. Aspects of the physician-patient privilege that are most significantly affected by this Tort Reform Act are highlighted, with recommendations for further refinement of the privilege in Ohio. Quotes Principles II and IV and Opinion 5.05. Note, *The Ohio Physician-Patient Privilege: Modified, Revised, and Defined*, 49 Ohio St. L. J. 1147, 1167 (1989).

Journal 1985 Focuses on the importance of patient autonomy in medical decision making. Initially describes how existing doctrines protect the value of autonomy in the context of the physician-patient relationship, then examines various problems in the current protective scheme. Case law is evaluated wherein enhanced protection is afforded to patient autonomy. Concludes by recommending the creation of an independent articulable protected interest in patient autonomy. Quotes Principles II and IV. Cites Opinions 4.04 (1984) [now Opinion 8.08] and 6.03 (1984) [now Opinion 6.02]. Shultz, *From Informed Consent to Patient Choice: A New Protected Interest*, 95 Yale L. J. 219, 275 (1985).

Journal 1983 Examines the evolution and impact of decisions in Tarasoff v. Regents of the University of California, 131 Cal. Rptr. 14 (Cal. 1976) and MacIntosh v. Milano, 403 A.2d 500 (N.J. Super. 1979) which established a duty on the part of a physician or psychotherapist to warn third parties foreseeably endangered by a patient. In establishing such a duty, the courts endeavored to balance the physician's duty to warn endangered third parties with the duty to maintain confidentiality within the physician-patient relationship. Much of the discussion centers on the vagueness of the concept of "dangerousness" which the courts use to establish the duty to warn and the manner in which a physician may fulfill this duty. Quotes Principle IV. Roth & Levin, *Dilemma of Tarasoff: Must Physicians Protect the Public or Their Patients?* 11 Law, Med. & Health Care 104, 106 (1983).

Journal 1981 Observes that a reevaluation of medicine and the medical profession is occurring on at least three levels: (1) theoretical; (2) educational; and (3) professional. Notes that physicians are facing various challenges to the exercise of many of their societal functions and emphasizes that physicians view law and the medical profession as the source most responsible for these challenges. Against the background of discussing the significant interface between law and medicine, describes how the Principles of Medical Ethics have significantly recognized a new professional role for physicians. Quotes Principle IV. Schwartz & Gibson, *Defining the Role of the Physician: Medical Education, Tradition, and the Legal Process*, 18 Houston L. Rev. 779, 791 (1981).

V.   A physician shall continue to study, apply and advance scientific knowledge, make relevant information available to patients, colleagues, and the public, obtain consultation, and use the talents of other health professionals when indicated.

S.D. Ind. 1992 Drug manufacturer sought protective order to prevent disclosure of patients' and physicians' names from adverse drug reaction reports. Plaintiff, quoting Principle V which requires that physicians "make relevant information available to ... the public," argued that requiring the disclosure of physicians' names would not deter physicians from reporting adverse drug reactions. The court held that the Principle notwithstanding, disclosure of physicians' names would seriously undermine the FDA's voluntary reporting system. *In re Eli Lilly & Co.*, 142 F.R.D. 454, 458.

D.S.C. 1968 Military dependent sued government physicians under Federal Tort Claims Act where child with acute abdominal pain was twice referred to naval hospital with diagnosis of possible appendicitis and twice sent home without treatment, eventually suffering ruptured appendix and serious complications. In finding for the plaintiff, the court quoted Principle 8 (1957) [now Principle V and Opinion 8.04] in considering whether the physicians had a duty to seek consultation in such a situation. *Steeves v. United States*, 294 F. Supp. 446, 454.

Tex. 1993 Estate of man who committed suicide after taking drug filed suit against manufacturer and sought adverse reaction or drug experience reports submitted to the FDA. These reports are voluntarily submitted by physicians and other health care providers and, according to 21 C.F.R. § 314.430(e)(4)(ii), the FDA must keep the identity of the reporters and the patients confidential. Noting the public interest in the voluntary reporting system and that the trial court had ordered disclosure of confidential information without applying the standard of relevance and need, the court denied disclosure of the reporters' identities. Quoting Principle V, the dissent declared that the decision adversely affected public health and safety by leaving drug manufacturers free to conceal important information. *Eli Lilly & Co. v. Marshall*, 850 S.W.2d 155, 163.

Journal 1997 Discusses physician frustration with managed care plans caused by gag clauses and cost-containment mechanisms. Reviews the development of managed care organizations and federal attempts at limiting the use of gag clauses. Concludes that gag clauses are "inherently flawed" and compromise quality health care. Quotes Principles II and V, Fundamental Elements (1), and Opinion 8.13. Note, *Physicians, Bound and Gagged: Federal Attempts to Combat Managed Care's Use of Gag Clauses*, 21 Seton Hall Legis. J. 567, 601-02 (1997).

Journal 1997 Discusses the need for balance between business ethics and medical ethics in the context of managed care. Explores two models for integrating ethics and managed care. Proposes the adoption of a collective responsibility model to improve quality of care. Quotes Principles I, II, III, IV, and V. Cites Preamble. References Opinion 8.13. Regan, *Regulating the Business of Medicine: Models for Integrating Ethics and Managed Care*, 30 Colum. J.L. & Soc. Probs. 635, 651, 656, 657 (1997).

Journal 1996 Discusses the trend toward conserving resources expended on health care by with-holding services absent a showing of necessity. Claims that the high standard of care physicians owe patients is jeopardized by medical treatment decisions based on coverage concerns. Concludes that the legal structure regarding health care plans should be changed. Quotes Preamble, Principles I, II, III, IV, V, VI, and VII and Opinion 2.03. Hirshfeld & Thomason, *Medical Necessity Determinations: The Need for a New Legal Structure*, 6 Health Matrix 3, 8-9 (1996).

Journal 1996 Considers the impact of gag clauses on the physician-patient relationship. Undertakes an extensive legal, ethical, and policy analysis. Concludes that gag clauses are viola-tive of legal and ethical principles. Quotes Principles II, V, and VI, and Fundamental Elements (1). Cites Preamble. Martin & Bjerknes, *The Legal and Ethical Implications of Gag Clauses in Physician Contracts*, XXII Am. J. Law & Med. 433, 465-66 (1996).

Journal 1994 Reviews the evolution of the physician-patient relationship. Describes legal responses to increasing awareness of the importance of ensuring patient autonomy. Examines the changing health care delivery environment. Concludes with a discussion of the impact of these changes on patient participation in medical decision-making. Quotes Preamble, Principles I, II, III, IV, V, and VI, Fundamental Elements (1) and (2), and Opinions 1.02 and 8.07 (1981) [now Opinion 8.08]. Cites Opinion 1.01. Szczygiel, *Beyond Informed Consent*, 21 Ohio N.U.L. Rev. 171, 217, 218, 220, 225, 226, 256 (1994).

Journal 1993 Discusses physicians' duty to disclose medical treatment alternatives to patients that are not readily available. Proposes that based on the historical development and legal requirements of the informed consent doctrine, physicians should be required to inform patients of nonreadily available alternatives or face liability for breach of such obligation. Quotes Principles I, II, III, IV, and V and Opinion 8.08. Note, *Informed Choice: Physicians' Duty to Disclose Nonreadily Available Alternatives*, 43 Case W. Res. L. Rev. 491, 491, 498-499, 508, 509 (1993).

Journal 1990 Discusses the moral dilemma in deciding whether to withdraw artificial nutrition and hydration from a patient and the appropriate role of the judiciary. States that part of the rea-son for judicial activism in this private area is because legislatures have not adequately expressed public policy. Concludes that judicial decisions do not represent the moral viewpoint of society and that moral pronouncements should not be made in the courtroom. Quotes Preamble, Principles I, II, III, IV, V, VI, and VII, and Opinion 2.20. Peccarelli, *A Moral Dilemma: The Role of Judicial Intervention in Withholding or Withdrawing Nutrition and Hydration*, 23 John Marshall L. Rev. 537, 539, 540, 541 (1990).

VI.   A physician shall, in the provision of appropriate patient care, except in emer-gencies, be free to choose whom to serve, with whom to associate, and the environment in which to provide medical services.

2d Cir. 1980 Appeal by hospital of National Labor Relations Board order to employ two part-time staff physicians on a full-time basis and to consider their applications for permanent admit-ting privileges. Physicians had joined picket line in sympathy with striking union employees without giving advance notice and were allegedly denied full-time positions in retaliation. The court held that support of the strike was activity protected by the National Labor Relations Act but that the physicians lost protection when they told patients the facility was unable to provide adequate care, in careless disregard of the truth. Further, the court noted that the failure to give notice before striking raised ethical questions under Principle 5 (1957) [now Principle VI]. *Montefiore Hosp. & Medical Ctr. v. NLRB*, 621 F.2d 510, 516.

4th Cir. 1984 Prisoner sued private physician under 42 U.S.C. Sec. 1983 for failure to provide medical treatment in violation of his eighth amendment rights. The court held that the exercise of the physician's medical judgment did not constitute action under color of state law. While not specifically referring to Principle VI (1980) the court cited the Principles for the general proposition that the physician-patient relationship is independent of state administrative supervision. This concept is apparently embodied in Principle VI. *Calvert v. Sharp*, 748 F.2d 861, 863, cert. denied, 471 U.S. 1132 (1975).

6th Cir. 1989 Plaintiff, a chiropractic association, alleged that the American Medical Association and several other professional associations violated antitrust law by conspiring to contain and ultimately eliminate the practice of chiropractic. The court provided an historical overview of the Association's gradual, but incomplete, recognition of chiropractors and "limited licensed practitioners" referring specifically to Principle 3 (1957) as well as to the Opinions and Reports of the Judicial Council Sec. 3, Para. 8 (1969) and to the Opinions and Reports 3.60 and 3.70 (1977) [now Principles VI and Opinions 3.01 and 3.04]. Based on its reading of these Principles and Opinions, the court reversed the trial court's grant of summary judgment to the Association because there remained a material issue of fact of whether it had continued to illegally boycott chiropractic. *Chiropractic Coop. Ass'n v. AMA*, 867 F.2d 270, 272-75.

W.D. Ark. 1989 Physician sued hospital alleging that it had acted in bad faith when it terminated his employment for failure to accept responsibility for "medical" as opposed to "surgical" patients. Plaintiff argued that the incorporation of the AMA's Principles of Medical Ethics into the hospital's by-laws gave him the right to choose which patients to serve, in apparent reference to Principle VI. While recognizing this right, the court held that the hospital had a corresponding right to consider such a refusal in its employment decisions. *Maxey v. United States*, 1989 U.S. Dist. LEXIS 5827.

N.D. Ga. 1981 Decedent's widow brought wrongful death action against hospital, treating physician, and physician supervising a group of emergency room physicians who had independent contracts with the hospital. Plaintiff claimed the supervising physician was vicariously liable in damages to her under the doctrine of respondeat superior. The court noted that the traditional control test used to identify agency relationships is ineffective in the context of physician-hospital relationships because physicians are bound by Principle 6 (1957) [now most closely embodied by the independent judgment aspects of Principle VI] which requires physicians to practice medicine according to their independent professional judgment. *Stewart v. Midani*, 525 F. Supp. 843, 848-49.

E.D. Mich. 1986 Plaintiff-chiropractors claimed violation of the Sherman Antitrust Act alleging that the American Medical Association conspired with others to injure them professionally and financially. In support of their claim, plaintiffs cited Principle 3 (1957) and the Opinions and Reports of the Judicial Council Sec.3, Para. 8 (1969) [now Principles VI and Opinions 3.01 and 3.04]. The court, noting the 1977 change in the Association's position regarding chiropractic reflected in the Opinions and Reports of the Judicial Council 3.60 and 3.70 (1977) [now Opinion 3.04] held that plaintiffs failed to demonstrate evidence of an overt act by the Association within the statutory limitations period. Summary judgment entered for Association. *Chiropractic Coop. Ass'n v. AMA*, 1986-2 Trade Cas. (CCH) ¶ 67,294, aff'd in part and rev'd in part, 867 F.2d 270 (6th Cir. 1989).

E.D. Mich. 1985 In an antitrust case brought by plaintiff-chiropractic association against the American Medical Association, plaintiffs presented the court with a motion in limine asking that the court strike defendant's affirmative defense of a good faith concern with public health and patient care. Plaintiffs argued that the defense was "unprecedented, in conflict with existing law and dramatically wrong." Plaintiffs referred to Principle 3 (1957) [now Principle VI and Opinions 3.01 and 3.04] as the source of the AMA's antitrust violations. The court denied plaintiffs' motion to strike, stating that under the "rule of reason" test, the Association had the right to present evidence that its actions furthered the public interest and patient care. *Chiropractic Coop. Ass'n v. AMA*, 617 F. Supp. 264, 266, aff'd in part and rev'd in part, 867 F.2d 270 (6th Cir. 1989).

D.N.M. 1987 In an antitrust action against major health insurance provider and state medical society, group of chiropractors alleged that a conspiracy existed in which the insurer refused to provide health cost reimbursement coverage for chiropractic services. Plaintiffs urged court to apply a "per se" analysis, rather than the "rule of reason" analysis to determine the legality of defendants' restrictive practices. The court declined to apply the "per se" test. In part, court's conclusion was based on view that concerns of defendant-physicians about relationship with chiropractors because of ethical restrictions imposed by Principle 3 (1957) [now Principle VI and Opinions 3.01 and 3.04] deserved more consideration than the "per se" test would afford. *Johnson v. Blue Cross/Blue Shield*, 677 F. Supp. 1112, 1118.

D. Vt. 1986 Prisoner sued prison officials and private physician under section 42 U.S.C. Sec. 1983, claiming cruel and unusual punishment in violation of his constitutional rights after physician allegedly frightened the prisoner while he was physically restrained, performed a colonoscopy with the examining room door open to a main hallway, and allowed guards to participate in the exam. The court held that although state law required the provision of medical care to inmates, the ethical canons upon which the physician-patient relationship was based were not derived from state law and the physician's actions did not constitute state action. In so holding, the court relied on Calvert v. Sharpe, 748 F.2d 861 (4th cir. 1984) which cites generally to the Principles for the proposition that the physician-patient relationship is independent of state supervision. Principle VI reflects this concept. *Nash v. Wennar, 645 F.Supp. 238, 242.*

Ariz. 1984 Mother sued hospital and physicians after minor son was transferred to another facility for solely financial reasons although emergency surgical care was medically indicated. In holding that the hospital's transfer policy pre-empted further care by the physicians and that the record revealed no physician negligence, the court stated that generally the standard of care for physicians is determined by "what is usually done by members of the profession." The court then cited Principle VI, apparently for the proposition that in emergency situations there may be an ethical, rather than legal, obligation to provide care. *Thompson v. Sun City Community Hosp., Inc., 141 Ariz. 597, 688 P.2d 605, 612 n.7.*

Ariz. App. 1980 Malpractice suit against a paid "on call" physician for refusal to treat decedent resulting in delay in treatment. The court quoted Principle 5 (1957) [now Principle VI and Opinion 8.11] as establishing an ethical duty to provide emergency care. However, court distinguished any such ethical obligation from its holding that physician had a contractual duty to treat emergency patients to the best of his ability. *Hiser v. Randolph, 126 Ariz. 608, 617 P.2d 774, 776 n.1, 777, 778.*

Cal. App. 1978 Surviving spouse sued physicians who were on emergency surgical call panel for malpractice where patient died during surgery. Although defendants claimed immunity under state Good Samaritan statute, the court held the statute inapplicable since the legislative purpose was to encourage physicians to render care on an irregular basis to unattended persons discovered by chance at the scene of an emergency. In so holding, the court noted that Principle 5 (1957) [now Principle VI and Opinions 8.11 and 9.06] imposed an ethical duty to render emergency medical care. *Colby v. Schwartz, 78 Cal. App. 3d 885, 144 Cal. Rptr. 624, 627 n.2.*

Ky. App. 1989 Malpractice suit was initiated against physician for failure to treat plaintiff's brother where defendant had repeatedly rebuffed plaintiff's request for emergency assistance and told him to "get in line" or "sign in." Plaintiff removed his brother to another hospital where he ubsequently died of heart attack. Plaintiff argued that defendant was under a duty to treat based upon, inter alia, the AMA "Code of Ethics" [apparently Principle VI and Opinion 8.11]. The court rejected the argument, finding that a breach of ethical standards may establish grounds for professional discipline, but not a civil cause of action, and held that defendant was under no legal duty to treat. *Noble v. Sartori, 1989 Ky. App. LEXIS 67.*

N.J. Super. 1994 Plaintiff-physician alleged that nursing home violated public policy when it terminated his at-will employment in retaliation for his refusal to see and treat patients in excess of his original work load. With apparent reference to Principle VI, physician argued that caring for excessive numbers of patients violated his ethical responsibilities and public policy. The court held that even though physician's objections to nursing home's practices may have supported a reasonable belief that public policy was violated, there was insufficient evidence that objections contributed to termination. *Fineman v. New Jersey Dept. of Human Servs., 272 N.J. Super. 606, 640 A.2d 1161, 1163, 1166, 1169-1170, cert. denied, 138 N.J. 267, 649 A.2d 1287 (1994).*

N.J. Super. 1960 Plaintiff, a graduate of a school of osteopathy and licensed to practice medicine and surgery in New Jersey, sought to compel the defendant medical society to admit him to full membership. Defendant claimed as an affirmative defense that to admit plaintiff would violate Principle 3 (1957) [now Principle VI and Opinion 3.01] because plaintiff possessed a degree in osteopathy rather than an M.D. The court noted that the defendant society had virtually monopolistic control of medical practice in the state and that exclusion from membership caused substantial injury. In view of this, the court ordered the defendant society to admit plaintiff to its membership. To bar membership of a licensed graduate of an approved school of osteopathy would, the court held, violate public policy. *Falcone v. Middlesex County Medical Soc'y, 62 N.J. Super. 184, 162 A.2d 324, 328-29, aff'd, 34 N.J. 582, 170 A.2d 791 (1961).*

N.Y. Sup. 1993 Defendant was charged with violating state statute imposing criminal sanction on a physician who refuses to treat a person seeking emergency medical care. Defendant sought dismissal of the charge challenging the constitutionality of the statute and arguing that it requires mens rea. The court denied defendant's motion for dismissal, concluding that the statute was constitutional and that the legislature clearly imposed strict liability. The court quoted Principle VI in support of its strict liability conclusion. *People v. Anyakora, 162 Misc. 2d 47, 616 N.Y.S.2d 149, 155.*

Ohio App. 1991 Medical corporation sought an injunction to enforce a covenant not to compete against defendant-physician. The lower court granted summary judgment based on a referee's report which concluded that, under Principle VI and Opinions 6.11, 9.02, and 9.06 (1989) restrictive covenants were *per se* unenforceable as a matter of public policy. While recognizing a strong public interest in allowing open access to health care, the appellate court in reversing held that Opinion 9.02, which applied specifically to restrictive covenants, only "discouraged" such covenants. *Ohio Urology, Inc. v. Poll, 72 Ohio. App. 446, 450, 451, 594 N.E.2d 1027, 1030, 1031.*

Wash. 1951 Plaintiff, a charitable, not for profit medical corporation, offered prepaid health care services to members and their families. Suit was filed against county medical society and others for damages and injunction for defendants' alleged efforts to monopolize prepaid medical care in area and unlawfully restrain competition by plaintiff and its physicians. Defendants alleged as affirmative defense that their efforts were designed to curb "unethical" prepaid contract practice by plaintiff. Court examined at length American Medical Association's position regarding "contract practice" including Principles Ch. III, Art. VI, Secs. 3 and 4 (1947) [now Principle VI and Opinions 8.05 and 9.06] concluding nothing in plaintiff's practice violated the Association's ethical guidelines. Further, quoting Principles Ch. III, Art. III, Sec.1 (1947) [now Opinion 8.04] dealing with consultations, court noted that defendants' efforts impeded plaintiff's physicians from obtaining consultations. Court concluded that defendants' actions constituted unlawful, monopolistic behavior and issued an injunction, although it declined to award damages. *Group Health Coop. v. King County Medical Soc'y, 39 Wash. 2d 586, 237 P.2d 737, 744, 750-51, 759-60.*

Wash. App. 1984 Plaintiff-pathologist sued his corporate employer and one of its subsidiaries for breach of his employment contract; defendants counterclaimed, alleging that plaintiff had tortiously interfered with defendants' business relationships. Plaintiff had discouraged the transfer of laboratory specimens for analysis at a distant lab because he allegedly believed that to do so would be a violation of medical ethics, particularly Principle 6 (1957) [now Principle VII]. In finding for plaintiff, the court acknowledged that a physician was bound to uphold duly prescribed medical ethical principles despite his employment status, especially where such a principle coincided with a public policy favoring acts that tend to prevent "a deterioration of the quality of medical care." *Wood v. Upjohn Co., No. 60931-II (Sept. 4, 1984) (LEXIS, States library, Wash. file).*

Journal 1997 Reports on a study of physician attitudes regarding expert witnesses. Notes that a majority of physicians believe that medical expert testimony should be subject to peer review and, when appropriate, medical licensing board discipline. Quotes Principles II and VI, and Opinion 9.07. Eitel, Hegeman, & Evans, *Medicine on Trial: Physicians' Attitudes about Expert Medical Witnesses, 18 J. Legal Med. 345, 355, 358 (1997).*

Journal 1997 Analyzes the prohibition against employment agreements between corporations and licensed physicians. Discusses the origins and development of the corporate practice of medicine doctrine. Proposes that state legislatures should adopt doctrinal modifications to aid in the movement toward managed care. Quotes Principle VI. Mars, *The Corporate Practice of Medicine: A Call for Action, 7 Heath Matrix 241, 267 (1997).*

Journal 1996 Discusses the trend toward conserving resources expended on health care by withholding services absent a showing of necessity. Claims that the high standard of care physicians owe patients is jeopardized by medical treatment decisions based on coverage concerns. Concludes that the legal structure regarding health care plans should be changed. Quotes Preamble, Principles I, II, III, IV, V, VI, and VII and Opinion 2.03. Hirshfeld & Thomason, *Medical Necessity Determinations: The Need for a New Legal Structure, 6 Health Matrix 3, 8-9 (1996).*

Journal 1996 Considers the impact of gag clauses on the physician-patient relationship. Undertakes an extensive legal, ethical, and policy analysis. Concludes that gag clauses are violative of legal and ethical principles. Quotes Principles II, V, and VI, and Fundamental Elements (1). Cites Preamble. Martin & Bjerknes, *The Legal and Ethical Implications of Gag Clauses in Physician Contracts, XXII Am. J. Law & Med. 433, 465-66 (1996).*

Journal 1996 Discusses commercialization of the medical industry. Addresses ethical and policy considerations that form the basis for the corporate practice of medicine doctrine. Observes that the doctrine is now outdated. Quotes Principle VI. Parker, *Corporate Practice of Medicine: Last Stand or Final Downfall?*, 29 J. Health & Hosp. L. 160, 167, 173 (1996).

Journal 1996 Examines the recent trend in health care laws and ethics to focus on the alleviation of suffering. Expresses concern that such a focus may result in the valuation of one life over another. Emphasizes the need to evaluate multiple, diverse responses to suffering. Quotes Principle VI. References Opinion 2.162. Shepherd, *Sophie's Choices: Medical and Legal Responses to Suffering*, 72 Notre Dame L. Rev. 103, 106, 133 (1996).

Journal 1995 Examines the rights of health care professionals to refuse to participate in patient care on the basis of conscientious objection. Discusses rights and duties of health care facilities in this context. Suggests steps that facilities may take when dealing with health care professionals who object to participating in patient care. Quotes Principles I and VI and Opinions 1.02, 2.035, and 9.055. Dellinger & Vickery, *When Staff Object to Participating In Care*, 28 J. Health & Hospital Law 269, 272, 276 (1995).

Journal 1995 Provides legal and medical definitions of physician-assisted suicide and euthanasia. Offers relevant historical perspectives and provides comprehensive ethical and legal discussion of these compelling social issues. Highlights important legislative developments, including the Oregon Death with Dignity Act, and analyzes significant judicial opinions. Advocates legal tolerance of physician-assisted suicide and euthanasia. Quotes Principles III, IV, and VI and Opinions 2.21 and 9.12. Cites Opinions 2.20 and 8.11. Stone & Winslade, *Physician-Assisted Suicide and Euthanasia in the United States: Legal and Ethical Observations*, 16 J. Legal Med. 481, 483, 490, 497, 498, 499 (1995).

Journal 1995 Examines the history of Medicaid physician reimbursement and physician participation. Discusses the debate over TennCare, Tennessee's Medicaid experiment. Concludes that states should facilitate tie-ins among Medicaid patients and privately insured patients rather than raising physician fees. Cites Principle VI. Watson, *Medicaid Physician Participation: Patients, Poverty, and Physician Self-Interest*, XXI Am. J. Law & Med. 191, 218 (1995).

Journal 1994 Analyzes the corporate practice of medicine doctrine. Asserts that viability of the doctrine is questionable in the modern health care industry. Quotes Principle VI. Dowell, *The Corporate Practice of Medicine Prohibition: A Dinosaur Awaiting Extinction*, 27 J. Health & Hospital Law 369, 370 (1994).

Journal 1994 Explores how the Americans with Disabilities Act has created, through federal civil rights mechanisms, a legal duty to treat HIV-infected patients. Discusses previous attempts to create a professional obligation to treat patients with AIDS. Quotes Principle VI and Opinion 9.131. Cites Opinion 9.12. Halevy & Brody, *Acquired Immunodeficiency Syndrome and the Americans with Disabilities Act: A Legal Duty to Treat*, 96 Am. J. Med. 282, 283, 284 (1994).

Journal 1994 Reviews the evolution of the physician-patient relationship. Describes legal responses to increasing awareness of the importance of ensuring patient autonomy. Examines the changing health care delivery environment. Concludes with a discussion of the impact of these changes on patient participation in medical decision-making. Quotes Preamble, Principles I, II, III, IV, V, and VI, Fundamental Elements (1) and (2), and Opinions 1.02 and 8.07 (1981) [now Opinion 8.08]. Cites Opinion 1.01. Szczygiel, *Beyond Informed Consent*, 21 Ohio N.U.L. Rev. 171, 217, 218, 220, 225, 226, 256 (1994).

Journal 1993 Examines challenges in New York to a lawyer's right to discriminate in the context of selecting clients. Explores the traditional view that lawyers have unfettered discretion to select clients and New York's antidiscrimination disciplinary rule, statutes, and case law. Concludes that the legal profession should prohibit invidious or improper discrimination. Quotes Principle VI and Opinions 9.12 and 9.131. Begg, *Revoking the Lawyers' License to Discriminate in New York: The Demise of a Traditional Professional Prerogative*, 7 Geo. J. Legal Ethics 275, 298, 299 (1993).

Journal 1993 Addresses both patient rights under California consent and confidentiality laws relating to AIDS and prohibitions on unreasonable searches and seizures under the United States Constitution. Concludes that any health care worker who can document an exposure to blood or body fluids should have the option of compelling a nonconsenting patient to be tested for HIV. Quotes Principle VI and Opinion 9.131. Comment, *Nonconsensual HIV Testing in the Health Care Setting: The Case for Extending the Occupational Protections of California Proposition 96 to Health Care Workers*, 26 Loy. L.A. L. Rev. 1251, 1269 (1993).

Journal 1993 Discusses physicians' duty to disclose medical treatment alternatives to patients that are not readily available. Proposes that based on the historical development and legal requirements of the informed consent doctrine, physicians should be required to inform patients of nonreadily available alternatives or face liability for breach of such obligation. Quotes Principles I, II, III, IV, and V and Opinion 8.08. Note, *Informed Choice: Physicians' Duty to Disclose Nonreadily Available Alternatives*, 43 Case W. Res. L. Rev. 491, 491, 498-499, 508, 509 (1993).

Journal 1993 Explores the idea of reverse informed consent, which would impose a duty on patients to inform health care professionals of their infectious status. Concludes that such a duty is justified. Quotes Principles IV and VI and Opinions 8.11 and 9.131. Oddi, *Reverse Informed Consent: The Unreasonably Dangerous Patient*, 46 Vand. L. Rev. 1417, 1449, 1463, 1465, 1479 (1993).

Journal 1992 Discusses the plight of undocumented aliens and their need for access to medical care. Considers existing systems for providing such care, as well as barriers to the receipt of medical attention. Concludes by examining remedies for this population and proposing alternative systems of delivery. Cites Principles VI and VII. Loue, *Access to Health Care and the Undocumented Alien*, 13 J. Legal Med. 271, 291 (1992).

Journal 1991 Considers whether physicians have an obligation to provide medical care to HIV-infected patients. Examines various sources for such a duty, including a moral obligation not to discriminate and a social responsibility to provide access to health care. Concludes that physicians have a duty to treat. Quotes Opinion 9.131. Cites Principle VI. Daniels, *Duty to Treat or Right to Refuse?*, 21 Hastings Center Rep. 36, 37, 42 (March/April 1991).

Journal 1991 Discusses the problem of noncompliant patients and whether a physician may deny treatment to these individuals. Notes relevant legal and ethical considerations. Concludes that physicians are not relieved of their duty to treat noncompliant patients, especially because these patients may not be able to adequately control their behavior. Cites Principle VI and Opinion 9.12. Orentlicher, *Denying Treatment to the Noncompliant Patient*, 265 J.A.M.A. 1579, 1581 (1991).

Journal 1990 Focuses on the concept of health care rationing. Examines the relationship between professional ethics and professional autonomy, perceived problems of rationing under a prospective payment versus a fee-for-service system, and the relationship between professional ethics and the problem of rationing. Concludes that rationing is inevitable, forcing important ethical questions to be addressed. Quotes Principles IV and VI. Agich, *Rationing and Professional Autonomy*, 18 Law, Med. & Health Care 77, 79, 82 (1990).

Journal 1990 Considers the propriety of HIV testing for hospital patients prior to non-emergency surgery. Discusses the medical aspects of AIDS and the risk of HIV transmission. Looks at available HIV tests, including reliability and cost. Concludes that testing of patients should be permitted so long as it is not done with the intent, nor the effect, of discriminating against individual patients. Quotes Principle VI and Opinion 9.131. Naccasha, *The Permissibility of Routine AIDS Testing in the Health Care Context*, 5 Notre Dame J.L. Ethics & Pub. Pol'y, 223, 241 (1990).

Journal 1990 Discusses a physician's duty to treat AIDS patients. Surveys applicable law and considers philosophical foundations underpinning ethical duty. Concludes that there is a weak basis for imposing an ethical duty to treat, but suggests that a legal duty may be fashioned. Quotes Principle V (1980) [now Principle VI]. Note, *Ethics and AIDS: A Summary of the Law and a Critical Analysis of the Individual Physician's Ethical Duty to Treat*, XVI Am. J. Law & Med. 249, 262 (1990).

Journal 1990 Discusses the moral dilemma in deciding whether to withdraw artificial nutrition and hydration from a patient and the appropriate role of the judiciary. States that part of the reason for judicial activism in this private area is because legislatures have not adequately expressed public policy. Concludes that judicial decisions do not represent the moral viewpoint of society and that moral pronouncements should not be made in the courtroom. Quotes Preamble, Principles I, II, III, IV, V, VI, and VII, and Opinion 2.20. Peccarelli, *A Moral Dilemma: The Role of Judicial Intervention in Withholding or Withdrawing Nutrition and Hydration*, 23 John Marshall L. Rev. 537, 539, 540, 541 (1990).

Journal 1989 Explores factors contributing to the stigmatization of HIV-infected individuals. Discusses the legal and ethical challenges that AIDS poses for health care providers. Proposes that health care providers actively participate in preventing HIV infection, providing care for HIV-infected individuals, and fighting AIDS and its associated stigma. Quotes Principle VI and Opinion 9.131. Forrester, *AIDS: The Responsibility to Care*, 34 Vill. L. Rev. 799, 811 (1989).

Journal 1989 Initially examines the significant factors that caused delay in the evolution of a legal duty to provide emergency care and treatment. Then discusses common law developments in the 1960s and 1970s that established a duty to provide such care. Observes that the common law met with only limited success in this regard and concludes that the Consolidated Omnibus Budget Reconciliation Act of 1985 offers the greatest likelihood for creating a nationally enforceable legal duty to provide emergency care. Quotes Principle VI. Rothenberg, *Who Cares? The Evolution of the Legal Duty to Provide Emergency Care, 26 Houston L. Rev. 21, 22 (1989).*

Journal 1988 Discusses the various biological hazards confronting health care workers caring for HIV seropositive patients. Noting that safety precautions have been recommended by CDC and OSHA, observes that, despite these measures, if health care providers believe that a risk of contagion exists, they may take steps to limit exposure by reducing care. Against this background, it is suggested that policies be developed to help ensure that the threat of AIDS does not limit access to care for HIV seropositive patients. Quotes Principle 5 (1980) [sic] [now Principle VII]. Brennan, *Ensuring Adequate Health Care for the Sick: The Challenge of the Acquired Immunodeficiency Syndrome as an Occupational Disease, 1988 Duke L. J. 29, 47.*

Journal 1988 Discusses the question of whether health professionals are obligated to subject themselves to the risks that attend treating patients with communicable diseases, particularly AIDS. Examines the ethical pronouncements and codes of the nursing and medical professions in this respect, noting that the most recent statements of professional values imply the existence of an obligation to treat HIV-infectious patients. Offers a discussion of the evolution of this viewpoint. Quotes Opinion 8.10 (1986) [now Opinion 8.11] and Principle VI. Cites Opinion 9.11 (1986) [now Opinion 9.12]. Freedman, *Health Professions, Codes, and the Right to Refuse to Treat HIV-Infectious Patients, 18 Hastings Center Rep. 20 (Supp.), 23, 24 (April/May 1988).*

Journal 1986 Addresses the problem of "patient dumping" and explores the various reasons underlying this practice. Examines applicable common law and statutory law, emphasizing the antidumping provisions of COBRA. Weaknesses in this federal legislative scheme are highlighted and recommendations for strengthening the statute and maximizing access to emergency medical care are offered. Quotes Principle VI and Opinion 8.10 (1986) [now Opinion 8.11]. Note, *Preventing Patient Dumping: Sharpening the COBRA's Fangs, 61 N. Y. U. L. Rev. 1186, 1189-90 (1986).*

VII. A physician shall recognize a responsibility to participate in activities contributing to an improved community.

Ariz. 1965 Physician appealed denial of medical license which was based on alleged violations of local medical society rules and Principles 3, 5, and 10 (1957) [now Principles III and VII, and Opinions 3.01, 8.11, and 9.06]. Alleged violations included treating a patient without first obtaining a prior treating physician's permission, inadequate patient care, performing operations without hospital privileges, and signing the medical record of a deceased patient who had been treated by interns. The court held that the evidence failed to show any clear violation of the Principles and that a local medical society had no right to prescribe a code of ethics for state licensing purposes. *Arizona State Bd. of Medical Examiners v. Clark, 97 Ariz. 205, 398 P.2d 908, 914-15, 915 n.3.*

Journal 1996 Discusses the trend toward conserving resources expended on health care by withholding services absent a showing of necessity. Claims that the high standard of care physicians owe patients is jeopardized by medical treatment decisions based on coverage concerns. Concludes that the legal structure regarding health care plans should be changed. Quotes Preamble, Principles I, II, III, IV, V, VI, and VII and Opinion 2.03. Hirshfeld & Thomason, *Medical Necessity Determinations: The Need for a New Legal Structure, 6 Health Matrix 3, 8-9 (1996).*

Journal 1996 Proposes an alternative method of capital punishment to allow for organ donation by executed prisoners. Provides justifications for this proposal. Concludes that physicians should be able to ethically participate in this process. Quotes Principle VII. Cites Opinion 2.06. References Opinion 2.162 (1994) [subsequently amended]. Patton, *A Call for Common Sense: Organ Donation and the Executed Prisoner, 3 Va. J. Soc. Pol'y & L. 387, 404, 405, 407-10 (1996).*

Journal 1995 Examines the conflict between medical ethics and patent laws. Explores the debates and commentaries regarding patenting medical instruments and processes. Concludes that current patent law fails to address the ethical concerns of physicians and their patients.

Quotes Principles of Medical Ethics § 10 (1971) [now Principle VII] and Principle § 2 (1971) [now Opinion 9.095] and Opinions 9.08 and 9.09. Reisman, *Physicians and Surgeons as Inventors: Reconciling Medical Process Patents and Medical Ethics*, 10 High Tech. L. J. 355, 356, 368-70, 385 (1995).

Journal 1992 Discusses the problem of discrimination based on HIV status, particularly among women and children. Examines medical and public health issues involving HIV. Looks at types of HIV discrimination, the degree of prevalence, and causes. Focuses on federal, state, and local laws. Cites Principle VII. References Opinion 9.131. Gittler & Rennart, *HIV Infection Among Women and Children and Antidiscrimination Laws: An Overview*, 77 Iowa L. Rev. 1313, 1363 (1992).

Journal 1992 Discusses the plight of undocumented aliens and their need for access to medical care. Considers existing systems for providing such care, as well as barriers to the receipt of medical attention. Concludes by examining remedies for this population and proposing alternative systems of delivery. Cites Principles VI and VII. Loue, *Access to Health Care and the Undocumented Alien*, 13 J. Legal Med. 271, 291 (1992).

Journal 1990 Discusses the moral dilemma in deciding whether to withdraw artificial nutrition and hydration from a patient and the appropriate role of the judiciary. States that part of the reason for judicial activism in this private area is because legislatures have not adequately expressed public policy. Concludes that judicial decisions do not represent the moral viewpoint of society and that moral pronouncements should not be made in the courtroom. Quotes Preamble, Principles I, II, III, IV, V, VI, and VII, and Opinion 2.20. Peccarelli, *A Moral Dilemma: The Role of Judicial Intervention in Withholding or Withdrawing Nutrition and Hydration*, 23 John Marshall L. Rev. 537, 539, 540, 541 (1990).

Fundamental Elements of the Patient-Physician Relationship

From ancient times, physicians have recognized that the health and well-being of patients depends upon a collaborative effort between physician and patient. Patients share with physicians the responsibility for their own health care. The patient-physician relationship is of greatest benefit to patients when they bring medical problems to the attention of their physicians in a timely fashion, provide information about their medical condition to the best of their ability, and work with their physicians in a mutually respectful alliance. Physicians can best contribute to this alliance by serving as their patients' advocate and by fostering these rights:

Journal 1997 Compares past ethical opinions to current opinions and notes the differences. Comments on the forces that have changed medical ethics through the years. Notes differing theories on the future course of medical ethics. Quotes Fundamental Elements (Preamble) and Opinions 5.05, 5.057, 7.01, 8.12, 9.12, and 9.131. Cites Fundamental Elements (5) and Opinions 8.115 and 8.13. Buchanan, *Medical Ethics at the Millennium: A Brief Retrospective*, 26 Colo. Law. 141, 142, 143, 144, 145 (1997).

1. The patient has the right to receive information from physicians and to discuss the benefits, risks, and costs of appropriate treatment alternatives. Patients should receive guidance from their physicians as to the optimal course of action. Patients are also entitled to obtain copies or summaries of their medical records, to have their questions answered, to be advised of potential conflicts of interest that their physicians might have, and to receive independent professional opinions.

Journal 1997 Discusses physician frustration with managed care plans caused by gag clauses and cost-containment mechanisms. Reviews the development of managed care organizations and federal attempts at limiting the use of gag clauses. Concludes that gag clauses are "inherently flawed" and compromise quality health care. Quotes Principles II and V, Fundamental Elements (1), and Opinion 8.13. Note, *Physicians, Bound and Gagged: Federal Attempts to Combat Managed Care's Use of Gag Clauses*, 21 Seton Hall Legis. J. 567, 601-02 (1997).

Journal 1994 Considers whether an exception should be made to physician-patient confidentiality that would allow a physician to reveal parental medical history to a child. Discusses whether parents should be required to divulge their medical history to their children. Concludes that such an exception would not completely erode physician-patient confidentiality. Quotes Principles IV, Fundamental Elements (4), and Opinion 5.05. Cites Principle I and Fundamental Elements (1). Friedland, *Physician-Patient Confidentiality: Time to Re-Examine a Venerable Concept in Light of Contemporary Society and Advances in Medicine*, 15 J. Legal Med. 249, 257, 264, 276 (1994).

Journal 1994 Reviews the evolution of the physician-patient relationship. Describes legal responses to increasing awareness of the importance of ensuring patient autonomy. Examines the changing health care delivery environment. Concludes with a discussion of the impact of these changes on patient participation in medical decision-making. Quotes Preamble, Principles I, II, III, IV, V, and VI, Fundamental Elements (1) and (2), and Opinions 1.02 and 8.07 (1981) [now Opinion 8.08]. Cites Opinion 1.01. Szczygiel, *Beyond Informed Consent*, 21 Ohio N.U.L. Rev. 171, 217, 218, 220, 225, 226, 256 (1994).

2.   The patient has the right to make decisions regarding the health care that is recommended by his or her physician. Accordingly, patients may accept or refuse any recommended medical treatment.

Journal 1996 Considers the ethical requirement for physicians to receive informed consent from patients before beginning treatment. Reviews the case of *Jacobson v. Massachusetts*, discussing its impact on informed consent and vaccination policy in the United States. Quotes Fundamental Elements (2). References Opinion 8.08. Severyn, *Jacobson v. Massachusetts: Impact on Informed Consent and Vaccine Policy*, 5 J. Pharmacy & L. 249, 253, 274 (1996).

Journal 1994 Reviews the evolution of the physician-patient relationship. Describes legal responses to increasing awareness of the importance of ensuring patient autonomy. Examines the changing health care delivery environment. Concludes with a discussion of the impact of these changes on patient participation in medical decision-making. Quotes Preamble, Principles I, II, III, IV, V, and VI, Fundamental Elements (1) and (2), and Opinions 1.02 and 8.07 (1981) [now Opinion 8.08]. Cites Opinion 1.01. Szczygiel, *Beyond Informed Consent*, 21 Ohio N.U.L. Rev. 171, 217, 218, 220, 225, 226, 256 (1994).

3.   The patient has the right to courtesy, respect, dignity, responsiveness, and timely attention to his or her needs.

4.   The patient has the right to confidentiality. The physician should not reveal confidential communications or information without the consent of the patient, unless provided for by law or by the need to protect the welfare of the individual or the public interest.

Journal 1997 Reviews ethical issues raised by genetic research. Explores the duty a physician may have to reveal the genetic diseases found in patients to their relatives. Considers case law and statutory law, and concludes that a limited duty to disclose exists. Quotes Fundamental Elements (4). Deftos, *Genomic Torts: The Law of the Future—The Duty of Physicians to Disclose the Presence of a Genetic Disease to the Relatives of Their Patients with the Disease*, 32 U.S.F. L. Rev. 105, 130 (1997).

Journal 1994 Considers whether an exception should be made to physician-patient confidentiality that would allow a physician to reveal parental medical history to a child. Discusses whether parents should be required to divulge their medical history to their children. Concludes that such an exception would not completely erode physician-patient confidentiality. Quotes Principles IV, Fundamental Elements (4), and Opinion 5.05. Cites Principle I and Fundamental Elements (1). Friedland, *Physician-Patient Confidentiality: Time to Re-Examine a Venerable Concept in Light of Contemporary Society and Advances in Medicine*, 15 J. Legal Med. 249, 257, 264, 276 (1994).

Journal 1994 Explores the ethical issues involved in a multidisciplinary team working with children in legal proceedings. Focuses on the relationships between professionals and the conflicts that arise regarding disclosure of confidential information and forced disclosure of non-privileged information. Examines theories supporting protection of client information. Quotes Principles III, IV, Fundamental Elements (4) and Opinions 1.02 (1992) and 5.07 (1992) [now Opinion 5.05]. Cites Opinions 2.02. Glynn, *Multidisciplinary Representation of Children: Conflicts Over Disclosures of Client Communications*, 27 J. Marshall L. Rev. 617, 625, 626, 630-32, 637, 639, 643 (1994).

Journal 1994 Discusses physician-patient confidentiality and the exception that permits breach of a patient's confidence if required by law. Argues that this is always a legitimate exception to the confidentiality rule. Quotes Principle IV and Fundamental Elements (4). McConnell, *Confidentiality and the Law*, 20 J. Med. Ethics 47, 47 (1994).

Journal 1994 Discusses the importance of confidentiality in the physician-patient relationship and under what circumstances patient information may be released. Examines unique considerations that apply when a physician provides medical care to a minor or an HIV-infected individual. Addresses medical record retention. Discusses threats to medical record privacy caused by new advances in communications technology. Quotes Principle IV and Fundamental Elements (4). Weiner & Wettstein, *Confidentiality of Patient-Related Information*, 112 Arch. Ophthalmology 1032, 1033 (1994).

5. The patient has the right to continuity of health care. The physician has an obligation to cooperate in the coordination of medically indicated care with other health care providers treating the patient. The physician may not discontinue treatment of a patient as long as further treatment is medically indicated, without giving the patient reasonable assistance and sufficient opportunity to make alternative arrangements for care.

Journal 1997 Compares past ethical opinions to current opinions and notes the differences. Comments on the forces that have changed medical ethics through the years. Notes differing theories on the future course of medical ethics. Quotes Fundamental Elements (Preamble) and Opinions 5.05, 5.057, 7.01, 8.12, 9.12, and 9.131. Cites Fundamental Elements (5) and Opinions 8.115 and 8.13. Buchanan, *Medical Ethics at the Millennium: A Brief Retrospective*, 26 Colo. Law. 141, 142, 143, 144, 145 (1997).

Journal 1996 Examines medically futile treatment in light of legislative enactments in Virginia and Maryland. Observes that the futility debate arises when requests for life-prolonging treatment are viewed as medically inappropriate by health care providers. Concludes that, while the ethical integrity of the medical profession justifies some legal recognition of futility, such recognition must be limited by respect for patient autonomy. References Fundamental Elements (5). Shiner, *Medical Futility: A Futile Concept?*, 53 Wash. & Lee L. Rev. 803, 834 (1996).

Journal 1995 Examines the impact of health care reform on physician-patient relationships. Observes that patients' primary relationships may be with their insurers (HMOs) rather than their physicians. Discusses how reform may threaten the physician's fiduciary duty of loyalty by forcing physicians to make rationing decisions and giving physicians financial incentives to limit use of health care resources. Considers how these potentially harmful effects may be mitigated. Quotes Fundamental Elements (5). Cites Opinion 5.05. Orentlicher, *Health Care Reform and the Patient-Physician Relationship*, 5 Health Matrix 141, 143, 148 (1995).

Journal 1993 Examines the legal, medical, and ethical issues involved when a patient or a patient's family demands treatment that the physician believes would be futile. Analyzes the implications of giving patients an absolute right to control medical treatment. Argues that courts should refrain from ordering physicians to treat patients when physicians believe that treatment would be ineffective. Quotes Fundamental Elements (5) and Opinions 2.11 (1982) [now Opinion 2.20] and 2.18 (1986) [now Opinion 2.20]. Comment, *Beyond Autonomy: Judicial Restraint and the Legal Limits Necessary to Uphold the Hippocratic Tradition and Preserve the Ethical Integrity of the Medical Profession*, 9 J. Contemp. Health L. & Pol'y 451, 467, 468 (1993).

6. The patient has a basic right to have available adequate health care. Physicians, along with the rest of society, should continue to work toward this goal. Fulfillment of this right is dependent on society providing resources so that no patient is deprived of necessary care because of an inability to pay for the care. Physicians should continue their traditional assumption of a part of the responsibility for the medical care of those who cannot afford essential health care. Physicians should advocate for patients in dealing with third parties when appropriate.

Journal 1997 Considers the current approach to health care in the United States. Examines financing mechanisms, and suggests that reform could be effected through a decentralized, community-based approach. Proposes use of volunteer systems in which medical personnel would care for certain patients free of charge or at reduced rates. Quotes Fundamental Elements (6). References Opinion 9.065. Solomon & Asaro, *Community-Based Health Care: A Legal and Policy Analysis*, 24 Fordham Urb. L. J. 235, 276-77 (1997).

Journal 1996 Describes the problem of lack of access to medical care by the indigent. Recognizes the commitment of the medical profession to providing care for indigent patients. Observes that state initiatives that provide physicians tort immunity in exchange for volunteer service can improve access to care by the indigent. Quotes Fundamental Elements (6). References Opinion 9.065. Comment, *Statutory Immunity for Volunteer Physicians: A Vehicle for Reaffirmation of the Doctor's Beneficent Duties—Absent the Rights Talk*, 1 Widener L. Symp. J. 425, 448, 449 (1996).

Report of the Council on Ethical and Judicial Affairs of the American Medical Association, June 1990.

Updated 1993.

Patient Responsibilities

It has long been recognized that successful medical care requires an ongoing collaborative effort between patients and physicians. Physicians and patients are bound in a partnership that requires both individuals to take an active role in the healing process. Such a partnership does not imply that both partners have identical responsibilities or equal power. While physicians have the responsibility to provide health care services to patients to the best of their ability, patients have the responsibility to communicate openly, to participate in decisions about the diagnostic and treatment recommendations, and to comply with the agreed upon treatment program.

Like patients' rights, patients' responsibilities are derived from the principle of autonomy. The principle of patient autonomy holds that an individual's physical, emotional, and psychological integrity should be respected and upheld. This principle also recognizes the human capacity to self-govern and choose a course of action from among different alternative options. Autonomous, competent patients assert some control over the decisions which direct their health care. With that exercise of self-governance and free choice come a number of responsibilities.

1. Good communication is essential to a successful patient-physician relationship. To the extent possible, patients have a responsibility to be truthful and to express their concerns clearly to their physicians.

    Journal 1994 Discusses notions of quality in health care, asking who is responsible to define quality, who is responsible to deliver it, and who is responsible for quality of care when it is unsatisfactory. Asserts that society has placed these responsibilities exclusively on physicians. Concludes that significant economic changes will require a reallocation of these responsibilities among patients, providers, and payers. References Patient Responsibilities (1), (4), and (5). Morreim, *Redefining Quality by Reassigning Responsibility*, 20 Am. J. Law & Med. 79, 103 (1994).

2. Patients have a responsibility to provide a complete medical history, to the extent possible, including information about past illnesses, medications, hospitalizations, family history of illness and other matters relating to present health.

3. Patients have a responsibility to request information or clarification about their health status or treatment when they do not fully understand what has been described.

4. Once patients and physicians agree upon the goals of therapy and a treatment plan, patients have a responsibility to cooperate with that treatment plan. Compliance with physician instructions is often essential to public and individual safety. Patients also have a responsibility to disclose whether previously agreed upon treatments are being followed and to indicate when they would like to reconsider the treatment plan.

Journal 1994 Discusses notions of quality in health care, asking who is responsible to define quality, who is responsible to deliver it, and who is responsible for quality of care when it is unsatisfactory. Asserts that society has placed these responsibilities exclusively on physicians. Concludes that significant economic changes will require a reallocation of these responsibilities among patients, providers, and payers. References Patient Responsibilities (1), (4), and (5). Morreim, *Redefining Quality by Reassigning Responsibility*, 20 Am. J. Law & Med. 79, 103 (1994).

5. Patients generally have a responsibility to meet their financial obligations with regard to medical care or to discuss financial hardships with their physicians. Patients should be cognizant of the costs associated with using a limited resource like health care and try to use medical resources judiciously.

Journal 1994 Discusses notions of quality in health care, asking who is responsible to define quality, who is responsible to deliver it, and who is responsible for quality of care when it is unsatisfactory. Asserts that society has placed these responsibilities exclusively on physicians. Concludes that significant economic changes will require a reallocation of these responsibilities among patients, providers, and payers. References Patient Responsibilities (1), (4), and (5). Morreim, *Redefining Quality by Reassigning Responsibility*, 20 Am. J. Law & Med. 79, 103 (1994).

6. Patients should discuss end of life decisions with their physicians and make their wishes known. Such a discussion might also include writing an advanced directive.

7. Patients should be committed to health maintenance through health-enhancing behavior. Illness can often be prevented by a healthy lifestyle, and patients should take personal responsibility when they are able to avert the development of disease.

8. Patients should also have an active interest in the effects of their conduct on others and refrain from behavior that unreasonably places the health of others at risk. Patients should inquire as to the means and likelihood of infectious disease transmission and act upon that information which can best prevent further transmission.

9. Patients should discuss organ donation with their physicians and, if donation is desired, make applicable provisions. Patients who are part of an organ allocation system and await a needed transplant should not try to go outside of or manipulate the system. A fair system of allocation should be answered with public trust and an awareness of limited resources.

10. Patients should not initiate or participate in fraudulent health care and should report illegal or unethical behavior by physicians and other providers to the appropriate medical societies, licensing boards, or law enforcement authorities.

Report of the Council on Ethical and Judicial Affairs of the American Medical Association, adopted June 1993.

Updated June 1998.

Introduction

1.01   Terminology

The term "ethical" is used in opinions of the Council on Ethical and Judicial Affairs to refer to matters involving (1) moral principles or practices and (2) matters of social policy involving issues of morality in the practice of medicine. The term "unethical" is used to refer to professional conduct which fails to conform to these moral standards or policies.

Many of the Council's opinions lay out specific duties and obligations for physicians. Violation of these principles and opinions represents unethical conduct and may justify disciplinary action such as censure, suspension, or expulsion from medical society membership.

Issued prior to April 1977.

Updated June 1996.

Journal 1994 Discusses the role of professional societies in establishing ethical guidelines for physicians in the context of using medical innovations and new technologies. Observes that these standards must be supplemented by additional external measures or incentives in order to be most effective. Concludes that professional societies are more successful at setting standards than ensuring acceptance and implementation of those standards by member professionals. Cites Opinions 1.01, 1.02, 8.061, 9.04, and 9.131. Orentlicher, *The Influence of a Professional Organization on Physician Behavior*, 57 Alb. L. Rev. 583, 592, 593, 594, 595, 596 (1994).

Journal 1994 Reviews the evolution of the physician-patient relationship. Describes legal responses to increasing awareness of the importance of ensuring patient autonomy. Examines the changing health care delivery environment. Concludes with a discussion of the impact of these changes on patient participation in medical decision-making. Quotes Preamble, Principles I, II, III, IV, V, and VI, Fundamental Elements (1) and (2), and Opinions 1.02 and 8.07 (1981) [now Opinion 8.08]. Cites Opinion 1.01. Szczygiel, *Beyond Informed Consent, 21 Ohio N.U.L. Rev. 171, 217, 218, 220, 225, 226, 256 (1994)*.

1.02   The Relation of Law and Ethics

The following statements are intended to clarify the relationship between law and ethics.

Ethical values and legal principles are usually closely related, but ethical obligations typically exceed legal duties. In some cases, the law mandates unethical conduct. In general, when physicians believe a law is unjust, they should work to change the law. In exceptional circumstances of unjust laws, ethical responsibilities should supersede legal obligations.

The fact that a physician charged with allegedly illegal conduct is acquitted or exonerated in civil or criminal proceedings does not necessarily mean that the physician acted ethically.

Issued prior to April 1977.

Updated June 1994.

Journal 1995 Examines the rights of health care professionals to refuse to participate in patient care on the basis of conscientious objection. Discusses rights and duties of health care facilities in this context. Suggests steps that facilities may take when dealing with health care professionals who object to participating in patient care. Quotes Principles I and VI and Opinions 1.02, 2.035, and 9.055. Dellinger & Vickery, *When Staff Object to Participating In Care*, 28 *J. Health & Hospital Law* 269, 272, 276 (1995).

Journal 1994 Explores the ethical issues involved in a multidisciplinary team working with children in legal proceedings. Focuses on the relationships between professionals and the conflicts that arise regarding disclosure of confidential information and forced disclosure of non-privileged information. Examines theories supporting protection of client information. Quotes Principles III, IV, Fundamental Elements (4) and Opinions 1.02 (1992) and 5.07 (1992) [now Opinion 5.05]. Cites Opinions 2.02. Glynn, *Multidisciplinary Representation of Children: Conflicts Over Disclosures of Client Communications*, 27 *J. Marshall L. Rev.* 617, 625, 626, 630-32, 637, 639, 643 (1994).

Journal 1994 Discusses the role of professional societies in establishing ethical guidelines for physicians in the context of using medical innovations and new technologies. Observes that these standards must be supplemented by additional external measures or incentives in order to be most effective. Concludes that professional societies are more successful at setting standards than ensuring acceptance and implementation of those standards by member professionals. Cites Opinions 1.01, 1.02, 8.061, 9.04, and 9.131. Orentlicher, *The Influence of a Professional Organization on Physician Behavior*, 57 *Alb. L. Rev.* 583, 592, 593, 594, 595, 596 (1994).

Journal 1994 Reviews the evolution of the physician-patient relationship. Describes legal responses to increasing awareness of the importance of ensuring patient autonomy. Examines the changing health care delivery environment. Concludes with a discussion of the impact of these changes on patient participation in medical decision-making. Quotes Preamble, Principles I, II, III, IV, V, and VI, Fundamental Elements (1) and (2), and Opinions 1.02 and 8.07 (1981) [now Opinion 8.08]. Cites Opinion 1.01. Szczygiel, *Beyond Informed Consent*, 21 *Ohio N.U.L. Rev.* 171, 217, 218, 220, 225, 226, 256 (1994).

Journal 1992 Considers the relationship between legal ethics and laws governing the legal profession. Argues that legal ethics and state laws governing attorney conduct are in conflict. Concludes that legal ethics continue to play a prominent role because states are "weakly committed" to regulation of the profession. Cites Opinion 1.02. Koniak, *The Law Between the Bar and the State*, 70 *No. Carolina L. Rev.* 1389, 1396 (1992).

Journal 1991 Explores ethical problems unique to the field of forensic psychiatry. Presents the results of a survey of members of the American Academy of Psychiatry and the Law (AAPL), asking their opinions regarding proposed ethical guidelines. Concludes that AAPL members are both interested in and sensitive to current ethical issues. Quotes Opinions 1.02 and 5.09. Weinstock, Leong, & Silva, *Opinions by AAPL Forensic Psychiatrists on Controversial Ethical Guidelines: A Survey*, 19 *Bull. Am. Acad. Psychiatry Law* 237, 238 (1991).

2.00 Opinions on Social Policy Issues

2.01 Abortion

The Principles of Medical Ethics of the AMA do not prohibit a physician from performing an abortion in accordance with good medical practice and under circumstances that do not violate the law. (III, IV)

Issued prior to April 1977.

U.S. 1973 Pregnant woman and physician sought declaratory relief and injunction against Texas criminal abortion statute. In holding that the constitutional right of privacy includes a woman's decision whether to terminate a pregnancy prior to viability, the Court reviewed the medical and legal history of abortion, including the AMA's lobbying efforts in support of criminal abortion statutes (1859, 1871), its opposition to induced abortion except when threat to life or health of mother exists (1967), its statement that lobbying efforts were consistent with the Principles of Medical Ethics (1957), and the Preamble, Sec. 10 (1971) [now Opinion 2.01], which stated that a physician was not prohibited from performing an abortion in accordance with good medical practice and consistent with local law. *Roe v. Wade, 410 U.S. 113, 144 n.39.*

Journal 1995 Examines four essential principles of bioethics: patient autonomy; nonmaleficence; beneficence; and justice. Describes the application of these principles in clinical settings according to bioethical norms and AMA opinions. Concludes that such an approach promotes compassionate medical caregiving and that laws should reflect these values. Quotes Opinions 2.01 and 8.18. References Opinion 2.211. Cohen, *Toward a Bioethics of Compassion, 28 Ind. L. Rev. 667, 673, 681-82, 683 (1995).*

2.015 Mandatory Parental Consent to Abortion

Physicians should ascertain the law in their state on parental involvement to ensure that their procedures are consistent with their legal obligations.

Physicians should strongly encourage minors to discuss their pregnancy with their parents. Physicians should explain how parental involvement can be helpful and that parents are generally very understanding and supportive. If a minor expresses concerns about parental involvement, the physician should ensure that the minor's reluctance is not based on any misperceptions about the likely consequences of parental involvement.

Physicians should not feel or be compelled to require minors to involve their parents before deciding whether to undergo an abortion. The patient, even an adolescent, generally must decide whether, on balance, parental involvement is advisable. Accordingly, minors should ultimately be allowed to decide whether parental involvement is appropriate. Physicians should explain under what circumstances (e.g., life-threatening emergency) the minor's confidentiality will need to be abrogated.

Physicians should try to ensure that minor patients have made an informed decision after giving careful consideration to the issues involved. They should encourage their minor patients to consult alternative sources if parents are not going to be involved in the abortion decision. Minors should be urged to seek the advice and counsel of those adults in whom they have confidence, including professional counselors, relatives, friends, teachers, or the clergy. (III, IV)

Issued June 1994 based on the report, "Mandatory Parental Consent to Abortion," adopted June 1992 (JAMA. 1993; 269: 82-86).

8th Cir. 1995 Court held several provisions of the South Dakota abortion law unconstitutional, including parental notice provision. In ruling that parental notice requirement, which lacked a bypass provision, unduly burdened liberty interests of some minors, the court cited AMA Council on Ethical and Judicial Affairs, Mandatory Parental Consent to Abortion, 269 JAMA 82 (1993) [now Opinion 2.015]. *Planned Parenthood v. Miller, 63 F.3d 1452, 1462.*

Mass. 1997 Plaintiffs brought suit seeking a declaration that statute prohibiting, with certain exceptions, a pregnant unmarried minor from obtaining an abortion unless either both parents consent or a judge authorizes the procedure, is unconstitutional. The court concluded that the statute did not facially violate due process or equal protection and was thus constitutional. However, the court struck down the provision requiring both parents' consent as lacking sufficient justification to overcome the minor's constitutional right to choose. The court cited AMA Council on Ethical and Judicial Affairs, Mandatory Parental Consent to Abortion, 269 JAMA 82 (1993) [now Opinion 2.015]. *Planned Parenthood League of Massachusetts, Inc. v. Attorney General, 424 Mass. 586, 596, 608, 677 N.E.2d 101, 107, 114.*

Journal 1997 Addresses the issue of teenage pregnancy. Examines governmental actions that have made it more difficult for teenagers to receive abortions. Suggests that parental consent and judicial bypass provisions are an infringement on their reproductive freedom. Advocates lawyer participation in abortion reform. References Opinion 2.015. Schiff, *The Lawyer's Role in Restoring Adolescents' Abortion Rights, 44 Fed. Law. 60, 62 (May 1997).*

Journal 1996 Reviews Supreme Court decisions that address parental involvement in the abortion decisions of mature minors. Suggests that the Court's position on parental involvement should be reevaluated. Posits that many young women are mature enough to make their own pregnancy decisions. References Opinion 2.015. O'Shaughnessy, *The Worst of Both Worlds?: Parental Involvement Requirements and the Privacy Rights of Mature Minors, 57 Ohio St. J. 1731, 1764-65 (1996).*

2.02*   Abuse of Spouses, Children, Elderly Persons, and Others at Risk

The following are guidelines for detecting and treating family violence:

Due to the prevalence and medical consequences of family violence, physicians should routinely inquire about physical, sexual, and psychological abuse as part of the medical history. Physicians must also consider abuse in the differential diagnosis for a number of medical complaints, particularly when treating women.

Physicians who are likely to have the opportunity to detect abuse in the course of their work have an obligation to familiarize themselves with protocols for diagnosing and treating abuse and with community resources for battered women, children and elderly persons.

Physicians also have a duty to be aware of societal misconceptions about abuse and prevent these from affecting the diagnosis and management of

---

* This opinion is currently under reconsideration by the Council, and may be amended in the next edition of the Code of Medical Ethics. Contact the Ethics Standards Division of the AMA for the most up-to-date version.

abuse. Such misconceptions include the belief that abuse is a rare occurrence; that abuse does not occur in "normal" families; that abuse is a private problem best resolved without outside interference; and that victims are responsible for the abuse.

In order to improve physician knowledge of family violence, physicians must be better trained to identify signs of abuse and to work cooperatively with the range of community services currently involved. Hospitals should require additional training for those physicians who are likely to see victims of abuse. Comprehensive training on family violence should be required in medical school curricula and in residency programs for specialties in which family violence is likely to be encountered.

The following are guidelines for the reporting of abuse:

Laws that require the reporting of cases of suspected abuse of children and elderly persons often create a difficult dilemma for the physician. The parties involved, both the suspected offenders and the victims, will often plead with the physician that the matter be kept confidential and not be disclosed or reported for investigation by public authorities.

Children who have been seriously injured, apparently by their parents, may nevertheless try to protect their parents by saying that the injuries were caused by an accident, such as a fall. The reason may stem from the natural parent-child relationship or fear of further punishment. Even institutionalized elderly patients who have been physically maltreated may be concerned that disclosure of what has occurred might lead to further and more drastic maltreatment by those responsible.

The physician who fails to comply with the laws requiring reporting of suspected cases of abuse of children and elderly persons and others at risk can expect that the victims could receive more severe abuse that may result in permanent bodily injury, emotional or psychological injury, or even death.

Public officials concerned with the welfare of children and elderly persons have expressed the opinion that the incidence of physical violence to these persons is rapidly increasing and that a very substantial percentage of such cases is unreported by hospital personnel and physicians. A child or elderly person brought to a physician with a suspicious injury is the patient whose interests require the protection of law in a particular situation, even though the physician may also provide services from time to time to parents or other members of the family.

The obligation to comply with statutory requirements is clearly stated in the Principles of Medical Ethics. In addition, physicians have an ethical obligation to report abuse even when the law does not require it. However, for mentally competent adult victims of abuse, physicians must not disclose an abuse diagnosis to spouses or any other third party without the consent of the patient. Physicians must discuss the problem of family violence with adult patients in privacy and safety. (I, III)

Issued December 1982.

Updated June 1994 based on the report, "Physicians and Family Violence: Ethical Considerations," adopted December 1991 (JAMA. 1992; 267: 3190-3193), and June 1996.

Cal. App. 1982 Defendant was convicted of lewd act with a child and child molestation or annoyance, after licensed clinical psychologist reported defendant's admission of sexual conduct to authorities. The court held that the psychologist's testimony was properly admitted since a statute requiring the reporting of actual or suspected child abuse expressly made the psychotherapist-patient privilege inapplicable. The court quoted Principle 9 (1957) [now Principle IV and Opinions 2.02 and 5.05] in concluding the disclosure was not a breach of professional ethics. *People v. Stritzinger, 137 Cal. App. 3d 126, 186 Cal. Rptr. 750, 752 rev'd 34 Cal. 3d 505, 668 p.2d 738, 194 Cal. Rptr. 431 (1983).*

Md. Att'y Gen. 1977 Opinion addresses the obligation of a psychiatrist to report child abuse information obtained from a parent-patient. Referring to state statutes and to Principle 9 (1957) [now Principle IV and Opinions 2.02 and 5.05] the opinion concludes that the question of whether to disclose suspected child abuse is a matter left to the individual psychiatrist's professional and moral judgment. *Maryland Att'y. Gen. Opinion, 62 Op. Att'y Gen. Md. 157, 160.*

Wis. Att'y Gen. 1987 Physicians may report cases of suspected child abuse or neglect when a patient discloses that he or she has abused a child in some manner. Where report is made in good faith, physicians are immune from any civil or criminal liability. Passing reference is made to Principle 9 (1957) [now Principle IV and Opinions 2.02 and 5.05] in support of this position. *Wisconsin Att'y Gen. Op. 10-87 (March 16, 1987) (LEXIS, States library, Wis. file).*

Journal 1997 Considers the best interests of children who are victims of domestic abuse. Advocates a rebuttable presumption against granting custody to a perpetrator. Concludes that courts should be educated about domestic violence. References Opinion 2.02. Comment, *Protecting Children Exposed to Domestic Violence in Contested Custody and Visitation Litigation*, 6 B.U. Pub. Int. L. J. 501, 502, 505 (1997).

Journal 1997 Reviews the historical treatment of domestic violence in tort law. Explores the difficulties victims of domestic violence suffer in pursuing traditional forms of relief. Considers this issue in the context of divorce proceedings. Offers practical guidance for achieving justice. References Opinion 2.02. Dalton, *Domestic Violence, Domestic Torts and Divorce: Constraints and Possibilities*, 31 New Eng. L. Rev. 319, 354 (1997).

Journal 1996 Considers means of combating spousal abuse problems. Suggests various schemes of liability to increase aid to victims and reporting of problems. Observes that physicians may play an important role in eliminating spousal abuse. Concludes that imposition of civil liability on physicians for failure to report abuse will help remedy problems. References Opinion 2.02. Jones, *Battered Spouses' Damage Actions Against Non-Reporting Physicians*, 45 DePaul L. Rev. 191 (1996).

Journal 1994 Explores the ethical issues involved in a multidisciplinary team working with children in legal proceedings. Focuses on the relationships between professionals and the conflicts that arise regarding disclosure of confidential information and forced disclosure of non-privileged information. Examines theories supporting protection of client information. Quotes Principles III, IV, Fundamental Elements (4) and Opinions 1.02 (1992) and 5.07 (1992) [now Opinion 5.05]. Cites Opinions 2.02. Glynn, *Multidisciplinary Representation of Children: Conflicts Over Disclosures of Client Communications*, 27 J. Marshall L. Rev. 617, 625, 626, 630-32, 637, 639, 643 (1994).

2.03 Allocation of Limited Medical Resources

A physician has a duty to do all that he or she can for the benefit of the individual patient. Policies for allocating limited resources have the potential to limit the ability of physicians to fulfill this obligation to patients. Physicians have a responsibility to participate and to contribute their professional expertise in order to safeguard the interests of patients in decisions made at the societal level regarding the allocation or rationing of health resources.

Decisions regarding the allocation of limited medical resources among patients should consider only ethically appropriate criteria relating to medical need. These criteria include likelihood of benefit, urgency of need, change in quality of life, duration of benefit, and, in some cases, the amount of resources required for successful treatment. In general, only very substantial differences among patients are ethically relevant; the greater the disparities, the more justified the use of these criteria becomes. In making quality of life judgments, patients should first be prioritized so that death or extremely poor outcomes are avoided; then, patients should be prioritized according to change in quality of life, but only when there are very substantial differences among patients. Non-medical criteria, such as ability to pay, age, social worth, perceived obstacles to treatment, patient contribution to illness, or past use of resources should not be considered.

Allocation decisions should respect the individuality of patients and the particulars of individual cases as much as possible. When very substantial differences do not exist among potential recipients of treatment on the basis of the appropriate criteria defined above, a "first-come-first-served" approach or some other equal opportunity mechanism should be employed to make final allocation decisions. Though there are several ethically acceptable strategies for implementing these criteria, no single strategy is ethically mandated. Acceptable approaches include a three-tiered system, a minimal threshold approach, and a weighted formula. Decision-making mechanisms should be objective, flexible, and consistent to ensure that all patients are treated equally.

The treating physician must remain a patient advocate and therefore should not make allocation decisions. Patients denied access to resources have the right to be informed of the reasoning behind the decision. The allocation procedures of institutions controlling scarce resources should be disclosed to the public as well as subject to regular peer review from the medical profession. (I,VII)

Issued March 1981.

Updated June 1994 based on the report, "Ethical Considerations in the Allocation of Organs and Other Scarce Medical Resources Among Patients," adopted June 1993 (*Arch Intern Med.* 1995; 155: 29-40).

Journal 1997 Posits that cost-containment schemes in managed care systems have eroded the fiduciary duty physicians owe patients. Notes that MCOs are prohibiting patients from trusting and relying on physicians. Concludes that patients must seek quality assurance from sources other than their physicians. Quotes Opinions 2.03, 2.09, and 8.13. Jacobi, *Patients at a Loss: Protecting Health Care Consumers through Data Driven Quality Assurance*, 45 U. Kan. L. Rev. 705, 720, 721, 759 (1997).

Journal 1996 Examines the role of physicians in managed health care. Posits that the new system of managed care is beneficial because it combines high performance with affordable outcomes. Concludes that outcome-based payment systems, with tort reform, will maximize results. Quotes Opinion 2.03 (1984) [subsequently amended]. Furrow, *Incentivizing Medical Practice: What (If Anything) Happens to Professionalism?*, 1 Widener L. Symp. J. 1, 9 (1996).

Journal 1996 Discusses the trend toward conserving resources expended on health care by withholding services absent a showing of necessity. Claims that the high standard of care physicians owe patients is jeopardized by medical treatment decisions based on coverage concerns. Concludes that the legal structure regarding health care plans should be changed. Quotes Preamble, Principles I, II, III, IV, V, VI, and VII and Opinion 2.03. Hirshfeld & Thomason, *Medical Necessity Determinations: The Need for a New Legal Structure*, 6 Health Matrix 3, 8-9 (1996).

Journal 1996 Considers whether the Oregon Health Plan discriminates on the basis of race by excluding coverage for obesity which disproportionately affects African-American women. Discusses discrimination in federally funded health care programs and the purpose of Title VI. Quotes Opinion 2.03. Jurevic, *Disparate Impact Under Title VI: Discrimination, By Any Other Name, Will Still Have the Same Impact*, 15 St. Louis U. Pub. L. Rev. 237, 253 (1996).

Journal 1996 Discusses conflicts of interest between health care professionals and patients created by managed health care and the drive toward reduction of costs. Suggests that a multi-disciplinary group of health professionals could act as patient advocates to help protect their interests. Quotes Opinion 2.03. Mehlman, *Medical Advocates: A Call for a New Profession*, 1 *Widener L. Symp. J.* 299, 314 (1996).

Journal 1996 Considers the change from traditional medical care systems to managed care, noting the conflicts of interest this creates between physicians' ethical obligations and financial concerns. Discusses these issues in the context of managed behavioral health care. Suggests community-based care and social supports as a solution. Quotes Opinion 2.03 and 4.04. Petrila, *Ethics, Money, and the Problem of Coercion in Managed Behavioral Health Care*, 40 *St. Louis U. L. J.* 359, 377 (1996).

Journal 1994 Considers how greater patient autonomy has led to situations in which medical care may be viewed as futile. Examines cases in which physicians' medical judgments conflict with requests for medical treatment by patients or families. Suggests that the law has intruded too far into this area of medicine. Quotes Opinion 2.035. Cites Opinions 2.03, 2.095, 2.17, 2.19, 2.20, and 2.22. Cultice, *Medical Futility: When Is Enough, Enough?*, 27 *J. Health & Hosp. Law* 225, 230, 256 (1994).

Journal 1994 Critiques ethical and public policy reasons for general assertion that physicians may never withhold beneficial treatment because of cost. Discusses the practice of physician rationing and how the principles of beneficence and autonomy are consistent with the practice. Explores the objection to using financial incentives, commonly adopted by HMOs, to promote rationing. Concludes that rationing should be allowed in some circumstances. Quotes Opinion 2.03. Hall, *Rationing Health Care at the Bedside*, 69 *N.Y.U. L. Rev.* 693, 704 (1994).

Journal 1994 Observes that health care reform proposals present significant challenges to the role and ethics of attending physicians. Emphasizes that reform proposals must set forth the role envisioned for physicians and must articulate an acceptable ethical framework within which physicians may fulfill that role. Quotes Opinions 4.04, 9.121, and 9.122. Cites Opinions 2.03, 2.09, 5.01, and 8.03. Wolf, *Health Care Reform and the Future of Physician Ethics*, 24 *Hastings Center Rep.* 28, 32, 40 (March/April 1994).

Journal 1992 Considers the problem of rising health care costs. Discusses two California cases focusing on the liability of physicians and third party payors when medically necessary care is denied. States that physicians and insurers may be liable in some circumstances. Concludes that physicians also may be obligated to advocate patient interests in attempting to secure payment from third parties when appropriate. Quotes Opinion 2.03. Comment, *Who's in Charge: The Doctor or the Dollar? Assessing the Relative Liability of Third Party Payors and Doctors After Wickline and Wilson*, 18 *J. Contemp. L.* 285, 301, 302 (1992).

Journal 1992 Examines the major health care rationing issues facing the United States including increasing costs and decreasing access. Considers the reasons for the rising cost of medical care as well as possible solutions. Explores the concept of the standard of care and considers whether it should be changed. Concludes that the standard of care should not be changed and that rationing should be a separate enterprise undertaken pursuant to explicit criteria. Quotes Opinions 2.03, 2.09, and 4.04. Hirshfeld, *Should Ethical and Legal Standards for Physicians Be Changed to Accommodate New Models for Rationing Health Care?*, 140 *Univ. Pa. L. Rev.* 1809, 1816 (1992).

Journal 1991 Focuses on the denial of insurance benefits for experimental medical procedures. Explains the de novo review process under ERISA. Asserts that courts are becoming less deferential to administrative rulings. Concludes that there is need for a structure that will permit greater objectivity in the context of data collection as well as judicial determination. Cites Opinions 2.03 and 2.09. Note, *Denial of Coverage for "Experimental" Medical Procedures: The Problem of De Novo Review Under ERISA*, 79 *Kentucky L.J.* 801, 824 (1990-91).

Journal 1990 Discusses economic considerations in clinical decision making, with emphasis on the standard of care. Considers the way in which the standard of care is defined, including the role of the physician. Concludes that organized medicine has made valuable contributions through development of practice parameters that offer guidance in the exercise of clinical judgment. Cites Opinions 2.03 and 2.09. Hirshfeld, *Economic Considerations in Treatment Decisions and the Standard of Care in Medical Malpractice Litigation*, 264 *J.A.M.A.* 2004, 2007 (1990).

Journal 1990 Discusses efforts of third party payors to control health care expenditures for beneficiaries. Focuses on use of financial incentives to encourage providers to minimize the amount of care provided. Also discusses monitoring of requests for payment to determine necessity of care provided. Raises questions regarding impact of cost control mechanisms on quality of care, observing that available evidence is equivocal. Evaluates importance of disclosure to beneficiaries of use of financial incentives to limit care as well as other cost control mechanisms. Concludes that financial incentives and other cost control techniques should be disclosed and that the rationale for such disclosure is compelling. Quotes Opinions 2.03, 2.09, and 8.03. Cites Opinions 2.19, 4.04, and 4.06. Hirshfeld, *Should Third Party Payors of Health Care Services Disclose Cost Control Mechanisms to Potential Beneficiaries?, 14 Seton Hall Legis. J. 115, 130, 131, 144, 145, 146 (1990).*

Journal 1988 Discusses various circumstances that have led to proposals for the rationing of health care by hospitals and other providers in order to contain health care costs. Because of the impact such proposals may have on older persons, focus is placed on the Age Discrimination Act of 1975 and its likely effect on the use of age as a criterion for rationing. In this context, discussion focuses on the availability of, and access to, heart transplantation. Quotes Opinion 2.02 (1982) [now Opinion 2.03]. Silver, *From Baby Doe to Grandpa Doe: The Impact of the Federal Age Discrimination Act on the "Hidden" Rationing of Medical Care, 37 Catholic Univ. L. Rev. 993, 1013 (1988).*

Journal 1985 Discusses recent medical technological advances that have substantially improved patient care. Notes that considerations of cost and availability of such advanced technology raise troublesome ethical and legal issues. In addressing these issues, examines potential mechanisms for rationing expensive lifesaving medical treatment, concluding that the cost of rationing probably exceeds the benefits. Further concludes that the issue of rationing in this context likely will lead to an increase in litigation. Accordingly, criteria are offered for use by the courts in addressing this difficult issue. Quotes Opinion 2.02 (1982) [now Opinion 2.03]. Mehlman, *Rationing Expensive Lifesaving Medical Treatments, 1985 Wisconsin L. Rev. 239, 250, 260 (1985).*

2.035   Futile Care

Physicians are not ethically obligated to deliver care that, in their best professional judgment, will not have a reasonable chance of benefiting their patients. Patients should not be given treatments simply because they demand them. Denial of treatment should be justified by reliance on openly stated ethical principles and acceptable standards of care, as defined in Opinions 2.03 and 2.095, not on the concept of "futility," which cannot be meaningfully defined. (I, IV)

Issued June 1994.

Journal 1997 Examines case law pertaining to medical futility disputes. Reviews hospital policies regarding futility and notes a variety of definitions and guidelines. Concludes that, absent a clear consensus, physicians should not act solely to decide questions of futility. References Opinions 2.035 and 2.22. Johnson, Gibbons, Goldner, Wiener, & Eton, *Legal and Institutional Policy Responses to Medical Futility, 30 J. Health & Hosp. L. 21, 26, 31, 35, 36 (1997).*

Journal 1995 Explores the role that physician autonomy plays in the medical futility debate. Considers how the judiciary, legislatures, and provider institutions balance the values of patients and their physicians. Recommends that physicians and hospitals promulgate written policies outlining their preferred treatment parameters in any given circumstance. Quotes Opinion 2.035. Daar, *Medical Futility and Implications for Physician Autonomy, XXI Am. J. Law & Med. 221, 234 (1995).*

Journal 1995 Examines the rights of health care professionals to refuse to participate in patient care on the basis of conscientious objection. Discusses rights and duties of health care facilities in this context. Suggests steps that facilities may take when dealing with health care professionals who object to participating in patient care. Quotes Principles I and VI and Opinions 1.02, 2.035, and 9.055. Dellinger & Vickery, *When Staff Object to Participating In Care, 28 J. Health & Hospital Law 269, 272, 276 (1995).*

Journal 1994 Considers how greater patient autonomy has led to situations in which medical care may be viewed as futile. Examines cases in which physicians' medical judgments conflict with requests for medical treatment by patients or families. Suggests that the law has intruded too far into this area of medicine. Quotes Opinion 2.035. Cites Opinions 2.03, 2.095, 2.17, 2.19, 2.20, and 2.22. Cultice, *Medical Futility: When Is Enough, Enough?*, 27 J. Health & Hosp. Law 225, 230, 256 (1994).

2.037 Medical Futility in End-of-Life Care

When further intervention to prolong the life of a patient becomes futile, physicians have an obligation to shift the intent of care toward comfort and closure. However, there are necessary value judgments involved in coming to the assessment of futility. These judgments must give consideration to the patient's or proxy's assessment of worthwhile outcome. They should also take into account the physician or other provider's perception of intent in treatment, which should not be to prolong the dying process without benefit to the patient or to others with legitimate interests. They may also take into account community and institutional standards, which in turn may have used physiological or functional outcome measures.

Nevertheless, conflicts between the parties may persist in determining what is futility in the particular instance. This may interrupt satisfactory decision-making and adversely affect patient care, family satisfaction, and physician-clinical team functioning. To assist in fair and satisfactory decision-making about what constitutes futile intervention:

(1) All health care institutions, whether large or small, should adopt a policy on medical futility; and

(2) Policies on medical futility should follow a due process approach. The following seven steps should be included in such a due process approach to declaring futility in specific cases.

   (a) Earnest attempts should be made in advance to deliberate over and negotiate prior understandings between patient, proxy and physician on what constitutes futile care for the patient, and what falls within acceptable limits for the physician, family, and possibly also the institution.

   (b) Joint decision-making should occur between patient or proxy and physician to the maximum extent possible.

   (c) Attempts should be made to negotiate disagreements if they arise, and to reach resolution within all parties' acceptable limits, with the assistance of consultants as appropriate.

   (d) Involvement of an institutional committee, such as the ethics committee, should be requested if disagreements are irresolvable.

   (e) If the institutional review supports the patient's position and the physician remains unpersuaded, transfer of care to another physician within the institution may be arranged.

   (f) If the process supports the physician's position and the patient/proxy remains unpersuaded, transfer to another institution may be sought and, if done, should be supported by the transferring and receiving institution.

   (g) If transfer is not possible, the intervention need not be offered. (I, V)

Issued June 1998 based on the report, "Medical Futility in End-of-Life Care," adopted December 1996.

2.04   Artificial Insemination by Known Donor

Any individual or couple contemplating artificial insemination by husband, partner, or other known donor should be counseled about the full range of infectious and genetic diseases for which the donor or recipient can be screened, including HIV infection. Full medical history disclosure and appropriate diagnostic screening should be recommended to the donor and recipient, but are not required.

Informed consent for artificial insemination should include disclosure of risks, benefits, and likely success rate of the method proposed and potential alternative methods. Individuals should receive information about screening, costs, and procedures for confidentiality, when applicable. The prospective parents or parent should be informed of the laws regarding the rights of children conceived by artificial insemination, as well as the laws regarding parental rights and obligations. If the donor is married to the recipient, resultant children will have all the rights of a child conceived naturally.

If the donor and recipient are not married, an appropriate legal rule would treat the situation as if the donor were anonymous: the recipient would be considered the sole parent of the child except in cases where both donor and recipient agree to recognize a paternity right.

Sex selection of sperm for the purposes of avoiding a sex-linked inheritable disease is appropriate. However, physicians should not participate in sex selection for reasons of gender preference. Physicians should encourage a prospective parent or parents to consider the value of both sexes.

If semen is frozen and the donor dies before it is used, the frozen semen should not be used or donated for purposes other than those originally intended by the donor. If the donor left no instructions, it is reasonable to allow the remaining partner to use the semen for artificial insemination but not to donate it to someone else. However, the donor should be advised of such a policy at the time of donation and be given an opportunity to override it. (I, V)

Issued June 1983.

Updated June 1993.

Colo. 1989 State statute prohibiting a sperm donor from asserting his parental status was held to be inapplicable where known donor and unmarried recipient agreed that the donor would have parental rights. Concurring opinion argued that the statute bars any non-husband donor, regardless of relationship to the recipient, from asserting parental rights. However, the concurring opinion found the statute inapplicable because its provision requiring "supervision" by a physician had not been met. In apparent reference to the standards set out under Opinions 2.04 and 2.05, the concurring opinion said that "supervision" should at the least require an examination to determine whether there are any health risks to the recipient as a result of the procedure and to protect the child from hereditary disease. *In re R.C., 775 P.2d 27, 37 n.3.*

Journal 1987 Examines various ethical issues surrounding surrogate motherhood, artificial insemination, in vitro fertilization and embryonic/fetal research. Reports on the positions of four ethics groups: the Warnock Committee of Inquiry into Human Fertilization and Embryology; the American Medical Association's Council on Ethical and Judicial Affairs; the Ethics Committee of the American Fertility Society; and the Ethics Committee of the American College of Obstetricians and Gynecologists. References Opinions 2.04, 2.05, and 2.13 (1986) [now Opinion 2.14]. Quotes Opinion 2.18. Rosner, Cassell, Friedland, Landolt, Loeb, Numann, Ora, Risemberg, & Sordillo, *Ethical Considerations of Reproductive Technologies,* 87 N.Y. State J. Med. 398, 399-400 (1987).

2.05 Artificial Insemination by Anonymous Donor

Thorough medical histories must be taken of all candidates for anonymous semen donation. All potential donors must also be screened for infectious or inheritable diseases which could adversely affect the recipient or the resultant child. Frozen semen should be used for artificial insemination because it enables the donor to be tested for HIV infection at the time of donation, and again after an interval before the original semen is used, thus increasing the likelihood that the semen is free of HIV infection. Physicians should rely on the guidelines formulated by relevant professional organizations, such as the American Society of Reproductive Medicine, the Centers for Disease Control and Prevention, and the Food and Drug Administration, in determining the interval between the initial and final HIV test, which disorders to screen for, and which procedures to use in screening.

Physicians should maintain a permanent record which includes both identifying and non-identifying health and genetic screening information. Other than exceptional situations where identifying information may be required, physicians should release only non-identifying health-related information in order to preserve the confidentiality of the semen donor. Physicians should maintain permanent records of donors to fulfill the following obligations: (1) to exclude individuals from the donor pool who test positive for infectious or inheritable diseases, (2) to limit the number of pregnancies resulting from a single donor source so as to avoid future consanguineous marriages or reproduction, (3) to notify donors of screening results which indicate the presence of an infectious or inheritable disease, and (4) to notify donors if a child born through artificial insemination has a disorder which may have been transmitted by the donor.

Informed consent for artificial insemination should include disclosure of risks, benefits, likely success rate of the method proposed and potential alternative methods, and costs. Both recipients and donors should be informed of the reasons for screening and confidentiality. They should also know the extent of access to non-identifying and identifying information about the donor. Participants should be advised to consider the legal ramifications, if any, of artificial insemination by anonymous donor.

The consent of the husband is ethically appropriate if he is to become the legal father of the resultant child from artificial insemination by anonymous donor. Anonymous donors cannot assume the rights or responsibilities of parenthood for children born through therapeutic donor insemination, nor should they be required to assume them.

In the case of single women or women who are part of a homosexual couple, it is not unethical to provide artificial insemination as a reproductive option.

Sex selection of sperm for the purposes of avoiding a sex-linked inheritable disease is appropriate. However, physicians should not participate in sex selection of sperm for reasons of gender preference. Physicians should encourage a prospective parent or parents to consider the value of both sexes.

In general, it is inappropriate to offer compensation to donors to encourage donation over and above reimbursement for time and actual expenses. (I, V)

Issued June 1983.

Updated June 1993.

Colo. 1989 State statute prohibiting a sperm donor from asserting his parental status was held to be inapplicable where known donor and unmarried recipient agreed that the donor would have parental rights. Concurring opinion argued that the statute bars any non-husband donor, regardless of relationship to the recipient, from asserting parental rights. However, the concurring opinion found the statute inapplicable because its provision requiring "supervision" by a physician had not been met. In apparent reference to the standards set out under Opinions 2.04 and 2.05, the concurring opinion said that "supervision" should at the least require an examination to determine whether there are any health risks to the recipient as a result of the procedure and to protect the child from hereditary disease. *In re R.C., 775 P.2d 27, 37 n.3.*

Journal 1987 Examines various ethical issues surrounding surrogate motherhood, artificial insemination, in vitro fertilization and embryonic/fetal research. Reports on the positions of four ethics groups: the Warnock Committee of Inquiry into Human Fertilization and Embryology; the American Medical Association's Council on Ethical and Judicial Affairs; the Ethics Committee of the American Fertility Society; and the Ethics Committee of the American College of Obstetricians and Gynecologists. References Opinions 2.04, 2.05, and 2.13 (1986) [now Opinion 2.14]. Quotes Opinion 2.18. Rosner, Cassell, Friedland, Landolt, Loeb, Numann, Ora, Risemberg, & Sordillo, *Ethical Considerations of Reproductive Technologies*, 87 N.Y. State J. Med. 398, 399-400 (1987).

2.06   Capital Punishment

An individual's opinion on capital punishment is the personal moral decision of the individual. A physician, as a member of a profession dedicated to preserving life when there is hope of doing so, should not be a participant in a legally authorized execution. Physician participation in execution is defined generally as actions which would fall into one or more of the following categories: (1) an action which would directly cause the death of the condemned; (2) an action which would assist, supervise, or contribute to the ability of another individual to directly cause the death of the condemned; and (3) an action which could automatically cause an execution to be carried out on a condemned prisoner.

Physician participation in an execution includes, but is not limited to, the following actions: prescribing or administering tranquilizers and other psychotropic agents and medications that are part of the execution procedure; monitoring vital signs on site or remotely (including monitoring electrocardiograms); attending or observing an execution as a physician; and rendering technical advice regarding execution.

In the case where the method of execution is lethal injection, the following actions by the physician would also constitute physician participation in execution: selecting injection sites; starting intravenous lines as a port for a lethal injection device; prescribing, preparing, administering, or supervising injection drugs or their doses or types; inspecting, testing, or maintaining lethal injection devices; and consulting with or supervising lethal injection personnel.

The following actions do not constitute physician participation in execution: (1) testifying as to medical diagnoses as they relate to competence to stand trial, testifying as to relevant medical evidence during trial, testifying as to medical aspects of aggravating or mitigating circumstances during the penalty phase of a capital case, or testifying as to medical diagnoses as they relate to the legal assessment of competence for execution; (2) certifying death, provided that the condemned has been declared dead by another person; (3) witnessing an execution in a totally nonprofessional capacity; (4) witnessing an execution at the specific voluntary request of the condemned person, provided that the physician observes the execution in a nonprofessional capacity; and (5) relieving the acute suffering of a condemned person while awaiting execution, including providing tranquilizers at the specific voluntary request of the condemned person to help relieve pain or anxiety in anticipation of the execution.

When a condemned prisoner has been declared incompetent to be executed, physicians should not treat the prisoner to restore competence unless a commutation order is issued. However, if the incompetent prisoner is undergoing extreme suffering as a result of psychosis or any other illness, medical intervention intended to mitigate the level of suffering is ethically permissible. Provision of medical testimony in the reevaluation of the prisoner's legal competence to be executed should be provided by an independent physician examiner. A physician cannot be compelled to provide medical testimony as it relates to legal competence for execution if it is contrary to the physician's personal beliefs.

Organ donation by condemned prisoners is permissible only if (1) the decision to donate was made before the prisoner's conviction, (2) the donated tissue is harvested after the prisoner has been pronounced dead and the body removed from the death chamber, and (3) physicians do not provide advice on modifying the method of execution for any individual to facilitate donation. (I)

Issued July 1980.

Updated June 1994 based on the report, "Physician Participation in Capital Punishment," adopted December 1992, (JAMA. 1993; 270: 365-368), and updated June 1996 based on the report, "Physician Participation in Capital Punishment: Evaluations of Prisoner Competence to be Executed; Treatment to Restore Competence to be Executed," adopted in June 1995.

La. 1992 State's attempt to circumvent prohibition against execution of insane prisoners by forcibly medicating prisoner was held to be a violation of the prisoner's right to privacy and constituted cruel and unusual punishment. Noting that a physician's administration of medication in order to facilitate the prisoner's execution is contrary to the AMA's ethical code, in apparent reference to Opinion 2.06, the court held that involuntary administration of medication is not medical treatment but constitutes a part of capital punishment. *State v. Perry, 610 So. 2d 746, 753.*

S.C. 1993 State sought to reverse order vacating death sentence and imposing life imprisonment. The court stated that the critical issue inherent in the state's contention of error was whether the state could forcibly medicate a prisoner solely to make prisoner competent enough to execute. Citing Opinion 2.06, the court held that the AMA's position reinforces the prohibition against the state's use of medication solely to facilitate an insane prisoner's execution. *Singleton v. State, 437 S.E. 2d 53, 61.*

Va. Att'y Gen. 1994 Attorney General responded in the negative when asked whether a physician employed by the Department of Corrections may be disciplined by the Board of Medicine for participating in the execution of a prisoner where "participating" was defined as "attending or observing an execution, for making a determination that death has occurred, for issuing a certificate of death, or for performing any other function that applicable state statutes lawfully require to be performed by a physician in connection with an execution." Citing Opinion 2.06, the Attorney General noted that such ethical opinions are not legally conclusive and that if they conflict with a state statute, the statute controls. *Va. Att'y Gen. Op., 1994 Va. AG LEXIS 12.*

Journal 1997 Explores the Eighth Amendment prohibition against cruel and unusual punishment in the context of capital punishment. Discusses widely used methods of execution. Suggests that execution methods may be unconstitutionally excessive. Concludes the death penalty should not be imposed until methods are more humane. Quotes Opinion 2.06. Denno, *Getting to Death: Are Executions Constitutional?, 82 Iowa L. Rev. 319, 385-86 (1997).*

Journal 1997 Describes capital punishment in the United States. Considers ethical and moral issues implicated by physician participation. Opines that executions constitute harm and that physician participation contravenes professional ethical obligations. Quotes Opinion 2.06. Michalos, *Medical Ethics and the Executing Process in the United States of America*, 16 Med. & Law 125, 131, 133 (1997).

Journal 1996 Examines how execution practices affect crime deterrence. Explores trend toward private and more humane executions. Discusses similarity between lethal injection and medical procedures. Concludes that deterrence is not served by current execution practices and should not be advanced as support for the death penalty. Cites Opinion 2.06. Abernethy, *The Methodology of Death: Reexamining the Deterrence Rationale*, 27 Colum. Hum. Rts. L. Rev. 379, 410-11 (1996).

Journal 1996 Examines the death penalty statute in New York. Discusses statutory provisions and notes it is unethical for medical personnel to assist with executions. Concludes that the death penalty statute fails to deter crime and may be unconstitutional. Quotes Opinion 2.06. Acker, *When the Cheering Stopped: An Overview and Analysis of New York's Death Penalty Legislation*, 17 Pace L. Rev. 41, 221-22 (1996).

Journal 1996 Discusses the current shortage of available organs for transplant patients. Suggests several new methods for increasing the supply. Includes among these suggestions a proposal that inmates sentenced to death should be allowed to donate organs. Quotes Opinion 2.06. Coleman, *"Brother, Can You Spare a Liver?" Five Ways to Increase Organ Donation*, 31 Val. U.L. Rev. 1, 30, 31 (1996).

Journal 1996 Discusses the involvement of psychiatrists in capital punishment. Posits that physicians should not aid legal executions. Expresses support for the ethical resolutions of psychiatric and medical associations regarding this issue. Quotes Opinion 2.06. Freedman & Halpern, *The Erosion of Ethics and Morality in Medicine: Physician Participation in Legal Executions in the United States*, 41 N.Y.L. Sch. L. Rev. 169, 174 (1996).

Journal 1996 Proposes an alternative method of capital punishment to allow for organ donation by executed prisoners. Provides justifications for this proposal. Concludes that physicians should be able to ethically participate in this process. Quotes Principle VII. Cites Opinion 2.06. References Opinion 2.162 (1994) [subsequently amended]. Patton, *A Call for Common Sense: Organ Donation and the Executed Prisoner*, 3 Va. J. Soc. Pol'y & L. 387, 404, 405, 407-10 (1996).

Journal 1996 Considers physician participation in execution of capital offenders. Observes that this practice is unethical and contrary to the physician's role as a healer. Concludes that physicians should not participate in any aspect of executions. Quotes Opinion 2.06. Schoenholtz, Freedman, & Halpern, *The "Legal" Abuse of Physicians in Deaths in the United States: The Erosion of Ethics and Morality in Medicine*, 42 Wayne L. Rev. 1505, 1542 (1996).

Journal 1996 Discusses the role psychiatrists play in capital punishment. Notes that the ethical prohibition against physician participation in the process creates complications for psychiatrists. References Opinion 2.06. Zwirn, *Professionalism, Mental Disability, and the Death Penalty*, 41 N.Y.L Sch. L. Rev. 163, 165 (1996).

Journal 1995 Summarizes the United States Supreme Court's capital punishment jurisprudence. Explores the history and methodology of the New York Court of Appeals' constitutional adjudication of capital punishment issues. Examines constitutional challenges to the death penalty in other states. Analyzes some of the challenges that will likely come before the New York Court of Appeals. Quotes Opinion 2.06. Falk & Cary, *Death-Defying Feats: State Constitutional Challenges To New York's Death Penalty*, 4 J. L. & Pol'y 161, 233, 234 (1995).

Journal 1995 Analyzes evolution of capital punishment in New York during the nineteenth century. Explores the relevance of this historical account to the contemporary debate regarding televised executions. Considers how the introduction of television cameras might destabilize the current practice of capital punishment. Concludes that increased publicity may give both the public and the condemned more power over how executions are conducted. Cites Opinion 2.06. Madow, *Forbidden Spectacle: Executions, the Public and the Press in Nineteenth Century New York*, 43 Buff. L. Rev. 461, 475 (1995).

Journal 1994 Considers the debate over assisted suicide. Argues that assisted suicide is not an implicit right under the fourteenth amendment's liberty guarantee. Examines the difficulty in establishing under what conditions assisted suicide would be protected. Suggests that giving physicians the authority to determine the appropriateness of assisted suicide furthers no legitimate state interest. Cites Opinion 2.06. References Opinion 2.211. Marzen, *"Out, Out Brief Candle": Constitutionally Prescribed Suicide for the Terminally Ill*, 21 Hastings Const. L.Q. 799, 821 (1994).

Journal 1994 Argues that physician aid-in-dying should be protected by the United States Constitution and that patients should have a federal cause of action to challenge prohibitive state statutes. Considers how such a cause of action might affect public policy. Quotes Principles I and III. References Opinion 2.06. Note, *Toward a More Perfect Union: A Federal Cause of Action for Physician Aid-In-Dying*, 27 U. Mich. J.L. Ref. 521, 538 (1994).

Journal 1993 Considers whether criminal penalties should be imposed on a physician who assists in the suicide of a competent, non-terminal patient who requested such assistance. Analyzes the actions of Dr. Jack Kevorkian and his views on physician-assisted suicide. Examines Dutch practices in this field and their value as a model for other countries. Presents the arguments for and against active euthanasia, with emphasis on the "slippery slope" argument. References Opinions 2.06 and 2.20. Persels, *Forcing the Issue of Physician-Assisted Suicide: Impact of the Kevorkian Case on the Euthanasia Debate*, 14 J. Legal Med. 93, 115 (1993).

Journal 1993 Explores the extent to which physicians may participate in capital punishment. Examines the various levels of physician involvement and the ethical implications of each. Explains the policy behind prohibiting physicians from taking part in executions. Cites Opinion 2.06. Truog & Brennan, *Participation of Physicians in Capital Punishment*, 329 New Eng. J. Med. 1346 (1993).

Journal 1991 Considers ethical issues raised by the case of *Perry v. Louisiana*, where the state attempted to treat an insane death row inmate in order to render him fit for execution. Examines medical and legal ethics and conflicts with goals of the criminal justice system. Explores various ethical questions involving mentally ill defendants/inmates. Proposes increased discussion and reform of ethical guidelines. Quotes Opinion 2.06. Note, *Perry v. Louisiana: Medical Ethics on Death Row—Is Judicial Intervention Warranted?*, 4 Georgetown J. Legal Ethics 707, 714 (1991).

Journal 1987 Considers arguments for and against active voluntary euthanasia, including arguments based on self-determination and various slippery-slope scenarios. Concludes that a policy or practice of active voluntary euthanasia is not desirable, linking a moral prohibition against active voluntary euthanasia to the moral prohibition against physicians actively participating in capital punishment. In place of any practice of active voluntary euthanasia, recommends increased use of hospices, greater emphasis on training physicians to care for the dying patient, and further research aimed at producing symptomatic relief in dying patients. Cites Opinions 2.06, 8.10 (1986) [now Opinion 8.11], and 9.06. Shewmon, *Active Voluntary Euthanasia: A Needless Pandora's Box*, 3 Issues in Law and Med. 219, 220, 222, 243 (1987).

Journal 1987 Focuses on the decision of the United States Supreme Court in Ford v. Wainwright, 106 S. Ct. 2595 (1986), wherein the Court ruled that the Eighth Amendment forbids the execution of a condemned inmate who has become "insane." Addresses the potential for significant involvement by mental health professionals in determining competency for purposes of execution in these types of cases. Noting that physicians should not ethically participate in a legally authorized execution, except to make a determination or certification of death, concludes that participation by mental health professionals in assessing competency for execution is incompatible with the general ethics of the profession. Cites Opinion 2.06. Wallace, *Incompetency for Execution: The Supreme Court Challenges the Ethical Standards of the Mental Health Professions*, 8 J. Legal Med. 265, 267 (1987).

Journal 1986 Observes that the AMA policy on capital punishment expressly forbids psychiatrists from making determinations of competency for execution. Such a practice places the psychiatrist in the position of a "double agent," employed by the state, yet required to serve the patient. Compares the psychiatrist's determination of competency for execution to the behavior of Nazi physicians, and condemns as inherently dishonest any therapy not grounded in the patient's best interests. References Principle I and Opinion 2.06. Sargent, *Treating the Condemned to Death*, 16 Hastings Center Rep. 5, 5 (Dec. 1986).

Journal 1983 Discusses the various methods of capital punishment among the states as well as the political and ethical impact of execution by lethal injection. Focuses on the medical-ethical dilemma inherent in the application of medical technology to bring about death and observes that medical professional organizations have done little to solve the dilemma. Concludes that there is a need for federal legislation preempting the multiplicity of state-sanctioned methods to reduce the potential of abuse of civil and human rights. Advocates lethal injection as the most appropriate method of execution. References 1980 American Medical Association Policy

Statement [now Opinion 2.06] prohibiting a physician from being a participant in an execution while allowing physician certification of the death of an executed prisoner. Finks, *Lethal Injection: An Uneasy Alliance of Law and Medicine*, 4 J. Legal Med. 383, 392, 394 (1983).

2.07 Clinical Investigation

The following guidelines are intended to aid physicians in fulfilling their ethical responsibilities when they engage in the clinical investigation of new drugs and procedures.

(1) A physician may participate in clinical investigation only to the extent that those activities are a part of a systematic program competently designed, under accepted standards of scientific research, to produce data which are scientifically valid and significant.

(2) In conducting clinical investigation, the investigator should demonstrate the same concern and caution for the welfare, safety, and comfort of the person involved as is required of a physician who is furnishing medical care to a patient independent of any clinical investigation.

(3) Minors or mentally incompetent persons may be used as subjects in clinical investigation only if:

   (a) The nature of the investigation is such that mentally competent adults would not be suitable subjects.

   (b) Consent, in writing, is given by a legally authorized representative of the subject under circumstances in which informed and prudent adults would reasonably be expected to volunteer themselves or their children as subjects.

(4) In clinical investigation primarily for treatment:

   (a) The physician must recognize that the patient-physician relationship exists and that professional judgment and skill must be exercised in the best interest of the patient.

   (b) Voluntary written consent must be obtained from the patient, or from the patient's legally authorized representative if the patient lacks the capacity to consent, following: (a) disclosure that the physician intends to use an investigational drug or experimental procedure, (b) a reasonable explanation of the nature of the drug or procedure to be used, risks to be expected, and possible therapeutic benefits, (c) an offer to answer any inquiries concerning the drug or procedure, and (d) a disclosure of alternative drugs or procedures that may be available. Physicians should be completely objective in discussing the details of the drug or procedure to be employed, the pain and discomfort that may be anticipated, known risks and possible hazards, the quality of life to be expected, and particularly the alternatives. Especially, physicians should not use persuasion to obtain consent which otherwise might not be forthcoming, nor should expectations be encouraged beyond those which the circumstances reasonably and realistically justify.

      (i) In exceptional circumstances, where the experimental treatment is the only potential treatment for the patient and full disclosure of information concerning the nature of the drug or experimental procedure or risks would pose such a serious psychological threat of detriment to the patient as to be medically contraindicated, such information may be withheld from the patient. In these circumstances, such information should be disclosed to a responsible relative or friend of the patient where possible.

(ii) Ordinarily, consent should be in writing, except where the physician deems it necessary to rely upon consent in other than written form because of the physical or emotional state of the patient.

(5) In clinical investigation primarily for the accumulation of scientific knowledge:

(a) Adequate safeguards must be provided for the welfare, safety and comfort of the subject. It is fundamental social policy that the advancement of scientific knowledge must always be secondary to primary concern for the individual.

(b) Consent, in writing, should be obtained from the subject, or from a legally authorized representative if the subject lacks the capacity to consent, following: (a) disclosure of the fact that an investigational drug or procedure is to be used, (b) a reasonable explanation of the nature of the procedure to be used and risks to be expected, and (c) an offer to answer any inquiries concerning the drug or procedure.

(6) No person may be used as a subject in clinical investigation against his or her will.

(7) The overuse of institutionalized persons in research is an unfair distribution of research risks. Participation is coercive and not voluntary if the participant is subjected to powerful incentives and persuasion.

(8) The ultimate responsibility for the ethical conduct of science resides within the institution (academic, industrial, public, or private) which conducts scientific research and with the individual scientist. Research institutions should assure that rigorous scientific standards are upheld by each of their faculty, staff, and students and should extend these standards to all reports, publications, and databases produced by the institution. All medical schools and biomedical research institutions should implement guidelines for a review process for dealing with allegations of fraud. These guidelines should ensure that (a) the process used to resolve allegations of fraud does not damage science, (b) all parties are treated fairly and justly with a sensitivity to reputations and vulnerabilities, (c) the highest degree of confidentiality is maintained, (d) the integrity of the process is maintained by an avoidance of real or apparent conflicts of interest, (e) resolution of charges is expeditious, (f) accurate and detailed documentation is kept throughout the process, and (g) responsibilities to all involved individuals, the public, research sponsors, the scientific literature, and the scientific community is met after resolution of charges. Academic institutions must be capable of, and committed to, implementing effective procedures for examining allegations of scientific fraud. No system of external monitoring should replace the efforts of an institution to set its own standards which fulfill its responsibility for the proper conduct of science and the training of scientists.

(9) With the approval of the patient or the patient's lawful representative, physicians should cooperate with the press and media to ensure that medical

news concerning the progress of clinical investigation or the patient's condition is available more promptly and more accurately than would be possible without their assistance. On the other hand, the Council does not approve of practices designed to create fanfare, sensationalism to attract media attention, and unwarranted expressions of optimism because of short term progress, even though longer range prognosis is known from the beginning to be precarious. With the approval of the patient or the patient's family, the Council, however, encourages the objective disclosure to the press and media of pertinent information. If at all possible, the identity of the patient should remain confidential if the patient or the patient's family so desires. The situation should not be used for the commercial ends of participating physicians or the institutions involved. (I, III, V)

Issued prior to April 1977.

Updated June 1994 and June 1998.

N.J. 1980 Physician employed to do research sued pharmaceutical company for wrongful discharge claiming that as an employee at will she had a cause of action for termination following her refusal to continue research she viewed as medically unethical. The court held that an employee has a cause of action when discharged contrary to a clearly mandated public policy. However, the court affirmed summary judgment because human testing was not imminent and because plaintiff failed to demonstrate the existence of a clear public policy based upon any statements of medical ethics to support her refusal to continue work on controversial drug. The dissent argued that the Opinions and Reports of the Judicial Council 5.03 and 5.18 (1979) [now Opinion 2.07] and other medical ethical statements did provide a clear expression of public policy and that plaintiff's failure to specifically cite them was merely a technical defect, and not fatal. *Pierce v. Ortho Pharmaceutical Corp., 84 N.J. 58, 417 A.2d 505, 516, 518.*

Journal 1997 Considers emergency room research informed consent standards. Reviews new federal regulations and related moral and ethical concerns. Concludes that regulations will require a case-by-case approach to balancing competing interests between research and ethics. References Opinion 2.07. Brody, *New Perspectives on Emergency Room Research*, 27 Hastings Center Rep. 7, 9 (Jan./Feb. 1997).

Journal 1997 Considers informed consent and the principle of self-determination. Analyzes the tradition of informed consent in medical research, with emphasis on international considerations. Concludes that research subjects need better protection. Cites Opinion 2.07. Note, *The Informed Consent Policy of the International Conference on Harmonization of Technical Requirements for Registrations of Pharmaceuticals for Human Use: Knowledge is the Best Medicine*, 30 Cornell Int'l L. J. 203, 209 (1997).

Journal 1993 Considers the legitimacy of neonatal HIV screening studies conducted without parental notice or consent. Asserts that such testing is morally and legally questionable. Quotes Opinion 2.07. Isaacman & Miller, *Neonatal HIV Seroprevalence Studies*, 14 J. Legal Med. 413, 428 (1993).

Journal 1989 Discusses various social control mechanisms that have an impact upon biomedical research. Emphasis is placed upon a comparison of the effectiveness of intra- and extraprofessional methods of control. Included among the control mechanisms discussed are the ethical pronouncements of the American Medical Association. References Opinion 2.07. Benson, *The Social Control of Human Biomedical Research: An Overview and Review of the Literature*, 29 Soc. Sci. Med. 1, 3 (1989).

2.075 The Use of Placebo Controls in Clinical Trials

Placebo controls are an important part of medicine's commitment to ensuring that the safety and efficacy of new drugs are sufficiently established. Used appropriately, placebo controls can safely provide valuable data and should continue to be considered in the design of clinical trials. The existence of an accepted therapy does not necessarily preclude the use of such controls; however, physician-investigators should adhere to the following guidelines to ensure that the interests of patients who participate in clinical trials are protected.

(1) Investigators must be extremely thorough in obtaining informed consent from patients. To the extent that research is dependent upon the willingness of patients to accept a level of risk, their understanding of the potential harms involved must be a top priority of any clinical investigation. The possibility presented in some studies that patients often do not fully understand the research protocol and therefore cannot truly give informed consent demonstrates a need to heighten the efforts of researchers to impress upon their subjects the nature of clinical research and the risks involved. Patients are capable of making decisions when presented with sufficient information and it is the responsibility of the institutional review board (IRB) and the individual investigators involved to ensure that each subject has been adequately informed and has given voluntary consent. Each patient must also be made aware that they can terminate their participation in a study at any time.

(2) Informed consent cannot be invoked to justify an inappropriate trial design. IRBs as well as investigators have an obligation to evaluate each study protocol to determine whether a placebo control is necessary and whether an alternative study design with another type of control would be sufficient for the purposes of research. Protocols that involve conditions causing death or irreversible damage cannot ethically employ a placebo control if alternative treatment would prevent or slow the illness progression. When studying illnesses characterized by severe or painful symptoms, investigators should thoroughly explore alternatives to the use of placebo controls. In general, the more severe the consequences and symptoms of the illness under study, the more difficult it will be to justify the use of a placebo control when alternative therapy exists. Consequently, there will almost certainly be conditions for which placebo controls cannot be justified. Similarly, the use of a placebo control will more easily be justified as the severity and number of negative side-effects of standard therapy increase.

(3) Researchers and IRBs should continue to minimize the amount of time patients are given placebo. The rationale provided by investigators for the length of study will give IRBs the opportunity to ensure that patients are given placebo therapy for as short a time as possible to provide verifiable results. Additionally, the interim data analysis and monitoring currently in practice will allow researchers to terminate the study because of either positive or negative results, thus protecting patients from remaining on placebo unnecessarily. (I, V)

Issued June 1998 based on the report, "Ethical Use of Placebos in Clinical Trials," adopted June 1996.

2.08 Commercial Use of Human Tissue

The rapid growth of the biotechnology industry has resulted in the commercial availability of numerous therapeutic and other products developed from human tissue. Physicians contemplating the commercial use of human tissue should abide by the following guidelines:

(1) Informed consent must be obtained from patients for the use of organs or tissues in clinical research.

(2) Potential commercial applications must be disclosed to the patient before a profit is realized on products developed from biological materials.

(3) Human tissue and its products may not be used for commercial purposes without the informed consent of the patient who provided the original cellular material.

(4) Profits from the commercial use of human tissue and its products may be shared with patients, in accordance with lawful contractual agreements.

(5) The diagnostic and therapeutic alternatives offered to patients by their physicians should conform to standards of good medical practice and should not be influenced in any way by the commercial potential of the patient's tissue. (II, V)

Issued June 1994 based on the report, "Who Should Profit from the Economic Value of Human Tissue? An Ethical Analysis," adopted June 1990.

2.09 Costs

While the physician should be conscious of costs and not provide or prescribe unnecessary services, concern for the quality of care the patient receives should be the physician's first consideration. This does not preclude the physician, individually or through medical or other organizations, from participating in policy-making with respect to social issues affecting health care. (I, VII)

Issued March 1981.

Updated June 1994 and June 1998.

Journal 1997 Posits that cost-containment schemes in managed care systems have eroded the fiduciary duty physicians owe patients. Notes that MCOs are prohibiting patients from trusting and relying on physicians. Concludes that patients must seek quality assurance from sources other than their physicians. Quotes Opinions 2.03, 2.09, and 8.13. Jacobi, *Patients at a Loss: Protecting Health Care Consumers through Data Driven Quality Assurance*, 45 U. Kan. L. Rev. 705, 720, 721, 759 (1997).

Journal 1996 Explores changing health care delivery environment and proposes a new approach to medical ethics. Suggests ways to improve the roles of care managers in capitated systems. Advocates disclosure of information to patients regarding coverage limitations and cost-containment policies. Quotes Opinion 2.09. Malinowski, *Capitation, Advances in Medical Technology, and the Advent of a New Era in Medical Ethics*, XXII Am. J. Law & Med. 331, 337 (1996).

Journal 1996 Discusses the health care system as it pertains to the elderly. Observes that age-based rationing decisions create significant value conflicts. Suggests that, in developing national health policy, decisions regarding resource allocation for the elderly must incorporate principles of ethical and moral reasoning. Quotes Opinion 2.09. Smith, *Our Hearts Were Once Young and Gay: Health Care Rationing and the Elderly*, 8 U. Fla. J.L. & Pub. Pol'y 1, 21 (1996).

Journal 1994 Considers how patients with insufficient financial resources place physicians in a conflict of interest situation with respect to patient needs and the financial interests of the physician, other patients, and society. Suggests that rules of contract and malpractice law do not provide satisfactory guidelines to resolve these conflicts. Concludes that legislative action may provide resolutions so long as physician-patient trust is preserved. Cites Opinions 2.09 and 2.095. Mehlman & Massey, *The Patient-Physician Relationship and the Allocation of Scarce Resources: A Law and Economics Approach*, 4 Kennedy Inst. Ethics J. 291, 292 (1994).

Journal 1994 Observes that health care reform proposals present significant challenges to the role and ethics of attending physicians. Emphasizes that reform proposals must set forth the role envisioned for physicians and must articulate an acceptable ethical framework within which physicians may fulfill that role. Quotes Opinions 4.04, 9.121, and 9.122. Cites Opinions 2.03, 2.09, 5.01, and 8.03. Wolf, *Health Care Reform and the Future of Physician Ethics*, 24 Hastings Center Rep. 28, 32, 40 (March/April 1994).

Journal 1993 Discusses the problem of physicians withholding needed medical treatment from HIV-infected infants. Explores the medical aspects of infant HIV infection. Considers ethical and legal issues involving nontreatment. Concludes that current law should be expanded to eliminate this discrimination. Quotes Opinions 2.09, 2.17, 2.20, 2.22, 4.04, and 8.03. Crossley, *Of Diagnoses and Discrimination: Discriminatory Nontreatment of Infants With HIV Infection*, 93 Columbia L. Rev. 1581, 1620, 1621 (1993).

Journal 1993 Examines the physician-patient relationship in the context of the need to control costs. Defines the physician-patient relationship within the framework of contract, tort, and fiduciary law. Considers whether a physician is required to provide care for the nonpaying patient. Concludes that the law does not require a physician to do so. Explores ways in which the law could be changed to ensure this result. Quotes Opinion 2.09. Mehlman, *The Patient-Physician Relationship in an Era of Scarce Resources: Is There a Duty to Treat?* 25 Conn. L. Rev. 349 (1993).

Journal 1992 Examines the major health care rationing issues facing the United States including increasing costs and decreasing access. Considers the reasons for the rising cost of medical care as well as possible solutions. Explores the concept of the standard of care and considers whether it should be changed. Concludes that the standard of care should not be changed and that rationing should be a separate enterprise undertaken pursuant to explicit criteria. Quotes Opinions 2.03, 2.09, and 4.04. Hirshfeld, *Should Ethical and Legal Standards for Physicians Be Changed to Accommodate New Models for Rationing Health Care?*, 140 Univ. Pa. L. Rev. 1809, 1816 (1992).

Journal 1991 Focuses on the denial of insurance benefits for experimental medical procedures. Explains the de novo review process under ERISA. Asserts that courts are becoming less deferential to administrative rulings. Concludes that there is need for a structure that will permit greater objectivity in the context of data collection as well as judicial determination. Cites Opinions 2.03 and 2.09. Note, *Denial of Coverage for "Experimental" Medical Procedures: The Problem of De Novo Review Under ERISA*, 79 Kentucky L.J. 801, 824 (1990-91).

Journal 1990 Discusses economic considerations in clinical decision making, with emphasis on the standard of care. Considers the way in which the standard of care is defined, including the role of the physician. Concludes that organized medicine has made valuable contributions through development of practice parameters that offer guidance in the exercise of clinical judgment. Cites Opinions 2.03 and 2.09. Hirsfeld, *Economic Considerations in Treatment Decisions and the Standard of Care in Medical Malpractice Litigation*, 264 J.A.M.A. 2004, 2007 (1990).

Journal 1990 Discusses efforts of third party payers to control health care expenditures for beneficiaries. Focuses on use of financial incentives to encourage providers to minimize the amount of care provided. Also discusses monitoring of requests for payment to determine necessity of care provided. Raises questions regarding impact of cost control mechanisms on quality of care, observing that available evidence is equivocal. Evaluates importance of disclosure to beneficiaries of use of financial incentives to limit care as well as other cost control mechanisms. Concludes that financial incentives and other cost control techniques should be disclosed and that the rationale for such disclosure is compelling. Quotes Opinions 2.03, 2.09, and 8.03. Cites Opinions 2.19, 4.04, and 4.06. Hirshfeld, *Should Third Party Payers of Health Care Services Disclose Cost Control Mechanisms to Potential Beneficiaries?*, 14 Seton Hall Legis. J. 115, 130, 131, 144, 145, 146 (1990).

2.095 The Provision of Adequate Health Care

Because society has an obligation to make access to an adequate level of health care available to all of its members regardless of ability to pay, physicians should contribute their expertise at a policy-making level to help achieve this goal. In determining whether particular procedures or treatments should be included in the adequate level of health care, the following ethical principles should be considered: (1) degree of benefit (the difference in outcome between treatment and no treatment), (2) likelihood of benefit, (3) duration of benefit, (4) cost, and (5) number of people who will benefit (referring to the fact that a treatment may benefit the patient and others who come into contact with the patient, as with a vaccination or antimicrobial drug).

Ethical principles require that a just process be used to determine the adequate level of health care. To ensure justice, the process for determining the adequate level of health care should include the following considerations: (1) democratic decision making with broad public input at both the developmental and final approval stages, (2) monitoring for variations in care that cannot be explained on medical grounds with special attention to evidence of discriminatory impact on historically disadvantaged groups, and (3) adjustment of the adequate level over time to ensure continued and broad public acceptance.

Because of the risk that inappropriate biases will influence the content of the basic benefits package, it may be desirable to avoid rigid or precise formulas to define the specific components of the basic benefits package. After applying the five ethical values listed above, it will be possible to designate some kinds of care as either clearly basic or clearly discretionary. However, for care that is not clearly basic or discretionary, seemingly objective formulas may result in choices that are inappropriately biased. For that care, therefore, it may be desirable to give equal consideration (e.g., through a process of random selection) to the different kinds of care when deciding which will be included in the basic benefits package.

The mechanism for providing an adequate level of health care should ensure that the health care benefits for the poor will not be eroded over time. (VII)

Issued June 1994 based on the report, "Ethical Issues in Health System Reform: The Provision of Adequate Health Care," adopted December 1993.

Journal 1996 Considers challenges to the psychiatrist-patient relationship that are triggered by managed care cost-containment methodologies. Offers guidance to psychiatrists for addressing these challenges. References Opinions 2.095, 8.13, and 8.132. Hoge, *APA Resource Document: I. The Professional Responsibilities of Psychiatrists in Evolving Health Care Systems*, 24 Bull. Am. Acad. Psychiatry Law 393, 405 (1996).

Journal 1994 Considers how greater patient autonomy has led to situations in which medical care may be viewed as futile. Examines cases in which physicians' medical judgments conflict with requests for medical treatment by patients or families. Suggests that the law has intruded too far into this area of medicine. Quotes Opinion 2.035. Cites Opinions 2.03, 2.095, 2.17, 2.19, 2.20, and 2.22. Cultice, *Medical Futility: When Is Enough, Enough?*, 27 J. Health & Hosp. Law 225, 230, 256 (1994).

Journal 1994 Considers how patients with insufficient financial resources place physicians in a conflict of interest situation with respect to patient needs and the financial interests of the physician, other patients, and society. Suggests that rules of contract and malpractice law do not provide satisfactory guidelines to resolve these conflicts. Concludes that legislative action may provide resolutions so long as physician-patient trust is preserved. Cites Opinions 2.09 and 2.095. Mehlman & Massey, *The Patient-Physician Relationship and the Allocation of Scarce Resources: A Law and Economics Approach*, 4 Kennedy Inst. Ethics J. 291, 292 (1994).

2.10 Fetal Research Guidelines

The following guidelines are offered as aids to physicians when they are engaged in fetal research:

(1) Physicians may participate in fetal research when their activities are part of a competently designed program, under accepted standards of scientific research, to produce data which are scientifically valid and significant.

(2) If appropriate, properly performed clinical studies on animals and non-gravid humans should precede any particular fetal research project.

(3) In fetal research projects, the investigator should demonstrate the same care and concern for the fetus as a physician providing fetal care or treatment in a non-research setting.

(4) All valid federal or state legal requirements should be followed.

(5) There should be no monetary payment to obtain any fetal material for fetal research projects.

(6) Competent peer review committees, review boards, or advisory boards should be available, when appropriate, to protect against the possible abuses that could arise in such research.

(7) Research on the so called "dead fetus," macerated fetal material, fetal cells, fetal tissue, or fetal organs should be in accord with state laws on autopsy and state laws on organ transplantation or anatomical gifts.

(8) In fetal research primarily for treatment of the fetus:
   (a) Voluntary and informed consent, in writing, should be given by the gravid woman, acting in the best interest of the fetus.
   (b) Alternative treatment or methods of care, if any, should be carefully evaluated and fully explained. If simpler and safer treatment is available, it should be pursued.

(9) In research primarily for treatment of the gravid female:
   (a) Voluntary and informed consent, in writing, should be given by the patient.
   (b) Alternative treatment or methods of care should be carefully evaluated and fully explained to the patient. If simpler and safer treatment is available, it should be pursued.
   (c) If possible, the risk to the fetus should be the least possible, consistent with the gravid female's need for treatment.

(10) In fetal research involving a fetus in utero, primarily for the accumulation of scientific knowledge:
   (a) Voluntary and informed consent, in writing, should be given by the gravid woman under circumstances in which a prudent and informed adult would reasonably be expected to give such consent.
   (b) The risk to the fetus imposed by the research should be the least possible.

(c) The purpose of research is the production of data and knowledge which are scientifically significant and which cannot otherwise be obtained.

(d) In this area of research, it is especially important to emphasize that care and concern for the fetus should be demonstrated. (I, III, V)

Issued March 1980.

Updated June 1994.

Journal 1991 Focuses on deliberations of the NIH Fetal Tissue Transplantation Research Panel. Explores arguments for and against fetal tissue transplantation research, including arguments for and against the use of federal funds to support such research. Considers whether the donation model is appropriate for the transfer of fetal tissue, and whether a woman who chooses elective abortion is an appropriate donor. References Opinion 2.10. Childress, *Ethics, Public Policy, and Human Fetal Tissue Transplantation Research*, Kennedy Inst. Ethics J. 93, 116 (June 1991).

Journal 1991 Considers how the use of in vitro fertilization (IVF) has blurred the distinction between medical practice and research. Suggests that extracorporeal embryos should be accorded the same respect as mature patients. Argues that medical-professional responsibility standards should be used to curtail the creation of life in vitro. Analyzes the need for limits on the use of IVF technology. Quotes Opinions 2.10 and 2.14. Comment, *Dangerous Relations: Doctors and Extracorporeal Embryos, The Need For New Limits To Medical Inquiry*, 7 J. Contemp. Health L. & Pol'y 307, 309 (1991).

2.11 Gene Therapy

Gene therapy involves the replacement or modification of a genetic variant to restore or enhance cellular function or to improve the reaction of non-genetic therapies.

Two types of gene therapy have been identified: (1) somatic cell therapy, in which human cells other than germ cells are genetically altered, and (2) germ line therapy, in which a replacement gene is integrated into the genome of human gametes or their precursors, resulting in expression of the new gene in the patient's offspring and subsequent generations. The fundamental difference between germ line therapy and somatic cell therapy is that germ line therapy affects the welfare of subsequent generations and may be associated with increased risk and the potential for unpredictable and irreversible results. Because of the far-reaching implications of germ line therapy, it is appropriate to limit genetic intervention to somatic cells at this time.

The goal of both somatic cell and germ line therapy is to alleviate human suffering and disease by remedying disorders for which available therapies are not satisfactory. This goal should be pursued only within the ethical tradition of medicine, which gives primacy to the welfare of the patient whose safety and well-being must be vigorously protected. To the extent possible, experience with animal studies must be sufficient to assure the effectiveness and safety of the techniques used, and the predictability of the results.

Moreover, genetic manipulation generally should be utilized only for therapeutic purposes. Efforts to enhance "desirable" characteristics through the insertion of a modified or additional gene, or efforts to "improve" complex human traits—the eugenic development of offspring—are contrary not only to the ethical tradition of medicine, but also to the egalitarian values of our society. Because of the potential for abuse, genetic manipulation to affect non-disease traits may never be acceptable and perhaps should never be pursued. If it is ever allowed, at least three conditions would have to be met before it could be deemed ethically acceptable: (1) there would have to be a clear and meaningful benefit to the person; (2) there would have to be no trade-off with other characteristics or traits; and (3) all citizens would have to have equal access to the genetic technology, irrespective of income or other socioeconomic characteristics. These criteria should be viewed as a minimal, not an exhaustive, test of the ethical propriety of non-disease-related genetic intervention. As genetic technology and knowledge of the human genome develop further, additional guidelines may be required.

As gene therapy becomes feasible for a variety of human disorders, there are several practical factors to consider to ensure safe application of this technology in society. First, any gene therapy research should meet the Council's guidelines on clinical investigation (Opinion 2.07) and investigators must adhere to the standards of medical practice and professional responsibility. The proposed procedure must be fully discussed with the patient and the written informed consent of the patient or the patient's legal representative must be voluntary. Investigators must be thorough in their attempts to eliminate any unwanted viral agents from the viral vector containing the corrective gene. The potential for adverse effects of the viral delivery system must be disclosed to the patient. The effectiveness of gene therapy must be evaluated fully, including the determination of the natural history of the disease and follow-up examination of subsequent generations. Gene therapy should be pursued only after the availability or effectiveness of other possible therapies is found to be insufficient. These considerations should be reviewed, as appropriate, as procedures and scientific information develop.

Issued December 1988. Updated June 1994 based on the report, "Prenatal Genetic Screening," adopted December 1992 (*Arch Fam Med.* 1994; 2: 633-642), and updated June 1996.

2.12   Genetic Counseling

Three primary areas of prenatal genetic testing are: (1) screening or evaluating prospective parents for genetic disease before conception to predict the likelihood of conceiving an affected child; (2) analysis of a pre-embryo at the preimplantation stage of artificial reproductive techniques; and (3) in utero testing after conception, such as ultrasonography, amniocentesis, fetoscopy, and chorionic villus sampling, to determine the condition of the fetus. Physicians engaged in genetic counseling are ethically obligated to provide prospective parents with the basis for an informed decision for childbearing. Counseling should include reasons for and against testing as well as discussion of inappropriate uses of genetic testing. Prenatal genetic testing is most appropriate for women or couples whose medical histories or family backgrounds indicate an elevated risk of fetal genetic disorders. Women or couples without an elevated risk of genetic disease may legitimately request prenatal diagnosis, provided they understand and accept the risks involved. When counseling prospective parents, physicians should avoid the imposition of their personal moral values and the substitution of their own moral judgment for that of the prospective parents.

The physician should be aware that where a genetic defect is found in the fetus, prospective parents may request or refuse an abortion. Physicians who consider the legal and ethical requirements applicable to genetic counseling to be in conflict with their moral values and conscience may choose to limit their services to preconception diagnosis and advice or not provide any genetic services. However, the physician who is so disposed is nevertheless obligated to alert prospective parents when a potential genetic problem does exist, so that the patient may decide whether to seek further genetic counseling from another qualified specialist.

Genetic selection refers to the abortion or discard of a fetus or pre-embryo with a genetic abnormality. In general, it is ethically permissible for physicians to participate in genetic selection to prevent, cure, or treat genetic disease. However, selection to avoid a genetic disease may not always be appropriate, depending on factors such as the severity of the disease, the probability of its occurrence, the age at onset, and the time of gestation at which selection would occur. It would not be ethical to engage in selection on the basis of non-disease related characteristics or traits. (II, IV, V, VI)

Issued June 1983.

Updated June 1994 based on the report, "Prenatal Genetic Screening," adopted December 1992 (*Arch Fam Med.* 1994; 3: 633-642).

Journal 1996 Discusses techniques and possibilities for genetic testing. Presents a series of problems designed as a starting point for understanding the conflicts surrounding genetic testing. Reviews the applications of state-of-the-art genetic research. Suggests potential difficulties that testing may cause in society. References Opinion 2.12. Underwood & Cadle, *Genetics, Genetic Testing, and the Specter of Discrimination: A Discussion Using Hypothetical Cases*, 85 Ky. L. J. 665, 684 (1996-97).

2.13 Genetic Engineering

Whatever form of regulation of gene splicing, recombinant DNA research, chemical synthesis of DNA molecules, or other genetic engineering research is eventually developed, there should be independent input from the scientific community, organized medicine, industry, and others, in addition to the federal government, to prevent abuse from any sector of society, private or public.

If and when gene replacement with normal DNA becomes a practical reality for the treatment of human disorders, the following factors should be considered:

(1) If procedures are performed in a research setting, reference should be made to the Council's guidelines on clinical investigation.

(2) If procedures are performed in a non-research setting, adherence to usual and customary standards of medical practice and professional responsibility would be required.

(3) Full discussion of the proposed procedure with the patient would be required. The consent of the patient or the patient's legal representative should be informed, voluntary and written.

(4) There must be no hazardous or other unwanted virus on the viral DNA containing the replacement or corrective gene.

(5) The inserted DNA must function under normal control within the recipient cell to prevent metabolic damage that could damage tissue and the patient.

(6) The effectiveness of the gene therapy should be evaluated as well as possible. This will include determination of the natural history of the disease and follow-up examination of subsequent generations.

(7) Such procedures should be undertaken in the future only after careful evaluation of the availability and effectiveness of other possible therapy. If simpler and safer treatment is available, it should be pursued.

(8) These considerations should be reviewed, as appropriate, as procedures and scientific information are developed in the future. (I, V, VII)

Issued March 1980.

Updated June 1996.

2.132 Genetic Testing by Employers

As a result of the human genome project, physicians will be able to identify a greater number of genetic risks of disease. Among the potential uses of the tests that detect these risks will be screening of potential workers by employers. Employers may want to exclude workers with certain genetic risks from the workplace because these workers may become disabled prematurely, impose higher health care costs, or pose a risk to public safety. In addition, exposure to certain substances in the workplace may increase the likelihood that a disease will develop in the worker with a genetic risk for the disease.

(1) It would generally be inappropriate to exclude workers with genetic risks of disease from the workplace because of their risk. Genetic tests alone do not have sufficient predictive value to be relied upon as a basis for excluding workers. Consequently, use of the tests would result in unfair discrimination against individuals who have positive test results. In addition, there are other ways for employers to serve their legitimate interests. Tests of a worker's actual capacity to meet the demands of the job can be used to ensure future employability and protect the public's safety. Routine monitoring of a worker's exposure can be used to protect workers who have a genetic susceptibility to injury from a substance in the workplace. In addition, employees should be advised of the risks of injury to which they are being exposed.

(2) There may be a role for genetic testing in the exclusion from the workplace of workers who have a genetic susceptibility to injury. At a minimum, several conditions would have to be met:

(a) The disease develops so rapidly that serious and irreversible injury would occur before monitoring of either the worker's exposure to the toxic substance or the worker's health status could be effective in preventing the harm.

(b) The genetic testing is highly accurate, with sufficient sensitivity and specificity to minimize the risk of false negative and false positive test results.

(c) Empirical data demonstrate that the genetic abnormality results in an unusually elevated susceptibility to occupational injury.

(d) It would require undue cost to protect susceptible employees by lowering the level of the toxic substance in the workplace. The costs of lowering the level of the substance must be extraordinary relative to the employer's other costs of making the product for which the toxic substance is used. Since genetic testing with exclusion of susceptible employees is the alternative to cleaning up the workplace, the cost of lowering the level of the substance must also be extraordinary relative to the costs of using genetic testing.

(e) Testing must not be performed without the informed consent of the employee or applicant for employment. (IV)

Issued June 1991 based on the report, "Genetic Testing by Employers" adopted June 1991 (JAMA. 1991; 266: 1827-1830).

Journal 1997 Explores the legality of pre-employment screening techniques. Considers legal reforms that would balance the interests of employers and job applicants. Offers suggestions that would enhance fairness and consistency in this screening process. References Opinion 2.132. Befort, *Pre-Employment Screening and Investigation: Navigating Between a Rock and a Hard Place*, 14 *Hofstra Lab. L. J.* 365, 391 (1997).

Journal 1997 Explores parents' legal rights to subject their children to genetic testing for untreatable, late-onset disorders or for carrier status. Examines potential negative aspects of genetic testing. Proposes that parents should not have the right to subject their children to such testing. References Opinion 2.132. Holland, *Should Parents Be Permitted to Authorize Genetic Testing for Their Children?*, 31 *Fam. L. Q.* 321, 346-47 (1997).

Journal 1997 Discusses the collection and storage of human tissues. Notes the use of genetic testing by employers. Examines whether those with biomedical experience perceive genetic research as dangerous. Considers problems of privacy and confidentiality raised by genetic technology and the storage of tissues. References Opinion 2.132. Merz, *Psychosocial Risks of Storing and Using Human Tissues in Research*, 8 *Risk: Health Safety & Env't* 235, 236 (1997).

Journal 1993 Discusses ethical issues created by the development of genetic tests to diagnose disease. Examines how these tests may be useful to private insurance companies in identifying persons for whom coverage will be provided. Considers the moral and social responsibilities of insurers in this context. Concludes that this issue should be considered as part of the national health care reform debate. References Opinion 2.132. Jecker, *Genetic Testing and the Social Responsibility of Private Health Insurance Companies*, 21 *J. Law, Med. & Ethics* 109, 112 (1993).

2.135 Insurance Companies and Genetic Information

Physicians should not participate in genetic testing by health insurance companies to predict a person's predisposition for disease. As a corollary, it may be necessary for physicians to maintain separate files for genetic testing results to ensure that the results are not sent to health insurance companies when requests for copies of patient medical records are fulfilled. Physicians who withhold testing results should inform insurance companies that, when medical records are sent, genetic testing results are not included. This disclosure should occur with all patients, not just those who have undergone genetic testing. (IV)

Issued June 1994 based on the report, "Physician Participation in Genetic Testing by Health Insurance Companies," adopted June 1993.

Updated June 1996.

2.137 Ethical Issues in Carrier Screening of Genetic Disorders

All carrier testing must be voluntary, and informed consent from screened individuals is required. Confidentiality of results is to be maintained. Results of testing should not be disclosed to third parties without the explicit informed consent of the screened individual. Patients should be informed as to potential uses for the genetic information by third parties, and whether other ways of obtaining the information are available when appropriate.

Carrier testing should be available uniformly among the at-risk population being screened. One legitimate exception to this principle is the limitation of carrier testing to individuals of childbearing age. In pursuit of uniform access, physicians should not limit testing only to patients specifically requesting testing. If testing is offered to some patients, it should be offered to all patients within the same risk category.

The direction of future genetic screening tests should be determined by well thought out and well-coordinated social policy. Third parties, including insurance companies or employers, should not be permitted to discriminate against carriers of genetic disorders through policies which have the ultimate effect of influencing decisions about testing and reproduction. (IV, V)

Issued June 1994 based on the report, "Ethical Issues in Carrier Screening of Cystic Fibrosis and Other Genetic Disorders," adopted June 1991.

2.138 Genetic Testing of Children

Genetic testing of children implicates important concerns about individual autonomy and the interest of the patients. Before testing of children can be performed, there must be some potential benefit from the testing that can reasonably be viewed as outweighing the disadvantages of testing, particularly the harm from abrogating the children's future choice in knowing their genetic status. When there is such a potential benefit, parents should decide whether their children will undergo testing. If parents unreasonably request or refuse testing of their child, physician should take steps to change or, if necessary, use legal means to override the parents' choice. Applying these principles to specific circumstances yields the following conclusions:

(1) When a child is at risk for a genetic condition for which preventive or other therapeutic measures are available, genetic testing should be offered or, in some cases, required.

(2) When a child is at risk for a genetic condition with pediatric onset for which preventive or other therapeutic measures are not available, parents generally should have discretion to decide about genetic testing.

(3) When a child is at risk for a genetic condition with adult onset for which preventive or other therapeutic measures are not available, genetic testing of children generally should not be undertaken. Families should still be informed of the existence of tests and given the opportunity to discuss the reasons why the tests are generally not offered for children.

(4) Genetic testing for carrier status should be deferred until either the child reaches maturity, the child needs to make reproductive decisions or, in the

case of children too immature to make their own reproductive decisions, reproductive decisions need to be made for the child.

(5) Genetic testing of children for the benefit of a family member should not be performed unless the testing is necessary to prevent substantial harm to the family member.

When a child's genetic status is determined incidentally, the information should be retained by the physician and entered into the patient record. Discussion of the existence of this finding should then be taken up when the child reaches maturity or needs to make reproductive decisions, so that the individual can decide whether to request disclosure of the information. It is important that physicians be consistent in disclosing both positive and negative results in the same way since if physicians raise the existence of the testing results only when the results are positive, individuals will know what the results must be. This information should not be disclosed to third parties. Genetic information should be maintained in a separate portion of the medical record to prevent mistaken disclosure.

When a child is being considered for adoption, the guidelines for genetic testing should be the same as for other children. (I, IV)

Issued June 1996 based on the report, "Testing Children for Genetic Status," adopted June 1995.

Journal 1997 Discusses the National Human Genome Research Institute and the activities of the Office of Genome Ethics. Offers an overview and evaluation, with emphasis on bioethical education and counsel that was provided to genetic researchers. References Opinion 2.138. Green, *NHGRI's Intramural Ethics Experiment*, 7 Kennedy Inst. of Ethics J. 181, 185, 188 (1997).

2.14   In Vitro Fertilization

The technique of in vitro fertilization and embryo transplantation enables certain couples previously incapable of conception to bear a child. It is also useful in the field of research directed toward an understanding of how genetic defects arise and are transmitted and how they might be prevented or treated. Because of serious ethical and moral concerns, however, any fertilized egg that has the potential for human life and that will be implanted in the uterus of a woman should not be subjected to laboratory research.

All fertilized ova not utilized for implantation and that are maintained for research purposes shall be handled with the strictest adherence to the Principles of Medical Ethics, to the guidelines for research and medical practice expressed in the Council's opinion on fetal research, and to the highest standards of medical practice. (I, V, VII)

Issued June 1983.

Journal 1991 Considers how the use of in vitro fertilization (IVF) has blurred the distinction between medical practice and research. Suggests that extracorporeal embryos should be accorded the same respect as mature patients. Argues that medical-professional responsibility standards should be used to curtail the creation of life in vitro. Analyzes the need for limits on the use of IVF technology. Quotes Opinions 2.10 and 2.14. Comment, *Dangerous Relations: Doctors and Extracorporeal Embryos, The Need For New Limits To Medical Inquiry*, 7 J. Contemp. Health L. & Pol'y 307, 309 (1991).

Journal 1987 Examines various ethical issues surrounding surrogate motherhood, artificial insemination, in vitro fertilization and embryonic/fetal research. Reports on the positions of four ethics groups: the Warnock Committee of Inquiry into Human Fertilization and Embryology; the American Medical Association's Council on Ethical and Judicial Affairs; the Ethics Committee of the American Fertility Society; and the Ethics Committee of the American College of Obstetricians and Gynecologists. References Opinions 2.04, 2.05, and 2.13 (1986) [now Opinion 2.14]. Quotes Opinion 2.18. Rosner, Cassell, Friedland, Landolt, Loeb, Numann, Ora, Risemberg, & Sordillo, *Ethical Considerations of Reproductive Technologies*, 87 N.Y. State J. Med. 398, 399-400 (1987).

2.141 Frozen Pre-embryos

The practice of freezing extra pre-embryos harvested during the in vitro fertilization (IVF) process has enhanced the ability of infertile couples to preserve embryos for future implantation. This practice has also posed a number of ethical and legal dilemmas, including questions regarding decision making authority over the pre-embryos and appropriate uses of pre-embryos.

This country's cultural and legal traditions indicate that the logical persons to exercise control over a frozen pre-embryo are the woman and man who provided the gametes (the ovum and sperm). The gamete providers have a fundamental interest at stake, their potential for procreation. In addition, the gamete providers are the parties most concerned with the interests of a frozen pre-embryo and most likely to protect those interests.

Gamete providers should be able to use the pre-embryos themselves or donate them for use by other parties, but not sell them. In addition, research on pre-embryos should be permitted as long as the pre-embryos are not destined for transfer to a woman for implantation and as long as the research is conducted in accordance with the Council's guidelines on fetal research. Frozen pre-embryos may also be allowed to thaw and deteriorate.

The gamete providers should have an equal say in the use of their pre-embryos and, therefore, the pre-embryos should not be available for use by either provider or changed from their frozen state without the consent of both providers. The man and woman each has contributed half of the pre-embryo's genetic code. In addition, whether a person chooses to become a parent and assume all of the accompanying obligations is a particularly personal and fundamental decision. Even if the individual could be absolved of any parental obligations, he or she may have a strong desire not to have offspring. The absence of a legal duty does not eliminate the moral duty many would feel toward any genetic offspring.

Advance agreements are recommended for deciding the disposition of frozen pre-embryos in the event of divorce or other changes in circumstances. Advance agreements can help ensure that the gamete providers undergo IVF and pre-embryo freezing after a full contemplation of the consequences, but should not be mandatory. (I, III, IV, V)

Issued March 1992 based on the report, "Frozen Pre-Embryos," adopted December 1989 (JAMA. 1990; 263: 2484-2487).

Updated June 1994.

Journal 1990 Discusses issues raised by technology allowing frozen preembryos to be preserved outside the human body. Considers ways in which the preembryo can be legally described and argues that it should not be considered either person or property. Evaluates the rights of "progenitors" relative to the preembryo and reviews state law concerning in vitro fertilization and IVF research. Concludes that IVF research is valuable to society and proposes research guidelines. References Opinion 2.141. Martin & Lagod, *The Human Preembryo, the Progenitors, and the State: Toward a Dynamic Theory of Status, Rights, and Research Policy*, 5 High Tech. L. J. 257, 304 (1990).

Journal 1990 Considers problems created by frozen preembryos that result from in vitro fertilization therapy. Explores problems with disposing of these preembryos and how prior agreements between couples have surfaced as a potential solution. Examines the enforceability and practical implications of these agreements. References Opinion 2.141. Robertson, *Prior Agreements for Disposition of Frozen Embryos*, 51 Ohio St. L. J. 407, 419 (1990).

2.145   Pre-embryo Splitting

The technique of splitting in vitro fertilized pre-embryos may result in multiple genetically identical siblings.

The procedure of pre-embryo splitting should be available so long as both gamete providers agree. This procedure may greatly increase the chances of conception for an infertile couple or for a couple whose future reproductive capacity will likely be diminished. Pre-embryo splitting also can reduce the number of invasive procedures necessary for egg retrieval and the necessity for hormonal stimulants to generate multiple eggs. The use and disposition of any pre-embryos that are frozen for future use should be consistent with the Council's opinion on frozen pre-embryos. (Opinion 2.141)

The use of frozen pre-embryo identical siblings many years after one child has been born raises new ethical issues. Couples might wait until they can discover the mental and physical characteristics of a child before transferring a genetically identical sibling for implantation, they might sell their frozen pre-embryos based upon the outcome of a genetically identical child, or they might decide to transplant a genetically identical sibling based on the need to harvest the child's tissue.

The Council does not find that these considerations are sufficient to prohibit pre-embryo splitting for the following reasons:

(1) It would take many years to determine the outcome of a child and most families want to complete their childbearing within a shorter time.

(2) The sale of pre-embryos can and should be prohibited.

(3) The small number of couples who might bear identical siblings solely for purposes of harvesting their tissue does not outweigh the benefits which might be derived from pre-embryo splitting. Additionally, it is not evident that a sibling would have negative psychological or emotional consequences from having acted as an organ or tissue donor. Indeed, the child may derive psychological benefits from having saved the life of a sibling.

To the extent possible, discussion of these issues should be had with gamete providers prior to pre-embryo splitting and freezing so as to inform the prospective parents of possible future ethical dilemmas. (I, III, IV, V)

Issued June 1994.

2.15 Financial Incentives for Organ Donation

The voluntary donation of organs in appropriate circumstances is to be encouraged. However, it is not ethical to participate in a procedure to enable a living donor to receive payment, other than for the reimbursement of expenses necessarily incurred in connection with removal, for any of the donor's non-renewable organs.

Procedures involving financial incentives for cadaveric organ donors should have adequate safeguards to ensure that the health of donors and recipients is in no way jeopardized, and that the quality of the organ supply is not degraded. Incentives should be limited to future contracts offered to prospective donors. By entering into a future contract, an adult would agree while still competent to donate his or her organs after death. In return, the donor's family or estate would receive some financial remuneration after the organs have been retrieved and judged medically suitable for transplantation. Several other conditions would apply:

(1) Only the potential donor, and not the donor's family or other third party, may be given the option of accepting financial incentives for cadaveric organ donation. In addition, the potential donor must be a competent adult when the decision to donate is made, and the donor must not have committed suicide.

(2) Any incentive should be of moderate value and should be the lowest amount that can reasonably be expected to encourage organ donation. By designating a state agency to administer the incentive, full control over the level of incentive can be maintained.

(3) Payment should occur only after the organs have been retrieved and judged medically suitable for transplantation. Suitability should continue to be determined in accordance with the procedures of the Organ Procurement and Transplantation Network.

(4) Incentives should play no part in the allocation of donated organs among potential transplant recipients. The distribution of organs for transplantation should continue to be governed only by ethically appropriate criteria relating to medical need. (I, III, V)

Issued June 1984.

Updated June 1994 based on the report, "Financial Incentives for Organ Procurement: Ethical Aspects of Future Contracts for Cadaveric Donors," adopted December 1993.

Journal 1995 Examines legal and ethical issues surrounding organ transplant procurement practices, with emphasis on a possible commercial system. Explores medical advances and industry regulations. Concludes that adequate market safeguards need to be developed to protect vulnerable donors and citizens. References Opinions 2.15 and 2.167. Banks, *Legal and Ethical Safeguards: Protection of Society's Most Vulnerable Participants in a Commercialized Organ Transplantation System, XXI Am. J. Law & Med. 45, 77, 79, 95-96, 103-04 (1995).*

Journal 1994 Examines the current system governing the transfer of transplantable organs. Proposes that a futures market in bodily organs would alleviate the shortage of available organs. Argues that existing organ transplantation laws must be amended to allow a futures market to operate. Quotes Opinion 2.15. Crespi, *Overcoming the Legal Obstacles to the Creation of a Futures Market in Bodily Organs, 55 Ohio St. L. J. 1, 74 (1994).*

2.155 Mandated Choice and Presumed Consent for Cadaveric Organ Donation

A system of mandated choice for organ donation, in which individuals are required to express their preferences regarding organ donation when renewing their drivers' licenses or performing some other state-mandated task, is an ethically appropriate strategy for encouraging donation and should be pursued. To be effective, information on the importance of organ donation and the success of organ transplantation should be provided when the donation decision is made.

A system of presumed consent for organ donation, in which individuals are assumed to consent to be organ donors after death unless they indicate their refusal to consent, raises serious ethical concerns. For presumed consent to be ethically acceptable, effective mechanisms for documenting and honoring refusals to donate must be in place. In addition, when there is no documented refusal by the individual decedent, the family of the decedent would have to be contacted to verify that they do not know of any objections to donation by the decedent while living. (I, III, V)

Issued June 1994 based on the report, "Strategies for Cadaveric Organ Procurement: Mandated Choice and Presumed Consent," adopted December 1993.

Journal 1997 Explores the current policies on cadaveric organ procurement in the United States. Offers improvements to help save lives and end the waste of suitable organs. Discusses pertinent ethical and legal issues. References Opinion 2.155. MacDonald, *Organ Donation: The Time Has Come to Refocus the Ethical Spotlight*, 8 Stan. L. & Pol'y Rev. 177, 179, 185 (1997).

2.157 Organ Procurement Following Cardiac Death

Given the increasing need for donor organs, protocols for procurement following cardiac death have been developed. In some instances, patients or their surrogate decision makers request withdrawal of life support and choose to serve as organ donors. In these cases, the organs can be preserved best by discontinuation of life support in the operating room so that organs can be removed two minutes following cardiac death. In other scenarios, patients who suffer unexpected cardiac death may be cannulated and perfused with cold preserving fluid (in situ preservation) to maintain organs. Both of these methods may be ethically permissible, with attention to certain safeguards.

(1) When securing consent for life support withdrawal and organ retrieval, the health care team must be certain that consent is voluntary. This is particularly true where surrogate decisions about life-sustaining treatment may be influenced by the prospect of organ donation. If there is any reason to suspect undue influence, a full ethics consultation should be required.

(2) In all instances, it is critical that there be no conflict of interest in the health care team. Those health care professionals providing care at the end of life must be separated from providers participating in the transplant team.

(3) Further pilot programs should assess the success and acceptability of organ removal following withdrawal of life-sustaining treatment.

(4) In cases of in situ preservation of cadaveric organs, the prior consent of the decedent or the consent of the decedent's surrogate decision maker makes perfusion ethically permissible. Perfusion without either prior specific consent to perfusion or general consent to organ donation violates requirements for informed consent for medical procedures and should not be permitted.

(5) The recipients of such procured organs should be informed of the source of the organs as well as any potential defects in the quality of the organs, so that they may decide with their physicians whether to accept the organs or wait for more suitable ones.

(6) Clear clinical criteria should be developed to ensure that only appropriate candidates, whose organs are reasonably likely to be suitable for transplantation, are considered eligible to donate organs under these protocols.

Issued June 1996 based on the reports, "Ethical Issues in the Procurement of Organs Following Cardiac Death: The Pittsburgh Protocol," and "Ethical Issues in Organ Procurement Following Cardiac Death: In Situ Preservation of Cadaveric Organs," adopted December 1994.

2.16   Organ Transplantation Guidelines

The following statement is offered for guidance of physicians as they seek to maintain the highest level of ethical conduct in the transplanting of human organs.

(1) In all professional relationships between a physician and a patient, the physician's primary concern must be the health of the patient. The physician owes the patient primary allegiance. This concern and allegiance must be preserved in all medical procedures, including those which involve the transplantation of an organ from one person to another where both donor and recipient are patients. Care must, therefore, be taken to protect the rights of both the donor and the recipient, and no physician may assume a responsibility in organ transplantation unless the rights of both donor and recipient are equally protected. A prospective organ transplant offers no justification for a relaxation of the usual standard of medical care for the potential donor.

(2) When a vital, single organ is to be transplanted, the death of the donor shall have been determined by at least one physician other than the recipient's physician. Death shall be determined by the clinical judgment of the physician, who should rely on currently accepted and available scientific tests.

(3) Full discussion of the proposed procedure with the donor and the recipient or their responsible relatives or representatives is mandatory. The physician should ensure that consent to the procedure is fully informed and voluntary, in accordance with the Council's guidelines on informed consent. Once such informed consent to donation has been given by the donor in accordance with applicable state law, it cannot be revoked by surviving family members. The physician's interest in advancing scientific knowledge must always be secondary to his or her concern for the patient.

(4) Transplant procedures of body organs should be undertaken (a) only by physicians who possess special medical knowledge and technical competence developed through special training, study, and laboratory

36

experience and practice, and (b) in medical institutions with facilities adequate to protect the health and well-being of the parties to the procedure.

(5) Recipients of organs for transplantation should be determined in accordance with the Council's guidelines on the allocation of limited medical resources.

(6) Organs should be considered a national, rather than a local or regional, resource. Geographical priorities in the allocation of organs should be prohibited except when transportation of organs would threaten their suitability for transplantation.

(7) Patients should not be placed on the waiting lists of multiple local transplant centers, but rather on a single waiting list for each type of organ. (I, III, V)

Issued prior to April 1977.

Updated June 1994 based on the report, "Ethical Considerations in the Allocation of Organs and Other Scarce Medical Resources Among Patients," adopted June 1993 (*Arch Intern Med.* 1995; 155: 29-40) and June 1998 based on the report, "Organ Procurement: Upholding Donor Decisions," adopted December 1996.

In addition, the 1986 Report of the U.S. Task Force on Organ Transplantation is an excellent resource for physicians involved in organ transplantation.

Journal 1987 Discusses the issue of the right of the individual to consent to organ removal and then examines the doctrine of informed consent as it is applied in the context of live organ donation. Evaluates the extent to which removal of non-regenerative organs disrupts the basis for application of the traditional informed consent model. Additional attention is devoted to special concerns regarding consent in cases of children and incompetent patients, with consideration of the role of judicial review in these types of cases. Quotes Opinion 2.15 (1986) [now Opinion 2.16]. Adams, *Live Organ Donors and Informed Consent: A Difficult Minuet, 8 J. Legal Med.* 555, 560-61 (1987).

2.161 Medical Applications of Fetal Tissue Transplantation

The principal ethical concern in the use of human fetal tissue for transplantation is the degree to which the decision to have an abortion might be influenced by the decision to donate the fetal tissue. In the application of fetal tissue transplantation the following safeguards should apply: (1) The Council's guidelines on clinical investigation and organ transplantation are followed, as they pertain to the recipient of the fetal tissue transplant (see Opinion 2.07, Clinical Investigation, and Opinion 2.16, Organ Transplantation Guidelines); (2) a final decision regarding abortion is made before initiating a discussion of the transplantation use of fetal tissue; (3) decisions regarding the technique used to induce abortion, as well as the timing of the abortion in relation to the gestational age of the fetus, are based on concern for the safety of the pregnant woman; (4) fetal tissue is not provided in exchange for financial remuneration above that which is necessary to cover reasonable expenses; (5) the recipient of the tissue is not designated by the donor; (6) health care personnel involved in the termination of a particular pregnancy do not participate in or receive any benefit from the transplantation of tissue from the abortus of the same pregnancy; and (7) informed consent on behalf of both the donor and the recipient is obtained in accordance with applicable law. (I, IV, V)

Issued March 1992 based on the report, "Medical Applications of Fetal Tissue Transplantation," adopted June 1989 (JAMA. 1990; 263: 565-570).

Updated June 1996.

Journal 1990 Presents an update on current medical research regarding Parkinson's disease. Discusses the relevance of fetal tissue transplantation to this research. Concludes that continued neurological research is necessary. References Opinion 2.161. Joynt, *Neurology,* 263 *J.A.M.A.* 2660 (1990).

2.162 Anencephalic Neonates as Organ Donors

Anencephaly is a congenital absence of major portion of the brain, skull, and scalp. Anencephalic neonates are thought to be unique from other brain-damaged beings because of a lack of past consciousness with no potential for future consciousness.

Physicians may provide anencephalic neonates with ventilator assistance and other medical therapies that are necessary to sustain organ perfusion and viability until such time as a determination of death can be made in accordance with accepted medical standards, relevant law and regional organ procurement organization policy. Retrieval and transplantation of the organs of anencephalic infants are ethically permissible only after such determination of death is made, and only in accordance with the Council's guidelines for transplantation.

Issued June 1988.

Reaffirmed in the report, "Anencephalic Infants as Organ Donors—Reconsideration," adopted December 1995.

Journal 1996 Explores courses of treatment for infants born with hypoplastic left heart syndrome. Discusses the various treatment options available to infants, and their frequency. Notes the controversy surrounding the AMA's opinion on anencephalic infants as organ donors. References Opinion 2.162 [subsequently amended]. Caplan, Cooper, Garcia-Prats, & Brody, *Diffusion of Innovative Approaches to Managing Hypoplastic Left Heart Syndrome,* 150 Arch. Pediatr. Adolesc. Med. 487, 490 (1996).

Journal 1996 Describes the impact of federal laws on medical decisions for anencephalic infants. Discusses selective nontreatment of such infants and the debate regarding availability of their organs for transplantation. Quotes Opinions 2.162 (1994) [subsequently amended] and 2.17. Crossley, *Infants with Anencephaly, the ADA, and the Child Abuse Amendments,* 11 Issues in Law & Med. 379, 385, 409 (1996).

Journal 1996 Proposes an alternative method of capital punishment to allow for organ donation by executed prisoners. Provides justifications for this proposal. Concludes that physicians should be able to ethically participate in this process. Quotes Principle VII. Cites Opinion 2.06. References Opinion 2.162 (1994) [subsequently amended]. Patton, *A Call for Common Sense: Organ Donation and the Executed Prisoner,* 3 Va. J. Soc. Pol'y & L. 387, 404, 405, 407-10 (1996).

Journal 1996 Examines the recent trend in health care laws and ethics to focus on the alleviation of suffering. Expresses concern that such a focus may result in the valuation of one life over another. Emphasizes the need to evaluate multiple, diverse responses to suffering. Quotes Principle VI. References Opinion 2.162. Shepherd, *Sophie's Choices: Medical and Legal Responses to Suffering,* 72 Notre Dame L. Rev. 103, 106, 133 (1996).

Journal 1994 Criticizes both the White House's proposed National Bioethics Advisory Commission and certain purely private ethical advisory bodies. Proposes that an appropriately organized new federal advisory body could provide essential guidance in developing public bioethical policies, particularly if the meaningful input of ethics scholars at universities, ethics centers, and other private organizations and public commissions were sought. Cites Opinion 2.162. Capron, *Ethics: Public and Private*, 24 Hastings Center Rep. 26, 27 (November/December 1994).

2.165 Fetal Umbilical Cord Blood

Human umbilical cord blood has been identified as a viable source of hematopoietic stem cells that can be used as an alternative to bone marrow for transplantation. It is obtained by clamping the umbilical cord immediately after delivery.

The use of umbilical cord blood raises two main ethical problems. First, the exact timing of the clamping has a significant impact on the neonate. Studies indicate that early clamping may cause an abrupt surge in arterial pressure, resulting in intraventricular hemorrhage (particularly in premature infants). Second, there is a risk that the infant donor will develop a need for his or her own cord blood later in life. If that child was a donor and this later need arises, he or she might be without blood, when he or she could have had his or her own blood stored.

To avoid health risks, normal clamping protocol should be followed and not altered in such a way that might endanger the infant. Additionally, parents of the infant must be fully informed of the risks of the donation and written consent should be obtained from them.

The second concern, that the child may need the blood later in life, is more complex. The possibility that an infant donor would be in need of his or her own umbilical cord blood is highly speculative. There are a number of reasons why the infant may not need the blood later. The diseases that are treated by bone marrow transplantation are not common, and there may be other treatment alternatives available, particularly in the future when the illness would occur. Additionally, the demand for fetal umbilical cord blood will increase as it becomes medically certain that the blood may be used in persons unrelated to the donor. This situation will reduce the need to store a particular infant's blood since umbilical cord blood from other donors would be available. If the blood is sufficient for use in unrelated individuals, then the donor may obtain the cord blood from another donor later in life, making the need to store his or her own blood unnecessary. These original donors, however, should be given priority in receipt of such blood if they need a donation later in life.

For all of these reasons, it would generally not be unethical to use the cord blood. However, if the child-donor is known to be at risk for an illness that is treated by bone marrow donation, the child should not be used as a donor, and his or her blood should be stored for future use. (I, V)

Issued June 1994.

Updated June 1996.

The Use of Minors as Organ and Tissue Donors

Minors need not be prohibited from acting as sources of organs, but their participation should be limited. Different procedures pose different degrees of risk and do not all require the same restrictions. In general, minors should not be permitted to serve as a source when there is a very serious risk of complications (e.g., partial liver or lung donation, which involve a substantial risk of serious immediate or longterm morbidity). If the safeguards in the remainder of this opinion are followed, minors may be permitted to serve as a source when the risks are low (e.g., blood or skin donation, in which the donated tissue can regenerate and spinal or general anesthesia is not required), moderate (e.g., bone marrow donation, in which the donated tissue can regenerate but brief general or spinal anesthesia is required) or serious (e.g., kidney donation, which involve more extensive anesthesia and major invasive surgery).

If a child is capable of making his or her own medical treatment decisions, he or she should be considered capable of deciding whether to be an organ or tissue donor. However, physicians should not perform organ retrievals of serious risk without first obtaining court authorization. Courts should confirm that the mature minor is acting voluntarily and without coercion.

If a child is not capable of making his or her own medical decisions, all transplantations should have parental approval, and those which pose a serious risk should receive court authorization. In the court authorization process, the evaluation of a child psychiatrist or psychologist must be sought and a guardian ad litem should be assigned to the potential minor donor in order to fully represent the minor's interests.

When deciding on behalf of immature children, parents and courts should ensure that transplantation presents a "clear benefit" to the minor source, which entails meeting the following requirements:

(1) Ideally the minor should be the only possible source. All other available sources of organs, both donor pools and competent adult family members, must be medically inappropriate or significantly inferior. An unwilling potential donor does not qualify him or her as medically inappropriate.

(2) For transplantations of moderate or serious risk, the transplantation must be necessary with some degree of medical certainty to provide a substantial benefit; that is, it both prevents an extremely poor quality of life and ensures a good quality of life for the recipient. A transplant should not be allowed if it merely increases the comfort of the recipient. If a transplant is not presently considered to provide a substantial benefit but is expected to do so within a period of time, the transplant need not be delayed until it meets this criterion, especially if the delay would significantly decrease the benefits derived from the transplant by the recipient.

(3) The organ or tissue transplant must have a reasonable probability of success in order for transplantation to be allowed. What constitutes a reasonable chance of success should be based on medical judgments about the physical condition of the recipient and the likelihood that the transplant will not be rejected, futile, or produce benefits which are very transient. Children should not be used for transplants that are considered experimental or nonstandard.

(4) Generally, minors should be allowed to serve as a source only to close family members.

(5) Psychological or emotional benefits to the potential source may be considered, though evidence of future benefit to the minor source should be clear and convincing. Possible benefits to a child include continued emotional bonds between the minor and the recipient, increased selfesteem, and prevention of adverse reaction to death of a sibling. Whether a child will capture these benefits depends upon the child's specific circumstances. A minor's assent or dissent to a procedure is an important piece of evidence that demonstrates whether the transplant will offer psychological benefits to the source. Dissent from incompetent minors should be powerful evidence that the donation will not provide a clear benefit, but may not present an absolute bar. Every effort should be made to identify and address the child's concerns in this case.

(6) It is essential to ensure that the potential source does not have any underlying conditions that create an undue individual risk. (I, V)

Issued June 1994 based on the report, "The Use of Minors as Organ and Tissue Donors," adopted December 1993.

Journal 1995 Examines legal and ethical issues surrounding organ transplant procurement practices, with emphasis on a possible commercial system. Explores medical advances and industry regulations. Concludes that adequate market safeguards need to be developed to protect vulnerable donors and citizens. References Opinions 2.15 and 2.167. Banks, *Legal and Ethical Safeguards: Protection of Society's Most Vulnerable Participants in a Commercialized Organ Transplantation System*, XXI Am. J. Law & Med. 45, 77, 79, 95-96, 103-04 (1995).

2.17   Quality of Life

In the making of decisions for the treatment of seriously disabled newborns or of other persons who are severely disabled by injury or illness, the primary consideration should be what is best for the individual patient and not the avoidance of a burden to the family or to society. Quality of life, as defined by the patient's interests and values, is a factor to be considered in determining what is best for the individual. It is permissible to consider quality of life when deciding about life-sustaining treatment in accordance with Opinions 2.20, 2.215, and 2.22. (I, III, IV)

Issued March 1981.

Updated June 1994.

N.J. Super. 1983 Guardian of elderly nursing home patient suffering from severe organic brain syndrome sought to remove nasogastric tube from patient. Trial court granted guardian's petition, and patient's guardian ad litem appealed. Appellate court reversed, in part based upon Opinions 2.11 (1981) and 5.17 (1979) [now Opinions 2.17 and 2.20], and held that it is improper and would violate medical ethics to allow dehydration and starvation in a "non-comatose, non-brain-dead patient not facing imminent death, not maintained by any life-support machine, and not able to speak for herself." *In re Conroy*, 190 N.J. Super. 453, 464 A.2d 303, 313-15, rev'd, 98 N.J. 321, 486 A.2d 1209 (1985).

Journal 1997 Considers percutaneous endoscopic gastrostomy tubes and the lack of standards for their placement. Discusses the medical and ethical problems involved, and creates a method for reconciling them. Recommends that patients in a persistent vegetative state not undergo the procedure. References Opinion 2.17. Rabeneck, McCullough, & Wray, *Ethically Justified, Clinically Comprehensive Guidelines for Percutaneous Endoscopic Gastrostomy Tube Placement*, 349 Lancet 496, 497, 498 (1997).

Journal 1996 Explores decision-making standards employed in the removal of medical treatment from incompetent patients. Suggests substituted judgment and best interests standards be replaced by a standard that focuses on patient dignity. Concludes that treatment should be removed when empirical evidence suggests a majority of individuals would want it removed. Cites Opinion 2.16 (1986) [now Opinion 2.17]. Cantor, *Discarding Substituted Judgment and Best Interests: Toward a Constructive Preference Standard for Dying, Previously Competent Patients Without Advance Instructions*, 48 Rutgers L. Rev. 1193, 1234, 1247 (1996).

Journal 1996 Examines the medical use of marijuana in a legal and ethical context. Posits that legal prohibitions against medical use of marijuana infringe upon patient autonomy and the physician-patient relationship. Concludes that societal laws should be modified to allow for regulated medical use of marijuana. Quotes Opinion 2.17. Comment, *Medical Use of Marijuana: Legal and Ethical Conflicts in the Patient-Physician Relationship*, 30 U. Rich. L. Rev. 249, 268-69 (1996).

Journal 1996 Describes the impact of federal laws on medical decisions for anencephalic infants. Discusses selective nontreatment of such infants and the debate regarding availability of their organs for transplantation. Quotes Opinions 2.162 (1994) [subsequently amended] and 2.17. Crossley, *Infants with Anencephaly, the ADA, and the Child Abuse Amendments*, 11 Issues in Law & Med. 379, 385, 409 (1996).

Journal 1994 Considers how greater patient autonomy has led to situations in which medical care may be viewed as futile. Examines cases in which physicians' medical judgments conflict with requests for medical treatment by patients or families. Suggests that the law has intruded too far into this area of medicine. Quotes Opinion 2.035. Cites Opinions 2.03, 2.095, 2.17, 2.19, 2.20, and 2.22. Cultice, *Medical Futility: When Is Enough, Enough?*, 27 J. Health & Hosp. Law 225, 230, 256 (1994).

Journal 1993 Discusses the problem of physicians withholding needed medical treatment from HIV-infected infants. Explores the medical aspects of infant HIV infection. Considers ethical and legal issues involving nontreatment. Concludes that current law should be expanded to eliminate this discrimination. Quotes Opinions 2.09, 2.17, 2.20, 2.22, 4.04, and 8.03. Crossley, *Of Diagnoses and Discrimination: Discriminatory Nontreatment of Infants With HIV Infection*, 93 Columbia L. Rev. 1581, 1620, 1621 (1993).

Journal 1993 Argues that society should not permit euthanasia because of lack of protection against potential abuses. Recommends that health care providers be taught to treat pain and more effectively care for dying patients, rather than to affirmatively end life. Quotes Opinions 2.17 and 2.20. Dickey, *Euthanasia: A Concept Whose Time Has Come?*, 8 Issues in Law & Med. 521, 523, 524 (1993).

Journal 1992 Examines the medical, ethical, and legal validity of selective nontreatment of severely handicapped newborns. Suggests that triage and cost-benefit analysis are the most effective means to evaluate issues associated with allocating scarce medical resources to disabled infants. Concludes both that selective treatment can never be considered murder and that governmental intrusion in this area should be minimal. Quotes Opinions 2.10 (1982) [now Opinion 2.17] and 2.18 (1986) [now Opinion 2.20]. Smith, *Murder, She Wrote or Was It Merely Selective Nontreatment?*, 8 J. Contemp. Health L. & Pol'y 49, 53 (1992).

Journal 1990 Considers the relation between Do-Not-Resuscitate orders and family preferences. Questions the value of medical treatment that is futile or may prolong suffering. Proposes that physicians be permitted to write DNR orders, in certain cases, without the consent of the family. Quotes Opinion 2.17. Hackler & Hiller, *Family Consent to Orders Not To Resuscitate: Reconsidering Hospital Policy*, 264 J.A.M.A. 1281, 1282 (1990).

Journal 1989 Examines the federal Baby Doe rule, contained in the Child Abuse Prevention and Treatment Act, 42 U.S.C. Secs. 5101-05. This statute, and its implementing regulations, require treatment of disabled infants in all but the most obviously hopeless cases. Discusses the federal requirements in relation to the moral issue of withholding treatment for disabled neonates and possible conflicts between the federal law and state constitutions. Concludes that the rule is insensitive to the complexities of the moral issue, and that state constitutions may prohibit local legislative adoption of the federal requirements. Quotes Opinion 2.14 (1984) [now Opinion

2.17]. Newman, *Baby Doe, Congress and the States: Challenging the Federal Treatment Standard for Impaired Infants*, XV Am. J. Law and Med. 1, 42, 47 (1989).

Journal 1985-86 Discusses the fact that the legal system has granted substantial professional autonomy to physicians. As a result, medical professionals have exerted dominance over individual health care decisions, particularly in the context of infanticide, or withholding of treatment from severely handicapped infants. Concludes that professional authority over health matters has been vastly overextended. Quotes Opinion 2.10 (1982) [now Opinion 2.17]. Malone, *Medical Authority and Infanticide*, 1 J. Law & Health 77, 94, 96 (1985-86).

Journal 1985 Discusses the constitutional rights of newborns with birth defects, noting that they are persons within the meaning of the fourteenth amendment. Observes that the fundamental right to life applies equally to healthy newborns as well as newborns with birth defects and concludes that the newborn's future quality of life with a disability should not be a factor in assessing whether medical treatment is in the child's best interest. Quotes from Opinion 2.10 (1982) [now Opinion 2.17]. Comment, *Withholding Life-saving Treatment From Defective Newborns: An Equal Protection Analysis*, 29 St. Louis Univ. L. J. 853, 854 (1985).

Journal 1982 Views the question of nontreatment of defective neonates from both a legal and moral perspective. From a legal viewpoint, focuses on the effect of abortion decisions on nontreatment issues as well as decisions that directly address the nontreatment issue. Also provides general discussion of the wide range of moral attitudes expressed by physicians on withholding treatment, the meaning of the terms "ordinary" and "extraordinary" care, and the question of who should bear the responsibility for deciding to treat or not to treat defective neonates. Quotes Opinion 2.10 (1981) [now Opinion 2.17]. Taub, *Withholding Treatment From Defective Newborns*, 10 Law, Med. & Health Care 4, 8 (Feb. 1982).

Journal 1981 Discusses a Danville, Illinois case in which the Illinois Department of Children and Family Services successfully opposed the decision of the physician and parents not to feed newborn Siamese twins. Focuses on both moral and legal aspects of nontreatment decisions, and discusses the common, yet controversial nature of decisions not to treat, categorization of birth defects for purposes of moral decision making, the importance of medical and social information in nontreatment decisions, the legal duty to treat such children, and substantive and procedural criteria for nontreatment decisions. Quotes Opinion 2.10 (1981) [now Opinion 2.17]. Robertson, *Dilemma in Danville*, 11 Hastings Center Rep. 5, 7 (Oct. 1981).

2.18   Surrogate Mothers

"Surrogate" motherhood involves the artificial insemination of a woman who agrees, usually in return for payment, to give the resulting child to the child's father by surrendering her parental rights. Often, the father's infertile wife becomes the child's adoptive mother. The woman bearing the child is in most cases genetically related to the child, though gestational surrogacy (in which the ovum is provided by the father's infertile wife or other donor) is possible as well.

Ethical, social, and legal problems may arise in surrogacy arrangements. Surrogate motherhood may commodify children and women's reproductive capacities, exploit poor women whose decision to participate may not be wholly voluntary, and improperly discourage or interfere with the formation of a natural maternal-fetal or maternal-child bond. Psychological impairment may occur in a woman who deliberately conceives with the intention of bearing a child which she will give up. In addition, the woman who has contracted to bear the child may decide to have an abortion or to refuse to relinquish her parental rights. Alternatively, if there is a subsequent birth of a disabled child, prospective parents and the birth mother may not want to or will be unable to assume the responsibilities of parenthood.

On the other hand, surrogate motherhood arrangements are often the last hope of prospective parents to have a child that is genetically related to at least one of them. In addition, most surrogacy arrangements are believed by the parties involved to be mutually beneficial, and most are completed without mishap or dispute. In light of the concerns expressed above, however, some safeguards are necessary to protect the welfare of the child and the birth mother. The Council believes that surrogacy contracts, while permissible, should grant the birth mother the right to void the contract within a reasonable period of time after the birth of the child. If the contract is voided, custody of the child should be determined according to the child's best interests.

In gestational surrogacy, in which the surrogate mother has no genetic tie to the fetus, the justification for allowing the surrogate mother to void the contract becomes less clear. Gestational surrogacy contracts should be strictly enforceable (i.e., not retractable by either party). (I, II, IV)

Issued December 1983.

Updated June 1994.

Journal 1990 Argues that gestational surrogacy, because of its inherent medical, ethical, and legal complications, is not an acceptable reproductive alternative. Discusses the California Superior Court case of *Johnson v. Calvert* in which a gestational surrogacy contract was held valid and the genetic parents were found to have exclusive custody and parental rights. Quotes Opinion 2.18 (1988). Rothenberg, *Gestational Surrogacy and the Health Care Provider: Put Part of the "IVF Genie" Back Into the Bottle, 18 Law, Med. & Health Care 345, 346 (1990).*

Journal 1987 Examines various ethical issues surrounding surrogate motherhood, artificial insemination, in vitro fertilization and embryonic/fetal research. Reports on the positions of four ethics groups: the Warnock Committee of Inquiry into Human Fertilization and Embryology; the American Medical Association's Council on Ethical and Judicial Affairs; the Ethics Committee of the American Fertility Society; and the Ethics Committee of the American College of Obstetricians and Gynecologists. References Opinions 2.04, 2.05, and 2.13 (1986) [now Opinion 2.14]. Quotes Opinion 2.18. Rosner, Cassell, Friedland, Landolt, Loeb, Numann, Ora, Risemberg, & Sordillo, *Ethical Considerations of Reproductive Technologies, 87 N.Y. State J. Med. 398, 399-400 (1987).*

2.19   Unnecessary Services

Physicians should not provide, prescribe, or seek compensation for services that they know are unnecessary. (II, VII)

Issued prior to April 1977.

Updated June 1994 and June 1996.

Journal 1994 Considers how greater patient autonomy has led to situations in which medical care may be viewed as futile. Examines cases in which physicians' medical judgments conflict with requests for medical treatment by patients or families. Suggests that the law has intruded too far into this area of medicine. Quotes Opinion 2.035. Cites Opinions 2.03, 2.095, 2.17, 2.19, 2.20, and 2.22. Cultice, *Medical Futility: When Is Enough, Enough?, 27 J. Health & Hosp. Law 225, 230, 256 (1994).*

Journal 1991 Discusses conflict of interest problems that sometimes arise in the doctor-patient relationship. Explores the impact of *Moore v. Regents of the University of California.* Looks at the physician as a fiduciary and the law governing fiduciary relationships. Concludes that fiduciary concepts are a valuable basis for establishing ethical and legal guidelines for physician behavior.

Quotes Opinions 2.19, 8.03 (1989) [now Opinion 8.032], and 8.06. Healey & Dowling, *Controlling Conflicts of Interest in the Doctor-Patient Relationship: Lessons From Moore v. Regents of the University of California*, 42 Mercer L. Rev. 989, 997, 998 (1991).

Journal 1991 Examines the issues surrounding judicial use of professional ethics codes in private litigation. Explores the history and major characteristics of the "professions." Explains how courts currently apply codes of ethics. Concludes that judges should more extensively use professional ethics codes to define public policy, standards of care, and legal causes of action. Quotes Principle II and Opinion 2.19. Note, *Professional Ethics Codes in Court: Redefining the Social Contract Between the Public and the Professions*, 25 Georgia L. Rev. 1327, 1335, 1351 (1991).

Journal 1990 Discusses efforts of third party payers to control health care expenditures for beneficiaries. Focuses on use of financial incentives to encourage providers to minimize the amount of care provided. Also discusses monitoring of requests for payment to determine necessity of care provided. Raises questions regarding impact of cost control mechanisms on quality of care, observing that available evidence is equivocal. Evaluates importance of disclosure to beneficiaries of use of financial incentives to limit care as well as other cost control mechanisms. Concludes that financial incentives and other cost control techniques should be disclosed and that the rationale for such disclosure is compelling. Quotes Opinions 2.03, 2.09, and 8.03. Cites Opinions 2.19, 4.04, and 4.06. Hirshfeld, *Should Third Party Payers of Health Care Services Disclose Cost Control Mechanisms to Potential Beneficiaries?*, 14 Seton Hall Legis. J. 115, 130, 131, 144, 145, 146 (1990).

Journal 1986 Discusses the Missouri living will statute and the Death-Prolonging Procedures Act. Examines the extent to which these laws ensure individuals the right to make choices regarding personal medical treatment in the event of terminal illness, even if they become incompetent. Also evaluates the protections afforded to physicians who comply with patient directives. Quotes Opinion 2.12 (1981) [now Opinion 2.19]. Johnson, *The Death-Prolonging Procedures Act and Refusal of Treatment in Missouri*, 30 St. Louis Univ. L. J. 805, 816 (1986).

2.20 Withholding or Withdrawing Life-sustaining Medical Treatment.

The social commitment of the physician is to sustain life and relieve suffering. Where the performance of one duty conflicts with the other, the preferences of the patient should prevail. The principle of patient autonomy requires that physicians respect the decision to forego life-sustaining treatment of a patient who possesses decision-making capacity. Life-sustaining treatment is any treatment that serves to prolong life without reversing the underlying medical condition. Life-sustaining treatment may include, but is not limited to, mechanical ventilation, renal dialysis, chemotherapy, antibiotics, and artificial nutrition and hydration.

There is no ethical distinction between withdrawing and withholding life-sustaining treatment.

A competent, adult patient may, in advance, formulate and provide a valid consent to the withholding or withdrawal of life-support systems in the event that injury or illness renders that individual incompetent to make such a decision. A patient may also appoint a surrogate decision maker in accordance with state law.

If the patient receiving life-sustaining treatment is incompetent, a surrogate decision maker should be identified. Without an advance directive that designates a proxy, the patient's family should become the surrogate decision maker. Family includes persons with whom the patient is closely associated. In the case when there is no person closely associated with the patient, but there are persons who both care about the patient and have sufficient relevant knowledge of the patient, such persons may be appropriate surrogates. Physicians should provide all relevant medical information and explain to surrogate decision makers that decisions regarding withholding or withdrawing life-sustaining treatment should be based on substituted judgment (what the patient would have decided) when there is evidence of the patient's preferences and values. In making a substituted judgment, decision makers may consider the patient's advance directive (if any); the patient's values about life and the way it should be lived; and the patient's attitudes towards sickness, suffering, medical procedures, and death. If there is not adequate evidence of the incompetent patient's preferences and values, the decision should be based on the best interests of the patient (what outcome would most likely promote the patient's well-being).

Though the surrogate's decision for the incompetent patient should almost always be accepted by the physician, there are four situations that may require either institutional or judicial review and/or intervention in the decision-making process: (a) there is no available family member willing to be the patient's surrogate decision maker, (b) there is a dispute among family members and there is no decision maker designated in an advance directive, (c) a health care provider believes that the family's decision is clearly not what the patient would have decided if competent, and (d) a health care provider believes that the decision is not a decision that could reasonably be judged to be in the patient's best interests. When there are disputes among family members or between family and health care providers, the use of ethics committees specifically designed to facilitate sound decision making is recommended before resorting to the courts.

When a permanently unconscious patient was never competent or had not left any evidence of previous preferences or values, since there is no objective way to ascertain the best interests of the patient, the surrogate's decision should not be challenged as long as the decision is based on the decision maker's true concern for what would be best for the patient.

Physicians have an obligation to relieve pain and suffering and to promote the dignity and autonomy of dying patients in their care. This includes providing effective palliative treatment even though it may foreseeably hasten death.

Even if the patient is not terminally ill or permanently unconscious, it is not unethical to discontinue all means of life-sustaining medical treatment in accordance with a proper substituted judgment or best interests analysis. (I, III, IV, V)

Issued March 1981 (former Opinion 2.11, "Terminal Illness") and December 1984 (former Opinion 2.21, "Withholding or Withdrawing Life-Prolonging Medical Treatment: Patient's Preferences").

Updated June 1994 based on the reports, "Decisions Near the End of Life" (JAMA. 1992; 267: 2229-2233) and "Decisions to Forgo Life-Sustaining Treatment for Incompetent Patients," both adopted June 1991, and updated June 1996.

[In March 1986, the Council on Ethical and Judicial Affairs adopted its policy statement, "Withholding or Withdrawing Life-Prolonging Medical Treatment." This statement was later included as Opinion 2.18 (1986), now Opinion 2.20. Numerous cases cited here simply note the March, 1986 statement, without specific reference to the Opinions.]

U.S. 1997 Several physicians and terminally ill patients sued the state seeking a declaration that its prohibition against physician-assisted suicide violates the Fourteenth Amendment's Equal Protection Clause. The trial court disagreed, but the Second Circuit reversed, holding that the state accords different treatment to those terminally ill patients who wish to hasten their death by self-administering prescribed drugs and to those patients who wish to do so by directing the removal of life support systems. The Supreme Court reversed holding that the prohibition against assisting suicide does not violate the Equal Protection Clause. The Court concluded that there is a distinction between assisting suicide and withdrawing treatment quoting reports of the AMA Council on Ethical and Judicial Affairs [now Opinions 2.20 and 2.211]. *Vacco v. Quill, 117 S. Ct. 2293, 2298, 138 L. Ed. 2d 834.*

U.S. 1990 Parents of patient in persistent vegetative state appealed denial of request to discontinue gastrotomy feeding tube. The Supreme Court held that the federal constitution did not forbid the state's requirement of clear and convincing evidence of an incompetent patient's wishes regarding the withdrawal of life-prolonging treatment. The Court acknowledged that a competent person has a liberty interest under the Due Process clause in refusing unwanted medical care; however, the Court assumed the existence of a constitutionally protected right to refuse artificial hydration and nutrition only for purposes of the case. In a concurring opinion, Justice O'Connor cited Opinion 2.20 for the proposition that artificial feeding cannot be distinguished from other forms of medical treatment. In his dissent, Justice Brennan likewise cited Opinion 2.20 for this point. *Cruzan v. Director, Missouri Department of Health, 497 U.S. 261.*

9th Cir. 1996 Suit was brought by several physicians and not-for-profit corporation which provides information, assistance, and counseling to competent terminally ill adult patients contemplating suicide, asserting that a state statute making it a crime to aid anyone in attempting to commit suicide unconstitutionally prevents terminally ill patients from exercising their protected liberty interests. Appeals court, en banc, held that the choice of how and when to die is a liberty interest and that the statute violates the due process rights of competent, terminally ill adults who wish to hasten their deaths by obtaining medication prescribed by their physicians. Stating that physician-assisted suicide runs counter to medical ethics, the dissent cited Opinions 2.20, 2.21, and 2.211 and quoted Opinion 2.211. *Compassion in Dying v. Washington, 79 F.3d 790, 840, 855, replacing 49 F.3d 586 (9th Cir. 1995).*

Ariz. 1987 Guardian of nursing home patient in persistent vegetative state sought removal of nasogastric tube and retention of "Do Not Resuscitate" and "Do Not Hospitalize" orders. Patient had not communicated desires regarding life-sustaining procedures while competent. In assessing whether safeguarding the integrity of the medical profession might be a state interest that outweighed the patient's right to refuse medical treatment, the court noted Opinion 2.18 (1986) [now Opinion 2.20] to support the view that the medical profession itself now recognizes that it is no longer obligated to provide medical treatment in all situations. Since the Opinion would allow the disputed orders for a patient suffering from an irreversible coma, the court concluded that the same action would be allowed in a case of irreversible chronic vegetative state and thus concluded that the case did not bring into disrepute the ethical integrity of the medical profession. *Rasmussen v. Fleming, 154 Ariz. 207, 741 P.2d 674, 684, 685.*

Ariz. App. 1986 Guardian of nursing home patient in persistent vegetative state sought removal of nasal gastric tube and retention of "Do Not Resuscitate" and "Do Not Hospitalize" orders. Patient had not communicated her desires regarding life-sustaining procedures while competent. The court quoted Opinion 2.18 (1986) [now Opinion 2.20] in holding that competing state interests, including the ethical integrity of the medical profession, did not outweigh patient's constitutional right to privacy and held that rights of incompetent patient could be asserted vicariously. *Rasmussen v. Fleming, 154 Ariz. 200, 741 P.2d 667, 671, 672, 673 n.4, aff'd in part and rev'd in part, 154 Ariz. 207, 741 P.2d 674 (1987).*

Cal. App. 1988 Conservator sought an injunction requiring physician to remove nasogastric feeding tube from a patient who was in a persistent vegetative state. The court held that while a conservator may authorize withdrawal or withholding of medical treatment, he may not force a physician to do so against the physician's personal moral objections if the patient can be transferred to the care of a physician who will follow the directive. Citing Opinion 2.18 (1986) [now Opinion 2.20], the court noted that the physician's compliance with the conservator's decision would not have violated the ethical code of the medical profession. *Morrison v. Abramovice, 206 Cal. App. 3d 304, 309, 253 Cal. Rptr. 530, 533.*

Cal. App. 1988 Conservator of patient in persistent vegetative state sought permission for removal of nasogastric feeding tube claiming such relief would serve the patient's best interests.

Patient had expressed a desire never to be kept alive through artificial means. The court held that a conservator is authorized to order that artificial life support be withdrawn after considering medical advice and the patient's best interests. In so holding, the court quoted Opinion 2.18 (1986) [now Opinion 2.20] showing support within the medical community for its analysis. *In re Drabick, 200 Cal. App. 3d 185, 245 Cal. Rptr. 840, 845 n.8.*

Cal. App. 1986 Mentally competent, physically debilitated patient sought authorization to discontinue forced feedings through nasogastric tube. Patient had dictated instructions to her lawyers and signed them with an "x" by means of a pen held in her mouth. In holding that a competent adult patient has the legal right to refuse medical treatment even though such refusal will hasten her death, the court quoted Opinion 2.18 (1986) [now Opinion 2.20]. *Bouvia v. Superior Court, 179 Cal. App. 3d 1127, 225 Cal. Rptr. 297, 303-04.*

Conn. 1989 Family of comatose, terminal patient in nursing home sought injunction to discontinue life support services. In holding that removal of a gastrostomy tube was authorized by statute and no compelling state interests outweighed the patient's rights, the court cited Opinion 2.18 (1986) [now Opinion 2.20] for its view that the provision of nutrition and hydration is a form of life-prolonging "medical treatment." *McConnell v. Beverly Enterprises-Connecticut, Inc., 209 Conn. 692, 553 A.2d 596, 603 n.13.*

Fla. App. 1986 Husband of terminally ill patient in persistent vegetative state sought declaratory judgment to permit removal of nasogastric feeding tube. In recognizing a right to allow the natural consequence of removal of artificial life sustaining measures, the court quoted Opinion 2.18 (1986) [now Opinion 2.20]. *Corbett v. D'Alessandro, 487 So. 2d 368, 371 n.1.*

Ill. 1989 Daughter of permanently unconscious patient petitioned to withdraw life-prolonging gastrotomy feeding tube. The court cited with approval Opinion 2.18 (1986) [now Opinion 2.20] that the American Medical Association considers artificial hydration and nutrition to be medical treatments which may be withdrawn under certain circumstances. The court based the right to refuse life-prolonging procedures upon the state's common law of informed consent, probate law, and power of attorney for health care statute. The court established guidelines for a guardian's exercise of this right. The patient must be terminally ill, in a persistent vegetative state, and the guardian must exercise the substituted judgment of the patient as shown through clear and convincing evidence in a judicial proceeding. *In re Longeway, 133 Ill. 2d 33, 549 N.E.2d 292, 295-96.*

Ill. App. 1988 Guardian of patient in persistent vegetative state petitioned to withdraw artificial feeding tube. Prior to her incompetence, the patient had stated in writing and in conversations with friends that she desired no artificial means of treatment if there was no hope for her recovery, and had completed a living will form, but had failed to obtain the requisite number of witness signatures. The trial court dismissed the case upon the patient's death. On appeal, the court held that the guardian, using the doctrine of substituted judgment, could consent to the removal of a feeding tube from a patient in a persistent vegetative state. In so holding, the court quoted Opinion 2.18 [now Opinion 2.20], noting that it was within a physician's ethical parameters to discontinue such treatment. *In re Prange, 166 Ill. App. 3d 1091, 520 N.E.2d 946, vacated, 121 Ill. 2d 570, 527 N.E.2d 303 (1988).*

Ind. 1991 State statute provided procedures by which parents of an incompetent patient, in consultation with the patient's physician, could withhold or withdraw life-prolonging medical treatment. The court held that barring any challenge from the treating physician or interested parties, the family could make these decisions without a court proceeding. Quoting Opinion 2.20 (1989), the court concluded that medical treatment includes artificial nutrition and hydration. *In re Lawrance, 579 N.E.2d 32, 40.*

Ky. 1993 In a declaratory judgment action, the court was asked to allow a surrogate to exercise the right to withdraw life-prolonging treatment for a patient who had orally expressed her wishes not to be sustained artificially. Since common law recognizes a patient's right to withdraw or withhold medical treatment, the court held that a surrogate could rely on the patient's statement of choice made before patient became incompetent to exercise "substituted judgment." The court quoted from guidelines for state courts deciding life-sustaining medical treatment cases issued by the National Center for State Courts. Citing Opinion 2.20 and other sources, the Guidelines stated that a consensus had already been reached on the primary ethical issues relating to life-prolonging treatment. *DeGrella v. Elston, 858 S.W.2d 698, 707 n.5.*

Me. 1987 Guardian sought to have nasogastric feeding tube withdrawn from patient in persistent vegetative state. Investigation by a state agency corroborated evidence of patient's prior statements that he desired no life-sustaining procedures if in a persistent vegetative state. The court noted that under state's common law an individual has a personal right to refuse medical treatment, including life-sustaining procedures. The court held that where the patient had clearly and convincingly expressed his desire not to be maintained by life-sustaining procedures if in a persistent vegetative state, health professionals had a duty to respect that decision. The court cited Opinion 2.18 (1986) [now Opinion 2.20] for the concept that artificial hydration and nutrition should be equated with other life-sustaining treatments in delineating the patient's right to reject such treatment. *In re Gardner, 534 A.2d 947, 954.*

Md. Att'y Gen. 1988 Attorney general was asked whether persons with capacity to decide about medical care have a right to instruct that artificially administered sustenance not be provided if they become terminally ill or permanently comatose. An opinion was also requested regarding decision making for incompetent persons who have given no prior instructions about artificial feeding. In response, Opinion 2.18 (1986) [now Opinion 2.20] is cited to support the view that no distinction should be drawn between artificial feeding and other forms of life-prolonging treatment. Further, in delineating procedures for deciding to forego treatment for an incompetent, terminally ill patient who has given no prior instructions, Opinion 2.18 (1986) [now Opinion 2.20] is also cited in terms of the physician's role in advising whether withdrawal is medically proper. Finally, while disallowing family members, without court approval, to terminate tube feeding for a nonterminal, permanently comatose patient, it is recognized that under this Opinion it is not unethical to discontinue life-sustaining treatment for such a patient. *Maryland Att'y Gen. Op. No. 88-046, 73 Op. Att'y Gen. 162.*

Mass. 1992 Request of parents of a patient in a persistent vegetative state to employ "substituted judgment" in order to withdraw medical treatment was granted. Citing Opinion 2.18 (1986) [now Opinion 2.20], the court noted that medical treatment includes artificial hydration and nutrition. *In re Doe, 411 Mass. 512, 517 n.11, 583 N.E.2d 1263, 1267 n.11.*

Mass. 1986 Guardian of patient in persistent vegetative state who, according to trial court, would have declined food and water, sued for declaratory judgment requesting authority to have artificial hydration and nutrition discontinued. The court held that while the hospital had a right to refuse to participate in the removal of the gastrostomy tube, the guardian was authorized to transfer the patient to other physicians who would honor the guardian's request. The court cited Opinion 2.18 (1986) [now Opinion 2.20] in finding that the patient's right to refuse medical treatment did not violate the state's interest in the maintenance of the ethical integrity of the medical profession as long as the hospital was not forced to participate in the removal or clamping of the gastronomy tube. *Brophy v. New England Sinai Hosp., Inc., 398 Mass. 417, 497 N.E.2d 626, 638-39 n.38.*

Mo. 1988 Parents-guardians of a nonterminal patient in a persistent vegetative state sought a declaratory judgment after a state hospital refused to terminate artificial hydration and nutrition. The court found that the patient's burden in being fed through gastronomy tube did not outweigh the state's interest in preserving life and that guardians could not order withdrawal of hydration and nutrition. The court, in refusing to classify artificial hydration and nutrition as medical treatment, rejected Opinion 2.18 (1986) [now Opinion 2.20] which expresses a contrary view. *Cruzan v. Harmon, 760 S.W.2d 408, 423 n.18, aff'd, 497 U.S. 261.*

N.J. 1987 Husband applied to court for authorization to discontinue wife's hydration and nutrition after nursing home refused his request to do so. The court held that the right of a patient in an irreversible vegetative state to refuse life-sustaining procedures may be exercised by the patient's family or close friend after two independent neurologists have confirmed the diagnosis and prognosis. The court further stated that the processes of surrogate decision-making should be substantially the same regardless of type of medical facility. In so holding, the court cited Opinion 2.18 (1986) [now Opinion 2.20] with approval. *In re Jobes, 108 N.J. 394, 529 A.2d 434, 446.*

N.J. 1987 Elderly nursing home patient was comatose in a persistent vegetative state. Patient's designee, under power of attorney for health care decisions, sought appointment as guardian and authorization for removal of patient's artificial nutrition and hydration. The court held that where there is clear and convincing proof that patient would refuse such treatment if competent, a surrogate may effect that decision regardless of the patient's life expectancy. The court quoted with approval Opinion 2.18 (1986) [now Opinion 2.20] stating that artificial hydration and nutrition is a form of medical treatment. *In re Peter, 108 N.J. 365, 529 A.2d 419, 427-28.*

N.J. 1987 Husband of competent, terminally ill patient applied to be special medical guardian to effectuate patient's desire to remove respirator. In holding that the right of a competent, terminally ill patient to decline medical treatment outweighed the state's interests in preserving life, preventing suicide, protecting innocent third parties, and safeguarding the integrity of the medical profession, the court cited as reflective of the views of the medical profession the Judicial Council's report at 253 J.A.M.A. 2424 (1985) [now Opinion 2.20]. *In re Farrell, 108 N.J. 335, 529 A.2d 404, 412.*

N.J. Super. 1983 Guardian of elderly nursing home patient suffering from severe organic brain syndrome sought to remove nasogastric tube from patient. Trial court granted guardian's petition, and patient's guardian ad litem appealed. Appellate court reversed, in part based upon Opinions 2.11 (1981) and 5.17 (1979) [now Opinions 2.17 and 2.20], and held that it is improper and would violate medical ethics to allow dehydration and starvation in a "non-comatose, non-brain-dead patient not facing imminent death, not maintained by any life-support machine, and not able to speak for herself." *In re Conroy, 190 N.J. Super. 453, 464 A.2d 303, 313-15, rev'd, 98 N.J. 321, 486 A.2d 1209 (1985).*

N.Y. 1990 Jehovah's Witness was given blood transfusion against her express wishes. The court held that the lower court erred in ordering the transfusions without giving the patient or her family notice and a hearing. Barring any superior interest of the state, the patient had a right to determine the course of her own treatment. Concurring opinion argued that the majority rule created an absolute right to refuse treatment. Quoting from Opinion 2.21 (1989) [now Opinion 2.20], the concurring opinion held that a physician had a corresponding ethical duty to render treatment which, in his judgment, benefits the patient. Note that Opinion 2.20 does not retain the specific language of former Opinion 2.21 relied on by concurring judge. *Fosmire v. Nicoleau, 75 N.Y.2d 218, 236 n.2, 551 N.E.2d 77, 87 n.2, 551 N.Y.S.2d 876, 886 n.2.*

N.Y. Sup. 1986 Plaintiff petitioned for judicial authorization to remove feeding tube from her 33-year-old husband, a patient in a permanent chronic vegetative state. In denying the petition, the court noted the American Medical Association's position set out in 245 JAMA 819 (1981), later included as Opinion 2.11 (1981) [now Opinion 2.20] that, in such cases, members of the family and physicians should decide whether to continue treatment. However, the court concluded that the legislature must resolve the issue and denied the petition. *Delio v. Westchester County Medical Center, 134 Misc. 2d 206, 510 N.Y.S.2d 415, 419, rev'd, 129 A.D. 2d 1, 516 N.Y.S. 2d 677 (1987).*

Ohio App. 1989 The divorced parents of a patient in a persistent vegetative state each petitioned to be appointed guardian of their son. The mother was initially appointed guardian and testified that it would be in the best interests of her son, and consistent with his wishes, to terminate nutrition and hydration. Over the father's objections, the probate court granted the mother, as guardian, the right to make decisions regarding her son's treatment and care. On appeal, the appellate court modified the lower court's order, pursuant to a state statute enacted after that order was entered. Although recognizing that the lower court's decision was consistent with the position of the American Medical Association as articulated in Opinion 2.20, the appellate court held that to allow termination of nutrition and hydration in this case would violate the public policy as expressed in recent legislation. *Couture v. Couture, 48 Ohio App. 3d 208, 549 N.E.2d 571, 574.*

Pa. Super. 1995 Parent of nursing home patient in persistent vegetative state sought removal of gastrostomy tube. Nursing home refused to comply with request without court order. Trial court, applying best interests test, authorized removal of tube. On appeal, court held that consent of close family member, with approval of two qualified physicians, is sufficient without court order to terminate life sustaining treatment for patient in a long-term persistent vegetative state. Court referred to In re Grant, 109 Wash. 2d 545, 747 P.2d 445 (1987) citing Opinion 2.18 [now Opinion 2.20] for proposition that medical ethical principles permit withdrawal of nutrition and hydration for patient in persistent vegetative state. *In re Fiori, 438 Pa. Super. 610, 652 A.2d 1350, 1354, app. granted, 655 A.2d 989 (Pa. 1995).*

Phila. Co. 1987 In a declaratory judgment action, the court held that a patient has a right to withhold or withdraw medical treatment. This right is subject to the state's interest in (1) the preservation of life, (2) protection of innocent third parties, (3) prevention of suicide, and (4) protecting the ethical integrity of the medical profession. The court held that the withholding or withdrawal of life support by a physician or hospital or their agents did not constitute a criminal act or give rise to any civil liability. Citing Opinion 2.18 (1986) [now Opinion 2.20]), the court noted that respect for a patient's autonomy and decision to withdraw life support was consistent with medical ethics. *In re Doe, 16 Phila. 229, 1987 Phila. Cty. Rptr. LEXIS 30 (1987).*

Va. Att'y Gen. 1990 Attorney general answered in the affirmative when asked whether a competent adult could create a document authorizing a surrogate to consent to the withholding or withdrawal of medical treatment if the person later enters a persistent vegetative state but is not terminally ill. Quoting Opinion 2.18 (1986) [now Opinion 2.20], the Attorney General concluded that medical treatment includes artificial hydration and nutrition. *Va. Att'y Gen. Op., 1990 Va. AG LEXIS 63.*

Wash. 1987 Court authorization sought by guardian to withhold mechanical or artificial life-sustaining procedures from incompetent patient with terminal disorder. Trial court denied request as premature because patient was not yet comatose or vegetative, and did not yet need intrusive medical procedures. Supreme court held that an incompetent patient in an advanced stage of a terminal illness has right to have life-sustaining treatment withheld, a right which stems from the constitutional right of privacy and the common law right to be free of bodily invasion. Court quoted Opinion 2.18 (1986) [now Opinion 2.20] in support of the right of a terminally ill, noncomatose patient to have life-sustaining procedures withheld including the right to withhold artificial means of nutrition and hydration. *In re Grant, 109 Wash. 2d 545, 747 P.2d 445, 450, 454.*

Wis. 1992 Guardian may consent to the withholding or withdrawal of life-prolonging medical treatment on behalf of an incompetent patient and/or a patient for whom the guardian cannot reasonably make a "substituted judgment" where (1) the patient is in a persistent vegetative state with no reasonable chance of recovery, and (2) the guardian in good faith determines that it is in the patient's "best interest." The court referred to the concurring opinion in Cruzan v. Director, Missouri Dept. of Health, 497 U.S. 261 (1990) which quoted Opinion 2.20 (1989) in holding that medical treatment includes nutrition and hydration. Further, citing Opinion 2.18 (1986) [now Opinion 2.20], the court found the actions here consistent with current medical ethics. Thus, the state's interest in protecting the integrity of the medical profession was not implicated. *L.W. v. L.E. Phillips Career Dev. Ctr., 167 Wis. 2d 53, 71, 72, 91, 482 N.W.2d 60, 66, 74.*

Journal 1997 Reviews the criminalization of physician-assisted suicide. Discusses informed consent, the "double effect," and the right to die. Explains the current state of the law and the position Illinois has taken. Advocates the adoption of a law authorizing physician-assisted suicide in Illinois. References Opinion 2.20. Comment, *An Illinois Physician-Assisted Suicide Act: A Merciful End to a Terminally Ill Criminal Tradition, 28 Loy. U. Chi. L. J. 763, 775 (1997).*

Journal 1997 Discusses Pennsylvania Supreme Court case of *In Re Fiori.* Explains that the court extended the right to refuse medical treatment to patients in permanent vegetative states. Notes that the court now allows family members to exercise this right on behalf of such patients. Quotes Opinion 2.20. Comment, *Surrogate Health Care Decision Making: The Pennsylvania Supreme Court Recognizes the Right of an Individual in a Permanent Vegetative State to Refuse Life-Sustaining Measures through a Surrogate Decision Maker, 35 Duq. L. Rev. 849, 859-60 (1997).*

Journal 1997 Discusses goals of care included in advance directives and whether they can be used to predict specific interventions and results. Offers insights provided by survey of physicians at Massachusetts General Hospital. Cites Opinions 2.20 and 2.21. Fischer, Alpert, Stoeckle, & Emanuel, *Can Goals of Care Be Used to Predict Intervention Preferences in an Advance Directive?, 157 Arch. Intern. Med. 801, 807 (1997).*

Journal 1997 Examines the evolution of the Indiana health care system. Discusses developments in Indiana jurisprudence regarding the physician-patient relationship. Explores various challenges facing the relationship and recognizes the need for legal rules to help address these challenges. Quotes Opinion 8.08. Cites Opinions 2.20, 9.06, and 9.12. Kinney & Selby, *History and Jurisprudence of the Physician-Patient Relationship in Indiana, 30 Ind. L. Rev. 263, 269, 272, 276 (1997).*

Journal 1996 Proposes a model state statute allowing and controlling physician-assisted suicide. Analyzes the constitutionality of the act and offers public policy justifications for the act's provisions. Concludes that proponents of physician-assisted suicide should provide precise, carefully tailored examples of regulations. Quotes Opinion 2.211. Cites Opinion 2.20. Baron, Bergstresser, Brock, Cole, Dorfman, Johnson, Schnipper, Vorenberg, & Wanzer, *A Model State Act to Authorize and Regulate Physician-Assisted Suicide, 33 Harv. J. on Legis. 1, 2, 7 (1996).*

Journal 1996 Explores the issue of legalizing physician-assisted suicide. Opines that the current state of technology increases life expectancy but with a concomitant decrease in dignity and autonomy surrounding one's death. Notes that the elderly are committing suicide at an increasing rate. Cites Opinions 2.20, 2.21, and 2.211. Morgan & Sutherland, *Last Rights? Confronting Physician-Assisted Suicide in Law and Society: Legal Liturgies on Physician-Assisted Suicide, 26 Stetson L. Rev. 481, 484 (1996).*

Journal 1996 Considers the right to death with dignity. Suggests that the AMA's position undermines mitigation of suffering and the individuals' right to self-determination. Concludes that restrictions on the right to death with dignity may be constitutionally impermissible. Quotes Opinion 2.211. Cites Opinion 2.20. Note, *Who Decides if There is "Triumph in the Ultimate Agony?" Constitutional Theory and the Emerging Right to Die With Dignity*, 37 Wm. & Mary L. Rev. 827, 829 (1996).

Journal 1996 Discusses the physician's duty to relieve pain. Considers current attitudes toward pain management. Concludes that, consistent with principles of beneficence, physicians are obligated to provide pain relief and palliation. Quotes Opinion 2.20. Post, Blustein, Gordon, & Dubler, *Pain: Ethics, Culture, and Informed Consent to Relief*, 24 J. Law, Med. & Ethics 348, 349, 356 (1996).

Journal 1996 Discusses children's rights to consent to or refuse life-sustaining medical treatment. Compares the rights of children to those of adults in a medical decision-making context. Proposes reforms to allow minors legal rights to make decisions regarding withdrawal of life-sustaining treatment. Quotes Opinion 2.20. Rosato, *The Ultimate Test of Autonomy: Should Minors Have a Right to Make Decisions Regarding Life-Sustaining Treatment?*, 49 Rutgers L. Rev. 1, 80-81, 82 (1996).

Journal 1995 Explores reluctance of long-term care facilities to allow patients to forgo life-sustaining tube feeding. Suggests that this reluctance cannot be supported by existing case law or statute. Concludes that policies must be adopted to ensure that patients' rights to refuse artificial nutrition and hydration are protected. Cites Opinion 2.20. Meisel, *Barriers to Forgoing Nutrition and Hydration in Nursing Homes*, XXI Am. J. Law & Med. 335, 353-54 (1995).

Journal 1995 Examines the problem of determining when a patient has lost decision-making capacity. Compares the authority of the treating physician with that of the patient's designated agent in making such a determination. Offers suggestions for resolving potential conflicts. Cites Opinion 2.20. Schneiderman, Teetzel, & Kalmanson, *Who Decides Who Decides? When Disagreement Occurs Between the Physician and the Patient's Appointed Proxy About the Patient's Decision-Making Capacity*, 155 Arch. Intern. Med. 793, 796 (1995).

Journal 1995 Provides legal and medical definitions of physician-assisted suicide and euthanasia. Offers relevant historical perspectives and provides comprehensive ethical and legal discussion of these compelling social issues. Highlights important legislative developments, including the Oregon Death with Dignity Act, and analyzes significant judicial opinions. Advocates legal tolerance of physician-assisted suicide and euthanasia. Quotes Principles III, IV, and VI and Opinions 2.21 and 9.12. Cites Opinions 2.20 and 8.11. Stone & Winslade, *Physician-Assisted Suicide and Euthanasia in the United States: Legal and Ethical Observations*, 16 J. Legal Med. 481, 483, 490, 497, 498, 499 (1995).

Journal 1994 Considers how greater patient autonomy has led to situations in which medical care may be viewed as futile. Examines cases in which physicians' medical judgments conflict with requests for medical treatment by patients or families. Suggests that the law has intruded too far into this area of medicine. Quotes Opinion 2.035. Cites Opinions 2.03, 2.095, 2.17, 2.19, 2.20, and 2.22. Cultice, *Medical Futility: When Is Enough, Enough?*, 27 J. Health & Hosp. Law 225, 230, 256 (1994).

Journal 1994 Discusses whether a patient's prior expression of treatment choices in an advance directive accurately represents future choices. Concludes that patients are capable of making stable scenario- and treatment-specific advance directives, that their choices become more stable with repeat consideration, and that illness has little effect on stability of choices. Suggests that periodic review of directives and discussion with physicians may improve stability. Cites Opinion 2.20. Emanuel, Emanuel, Stoeckle, Hummel, & Barry, *Advance Directives: Stability of Patients' Treatment Choices*, 154 Arch. Intern. Med. 209, 217 (1994).

Journal 1994 Analyzes physicians' attitudes about whether to initiate or withhold tube feeding when patients' preferences are unknown. Recognizes that some physicians consider tube feeding to be basic humane care, not medical therapy. Concludes that patient prognosis and quality of life are the most important influences on physician decisions about tube feeding. Cites Opinion 2.20. Hodges, Tolle, Stocking, & Cassel, *Tube Feeding: Internists' Attitudes Regarding Ethical Obligations*, 154 Arch. Intern. Med. 1013, 1020 (1994).

Journal 1994 Examines the various types of advance health care directives and reviews pertinent Arkansas law. Provides a model directive and guidelines for preparing an advance directive.

Concludes that directives should conform to each person's values, health status, and medical prognosis. Cites Opinion 2.20. Leflar, *Advance Health Care Directives Under Arkansas Law*, 1994 *Ark. L. Notes 37, 42.*

Journal 1994 Examines how state laws have accommodated medical developments in the area of treatment decisions and how they serve to resolve and encourage conflict in health care decision making. Considers the roles of physicians, hospitals, and families and how their wishes may conflict with those of the patient. Proposes solutions for preventing disagreeable legal and ethical conflicts. Cites Opinion 2.20. Tarantino, *Withdrawal of Life Support: Conflict Among Patient Wishes, Family, Physicians, Courts and Statutes, and the Law, 42 Buff. L. Rev. 623, 638, 639, 646 (1994).*

Journal 1994 Examines the assertion that advance directives enhance physician-patient communications about end-of-life medical treatment. Determines that physicians are not taking the responsibility for initiating such discussions and that many patients falsely assume that their physicians would know what kind of treatments they would want. Concludes that physician-patient communication is improved slightly when there is an advance directive, but that there is still a lack of detailed discussion about end-of-life treatments. Cites Opinion 2.20. Virmani, Schneiderman, & Kaplan, *Relationship of Advance Directives to Physician-Patient Communication, 154 Arch. Intern. Med. 909, 913 (1994).*

Journal 1993 Examines the legal, medical, and ethical issues involved when a patient or a patient's family demands treatment that the physician believes would be futile. Analyzes the implications of giving patients an absolute right to control medical treatment. Argues that courts should refrain from ordering physicians to treat patients when physicians believe that treatment would be ineffective. Quotes Fundamental Elements (5) and Opinions 2.11 (1982) [now Opinion 2.20] and 2.18 (1986) [now Opinion 2.20]. Comment, *Beyond Autonomy: Judicial Restraint and the Legal Limits Necessary to Uphold the Hippocratic Tradition and Preserve the Ethical Integrity of the Medical Profession, 9 J. Contemp. Health L. & Pol'y 451, 467, 468 (1993).*

Journal 1993 Discusses Ohio's living will statute in light of the *Cruzan* decision. Presents the medical implications of the persistent vegetative state patient. Discusses the *Cruzan* decision and relevant constitutional guarantees. Considers whether the Ohio statute is constitutional in light of *Cruzan*. Examines the practical implications of the Ohio statute. Quotes Opinion 2.18 (1986) [now Opinion 2.20]. Comment, *One Step Forward, Two Steps Back: A Constitutional and Critical Look at Ohio's New Living Will Statute, 54 Ohio St. L. J. 445, 447, 460, 470 (1993).*

Journal 1993 Discusses the problem of physicians withholding needed medical treatment from HIV-infected infants. Explores the medical aspects of infant HIV infection. Considers ethical and legal issues involving nontreatment. Concludes that current law should be expanded to eliminate this discrimination. Quotes Opinions 2.09, 2.17, 2.20, 2.22, 4.04, and 8.03. Crossley, *Of Diagnoses and Discrimination: Discriminatory Nontreatment of Infants With HIV Infection, 93 Columbia L. Rev. 1581, 1620, 1621 (1993).*

Journal 1993 Discusses the relationship between a physician's professional conscience and end of life decision making. Considers the issue of futile medical treatment—and a physician's responsibility to provide such treatment. Examines case law concerning a patient's right to demand treatment and a physician's obligation to provide it. Proposes a model for resolving physician-patient conflicts in this context. References Opinions 2.20 and 2.22. Daar, *A Clash at the Bedside: Patient Autonomy v. A Physician's Professional Conscience, 44 Hastings L. J. 1241, 1257, 1268, 1286 (1993).*

Journal 1993 Argues that society should not permit euthanasia because of lack of protection against potential abuses. Recommends that health care providers be taught to treat pain and more effectively care for dying patients, rather than to affirmatively end life. Quotes Opinions 2.17 and 2.20. Dickey, *Euthanasia: A Concept Whose Time Has Come?, 8 Issues in Law & Med. 521, 523, 524 (1993).*

Journal 1993 Discusses the legal distinction between "the right to die" and physician-assisted suicide. Examines how the law is applied and whether it should be reformed. Considers the significance of public opinion and changing ethical standards. References Opinion 2.20. Gostin, *Drawing a Line Between Killing and Letting Die: The Law, and Law Reform, on Medically Assisted Dying, 21 J. Law, Med. & Ethics 94, 98 (1993).*

Journal 1993 Considers how life-sustaining treatments have led to prolonged life under unacceptable circumstances. Discusses situations in which patients would prefer to die rather than to stay alive. Recommends quality assurance programs that promote discussion between physicians and patients regarding life-sustaining treatment problems. Cites Opinions 2.20 and 2.21. Pearlman, Cain, Patrick, Appelbaum-Maizel, Starks, Jecker, & Uhlmann, *Insights Pertaining to Patient Assessments of States Worse than Death, 4 J. Clinical Ethics 33, 40 (1993).*

Journal 1993 Considers whether criminal penalties should be imposed on a physician who assists in the suicide of a competent, non-terminal patient who requested such assistance. Analyzes the actions of Dr. Jack Kevorkian and his views on physician-assisted suicide. Examines Dutch practices in this field and their value as a model for other countries. Presents the arguments for and against active euthanasia, with emphasis on the "slippery slope" argument. References Opinions 2.06 and 2.20. Persels, *Forcing the Issue of Physician-Assisted Suicide: Impact of the Kevorkian Case on the Euthanasia Debate, 14 J. Legal Med. 93, 115 (1993).*

Journal 1993 Discusses legal and ethical issues raised by physician aid-in-dying. Concludes that passive euthanasia for competent, terminal adults is the accepted norm and physician aid-in-dying is the new frontier. Quotes Opinion 2.18 (1986) [now Opinion 2.20]. Risley, *Ethical and Legal Issues in the Individual's Right to Die, 20 Ohio N.U.L. Rev. 597, 605 (1993).*

Journal 1992 Considers when it is appropriate to withdraw artificial food and nutrition from an incompetent patient under the Indiana "Living Wills" statute. Attempts to define "appropriate nutrition and hydration." Concludes that, in Indiana, it is appropriate to remove artificial nutrition and hydration that only "prolongs the dying process." Quotes Opinion 2.20. Anderson, *A Medical-Legal Dilemma: When Can "Inappropriate" Nutrition and Hydration Be Removed in Indiana? 67 Ind. L. J. 479, 480 (1992).*

Journal 1992 Analyzes the arguments for and against active euthanasia, including ethical concerns, the slippery slope argument, and the proper role of the physician. Suggests that active euthanasia may be acceptable when its administration is restricted to physicians. References Opinions 2.20 and 2.21. Brock, *Voluntary Active Euthanasia, 22 Hastings Center Rep. 10 (March/April 1992).*

Journal 1992 Examines several issues regarding persistent vegetative state (PVS) patients, including whether PVS patients are really dead, whether nutrition and hydration should be withheld, whether life-sustaining treatments are futile or medically inappropriate, and whether ordinary standards for decision making should be applied to PVS patients. Concludes that life-sustaining therapy may be withheld or continued, but that withdrawal of nutrition and hydration, as well as active euthanasia, present more difficult questions. References Opinions 2.20 and 2.22. Brody, *Special Ethical Issues in the Management of PVS Patients, 20 Law, Med. & Health Care 104, 109 (1992).*

Journal 1992 Examines ethical issues surrounding cardiopulmonary resuscitation and emergency cardiac care. Discusses advance directives and proxy decision making, medical futility, resource allocation, and Do-Not-Resuscitate orders. Concludes with a discussion of legal considerations. References Opinions 2.20 and 2.22. Comment, *Ethical Considerations in Resuscitation, 268 J.A.M.A. 2282, 2283, 2287 (1992).*

Journal 1992 Discusses the rights of terminally ill, competent patients to die with the assistance of a physician. Defines this right and argues that it is essentially the same as the right to die by refusing life-sustaining medical treatment. Concludes that courts should balance patients' rights with compelling state interests in assessing the scope of this right. Cites Opinion 2.20. Comment, *Physician Assisted Suicide and the Right to Die With Assistance, 105 Harvard L. Rev. 2021, 2027, 2035 (1992).*

Journal 1992 Discusses the Iowa living will statute, comparing it to similar laws in other states. Considers possible problems with the Iowa statute in light of recent court decisions. Proposes a revised statute to address these problems. References Opinion 2.20. Goldman, *Revising Iowa's Life-Sustaining Procedures Act: Creating a Practical Guide to Living Wills in Iowa, 76 Iowa L. Rev. 1137, 1149 (1992).*

Journal 1992 Explores various health policy issues addressed by the Indiana state legislature. Considers lawmakers' responses to the following concerns: health care access; tort reform; the right to die; medicaid reimbursements; and discrimination against AIDS patients. Notes that Indiana has created a commission on health policy and that this commission is grappling with these important issues. Cites Opinion 2.18 (1986) [now Opinion 2.20]. Kumar & Kinney, *Indiana Lawmakers Face National Health Policy Issues, 25 Indiana L. Rev. 1271, 1275, 1276 (1992).*

Journal 1992 Discusses the need for a policy governing life-sustaining treatment decisions for incompetent adult wards of the state. Addresses relevant statutory and case law. Provides a basic outline for such a policy and proposes a model policy statement. Quotes Opinion 2.20. McKnight & Bollis, *Foregoing Life-Sustaining Treatment for Adult Developmentally Disabled, Public Wards: A Proposed Statute*, XVIII Am. J. Law & Med. 203, 206, 220, 227 (1992).

Journal 1992 Examines several aspects of the legal consensus concerning the withdrawing or withholding of life-sustaining treatment prior to the *Cruzan* decision. Discusses the viability of this consensus in light of *Cruzan* and subsequent cases. Observes that the fundamental question in *Cruzan* was whether there should be judicial oversight regarding decisions to forego life-sustaining treatment. Concludes that *Cruzan* did not resolve this issue. Cites Opinion 2.18 (1986) [now Opinion 2.20]. Meisel, *A Retrospective on Cruzan*, 20 Law, Med. & Health Care 340, 345 (1992).

Journal 1992 Explores evolution of the legal consensus that terminating life support is legitimate under some circumstances. Suggests that the consensus will continue to spread in the absence of opposition. Considers how the consensus might extend to mercy killing and futility cases. Quotes Opinion 2.18 (1986) [now Opinion 2.20]. Meisel, *The Legal Consensus About Forgoing Life-Sustaining Treatment: Its Status and Its Prospects*, 2 Kennedy Inst. Ethics J. 309, 325 (1992).

Journal 1992 Considers the debate surrounding medical futility. Observes that this debate is encouraging reexamination of the nature of patient entitlement to medical care as well as the "ends of medicine." References Opinions 2.20, 2.21, and 2.22. Miles, *Medical Futility*, 20 Law, Med. & Health Care 310, 311, 313 (1992).

Journal 1992 Analyzes North Carolina's living will and health care power of attorney statutes in light of the *Cruzan* case. Notes recent changes to both statutes and problems that continue to exist. Concludes that both statutes need to be reformed and clarified. Quotes Opinion 2.21 (1992) [now Opinion 2.20]. Note, *Exercising the Right to Die: North Carolina's Amended Natural Death Act and the 1991 Health Care Power of Attorney Act*, 70 No. Carolina L. Rev. 2108, 2116 (1992).

Journal 1992 Examines the significance of natural death acts in light of the *Cruzan* decision. Explains how the "terminal condition" requirement in these statutes may reduce the number of people who fall within the scope of coverage. Also indicates that omission of nutrition and hydration from the list of treatments that may be withdrawn limits patient choices. Concludes with a discussion of practical problems faced by persons executing living wills. Quotes Opinion 2.20. References Opinion 2.22. Note, *State Natural Death Acts: Illusory Protection of Individuals' Life-Sustaining Treatment Decisions*, 29 Harvard J. Legis. 175, 186, 194, 195, 201 (1992).

Journal 1992 Examines the issue of physician-assisted suicide, noting the current ethical and legal debate issue. Contrasts physician-assisted suicide and voluntary euthanasia. Recommends legalization of physician-assisted suicide and proposes guidelines for implementation. References Opinion 2.20. Quill, Cassel, & Meier, *Care of the Hopelessly Ill: Proposed Clinical Criteria for Physician-Assisted Suicide*, 327 New Eng. J. Med. 1380, 1381 (1992).

Journal 1992 Examines the medical, ethical, and legal validity of selective nontreatment of severely handicapped newborns. Suggests that triage and cost-benefit analysis are the most effective means to evaluate issues associated with allocating scarce medical resources to disabled infants. Concludes both that selective treatment can never be considered murder and that governmental intrusion in this area should be minimal. Quotes Opinions 2.10 (1982) [now Opinion 2.17] and 2.18 (1986) [now Opinion 2.20]. Smith, *Murder, She Wrote or Was It Merely Selective Nontreatment?*, 8 J. Contemp. Health L. & Pol'y 49, 53 (1992).

Journal 1991 Examines the right to refuse life-sustaining medical treatment. Discusses the manner in which competent and incompetent patients could exercise this right prior to *Cruzan*. Analyzes the effect *Cruzan* had on these rights. Concludes that *Cruzan* had limited far-reaching impact and failed to answer several important questions. Cites Opinion 2.20. Albert, *Cruzan v. Director, Missouri Department of Health: Too Much Ado*, 12 J. Legal Med. 331, 338, 343 (1991).

Journal 1991 Discusses why families of persistent vegetative state (PVS) patients should not make decisions regarding whether to withdraw life support. Explains that patients probably would be in favor of withdrawing such support. Observes that leaving decisions to families creates the possibility they will erroneously decide otherwise. References Opinion 2.20. Baron, *Why Withdrawal of Life-Support for PVS Patients Is Not A Family Decision*, 19 Law, Med. & Health Care 73 (1991).

Journal 1991 Considers the issue of how courts should decide right-to-die cases in Massachusetts. Analyzes the case of *Cruzan v. Director, Missouri Department of Health*. Concludes that there are no clear standards for physicians to follow and recommends that physicians obtain court approval before withdrawing artificial nutrition and hydration from a patient in a persistent vegetative state. Quotes Opinion 2.20. Comment, *A Right to Die: Can a Massachusetts Physician Withdraw Artificial Nutrition and Hydration From a Persistently Vegetative Patient Following Cruzan v. Director, Missouri Department of Health?* 26 New Eng. L. Rev. 199, 216, 220 (1991).

Journal 1991 Discusses disabling neurologic conditions, with emphasis on the propriety of withdrawing or withholding artificial hydration and nutrition. Discusses major neurologic syndromes in life-sustaining medical treatment decisions. Concludes with a survey of the major legal developments in the area since *Cruzan*. References Opinion 2.20. Cranford, *Neurologic Syndromes and Prolonged Survival: When Can Artificial Nutrition and Hydration Be Foregone?* 19 Law, Med. & Health Care 13, 14, 16, 17 (1991).

Journal 1991 Discusses the issue of advance medical directives and proxy decision-making. Presents the results of a study in which individuals are asked about attitudes regarding advance directives, possible obstacles to such planning, and treatment preferences if faced with a poor medical prognosis. Reports that most individuals favor use of advance directives and would not desire life-sustaining treatment if faced with a poor prognosis. Recommends that physicians routinely discuss advance directives with patients. Cites Opinion 2.20. Emanuel, Barry, Stoeckle, Ettelson, & Emanuel, *Advance Directives for Medical Care—A Case for Greater Use*, 324 New Eng. J. Med. 889 (1991).

Journal 1991 Discusses the "slippery slope" argument against expanding the right to die. Considers the history of this right and how it has been expanded over the years. Explores when the right to die and the right to live exist. Concludes that society seems to be sliding down the slippery slope toward euthanasia. Cites Opinion 2.18 (1986) [now Opinion 2.20]. Kamisar, *When is There A Constitutional "Right to Die"? When is There No Constitutional "Right to Live"?* 25 Georgia L. Rev. 1203, 1207, 1208, 1222 (1991).

Journal 1991 Discusses common misperceptions about legal implications of terminating life support. Emphasizes importance of educating physicians about these medical legal considerations. References Opinion 2.20. Meisel, *Legal Myths About Terminating Life Support*, 151 Arch. Intern. Med. 1497, 1499 (1991).

Journal 1991 Discusses health care decision making for terminally ill incompetent patients in Ohio. Considers Ohio law in relation to that of other states. Argues that Ohio is one of the few remaining states that does not adequately protect the rights of incompetent terminally ill patients. Proposes legal reforms, that would better protect autonomous medical decision making in this context. Cites Opinion 2.18 (1986) [now Opinion 2.20]. Mullins, *The Need for Guidance in Decision Making for Terminally Ill Incompetents: Is the Ohio Legislature in a "Persistent Vegetative State"?*, 17 Ohio No. Univ. L. Rev. 827, 844 (1991).

Journal 1991 Discusses the major issues contained in the *Cruzan* decision. Analyzes the legal predicates for an incompetent patient's right to refuse life-sustaining treatment. Also surveys relevant state cases. Concludes with a discussion of living wills. References Opinion 2.20. Note, *Cruzan v. Director, Missouri Department of Health: To Die or Not to Die: That is the Question—But Who Decides?*, 51 Louisiana L. Rev. 1307, 1327, 1333 (1991).

Journal 1991 Explores the growth of "right to die" jurisprudence with particular emphasis on post-*Cruzan* developments. Focuses on the New York "Health Care Proxy Law." Notes that the statute does not apply to situations in which a patient is incompetent, but did not appoint an agent. Proposes alternative provisions that would apply in these situations. References Opinion 2.20. Note, *Health Care Proxies: New York's Attempt to Resolve the Right to Die Dilemma*, 57 Brooklyn L. Rev. 145, 168 (1991).

Journal 1991 Analyzes the Illinois Supreme Court case of *In re Estate of Longeway*, where the court decided that, absent an advance directive, the guardian of an incompetent patient could authorize the withdrawal of artificial nutrition and hydration. Discusses the importance of using advance medical directives. Concludes that written directives other than living wills may best secure patients' rights. Cites Opinion 2.18 (1986) [now Opinion 2.20]. Note, *Redefining the Right to Die in Illinois*, 15 So. Ill. Univ. L. J. 1261, 1273 (1991).

Journal 1991 Discusses applicable law regarding patients in a persistent vegetative state. Examines the *Cruzan* case, including the "clear and convincing" evidence standard used by the Court. Compares *Cruzan* with other right-to-die cases, arguing that the *Cruzan* decision makes it more difficult for individuals to secure this right. Concludes by discussing various advance medical directives. Quotes Opinion 2.20. Note, *Something Worth Writing Home About: Clear and Convincing Evidence, Living Wills, and Cruzan v. Director, Missouri Department of Health,* 22 Univ. Toledo L. Rev. 871, 879 (1991).

Journal 1991 Examines the living will and durable power of attorney as health care planning devices in South Carolina. Considers both statutory and non-statutory forms of the living will. Provides practical information and drafting guidelines. Encourages lawyers to look at various health care planning options with clients. References Opinion 2.20. Patterson, *Planning for Health Care Using Living Wills and Durable Powers of Attorney: A Guide for the South Carolina Attorney,* 42 So. Carolina L. Rev. 525, 535, 541, 547, 548 (1991).

Journal 1991 Discusses the issue of privacy in medical decision making. Explains the contractual nature of the physician-patient relationship and how it has been ignored by many courts in right-to-die cases. Examines state interests in these cases and argues that they should not be dispositive. Concludes there is a constitutional right to privacy in health care decision making. Cites Opinion 2.18 (1986) [now Opinion 2.20]. Rich, *The Assault on Privacy on Healthcare Decision Making,* 68 Denver L. Rev. 1, 10 (1991).

Journal 1991 Considers the limits of patient autonomy in demanding treatment that the physician feels provides no medical benefit. Discusses these issues in light of the Helga Wanglie case. Concludes that courts should define limits to patient autonomy in these situations. References Opinion 2.20. Rie, *The Limits of a Wish,* 21 Hastings Center Rep. 24 (July/August 1991).

Journal 1991 Analyzes three important right-to-die cases: *Cruzan; Wanglie;* and *Busalacchi.* Examines recent state legislation concerning advance medical directives. Concludes that there should be a nationwide system to address right-to-die cases. Proposes a state/federal cooperative framework to fill this need. References Opinion 2.20. Roach, *Paradox and Pandora's Box: The Tragedy of Current Right-to-Die Jurisprudence,* 25 Univ. Mich. J. Law Reform 133, 137, 158 (1991).

Journal 1990 Examines the constitutional right to privacy in relation to the physician-patient relationship. Argues that *Roe v. Wade* not only protects a woman's right to choose, but also preserves a doctor's right to treat. Observes that this protected relationship extends into the arena of right-to-die cases. Cites Opinion 2.20. Annas, Glantz, & Mariner, *The Right of Privacy Protects the Doctor-Patient Relationship,* 263 J.A.M.A. 858, 861 (1990).

Journal 1990 Discusses the connection between law and medicine in the context of health care decision making. Presents several illustrations, noting the involvement of courts and judges. Explains relevant law in this field, and predicts how the law is likely to change. Quotes Opinion 2.18 [now Opinion 2.20]. Bellacosa, *The Fusion of Medicine and Law for In Extremis Health and Medical Decisions: Does It Produce Energy and Light or Just Cosmic Debris?,* 18 Bull. Am. Acad. Psychiatry Law 5, 9 (1990).

Journal 1990 Examines cardiopulmonary resuscitation policies in North Carolina nursing homes. Finds that a vast majority of nursing homes have written policies, but that there is substantial variation among them. Concludes that such variations risk limiting or ignoring the personal rights of residents. References Opinions 2.20 and 2.22. Brunetti, Weiss, Studenski, & Clipp, *Cardiopulmonary Resuscitation Policies and Practices: A Statewide Nursing Home Study,* 150 Arch. Intern. Med. 121, 122 (1990).

Journal 1990 Discusses the importance of living wills and society's acceptance of terminating medical care in appropriate situations. Notes the shortcomings of current living will statutes. Proposes a living will that addresses these problems. Cites Opinion 2.18 (1986) [now Opinion 2.20]. Cantor, *My Annotated Living Will,* 18 Law, Med. & Health Care 114 (1990).

Journal 1990 Discusses the "living will" and its role in American society. Explains the shortcomings of living will statutes and the need for legislative reform. Lists specific problems that should be addressed. Concludes that legislators need to be more aware of the goals of living wills when drafting these statutes. Quotes Opinion 2.20. Comment, *The Living Will: Preservation of the Right-To-Die Demands Clarity and Consistency,* 95 Dickinson L. Rev. 209, 217 (1990).

Journal 1990 Discusses the right to die in Oklahoma. Examines the development of the common law right to refuse life-sustaining treatment. Explores current law governing the right of a person to withdraw artificial hydration and nutrition, with emphasis on Oklahoma law, which omits artificial nutrition and hydration from the list of treatments that may be withdrawn. Concludes that individuals have a right to withdraw such treatment and that Oklahoma law may be unconstitutional. Quotes Opinion 2.18 (1986) [now Opinion 2.20]. Comment, *Right to Die: Oklahoma's Position on Nutrition and Hydration: Confusing or Unconstitutional?* 43 Okla. L. Rev. 143, 151 (1990).

Journal 1990 Examines the right of competent patients to refuse treatment on the basis of a common law right of bodily integrity, the right to privacy, and statutory provisions such as natural death acts. Explains how this right has been extended to incompetent patients who are terminally ill. Concludes that the law is unsettled with respect to the right of incompetent, nonterminal patients to refuse medical care. Quotes Opinion 2.18 (1986) [now Opinion 2.20]. Comment, *The Right to Refuse Life Sustaining Medical Treatment and the Nonterminally Ill Patient: An Analysis of Abridgment and Anarchy*, 17 Pepperdine L. Rev. 461, 462 (1990).

Journal 1990 Discusses how the imprecise language of euthanasia muddles public discussion of the issue. Concludes that medical ethics must distinguish between acts and omissions undertaken to cause death and those considered reasonable treatment under the circumstances. Quotes Opinion 2.20 (1989). Devettere, *The Imprecise Language of Euthanasia and Causing Death*, 1 J. Clinical Ethics 268, 268 (1990).

Journal 1990 Discusses the proposition that an objective standard should govern end-of-life decision making instead of living wills or similar instruments. Considers the arguments in favor of allowing living wills to control and against objective standards. Concludes that an objective standard is preferable and recommends that courts adopt such a standard. References Opinion 2.20. Dresser, *Relitigating Life and Death*, 51 Ohio St. L. J. 425, 436 (1990).

Journal 1990 Considers the right to die in light of the *Cruzan* case. Discusses the development of the law regarding the withdrawal of life-sustaining medical treatment from incompetent patients since the *Quinlan* case. Summarizes the facts of *Cruzan* and examines the basis of the decision with emphasis on the opinions of the individual justices. Concludes that *Cruzan* did not resolve a number of important questions concerning the right to die. Quotes Opinion 2.18 (1986) [now Opinion 2.20]. McNoble, *The* Cruzan *Decision—A Surgeon's Perspective*, 20 Memphis State Univ. L. Rev. 569, 581, 600, 601 (1990).

Journal 1990 Explains the ruling of the Supreme Court in the *Cruzan* case. Considers how the case may be misperceived. Proposes that health care professionals should routinely advise patients of the necessity of making their wishes about life-sustaining treatment known. Quotes Opinion 2.18 (1986) [now Opinion 2.20]. Meisel, *Lessons from* Cruzan, 1 J. Clinical Ethics 245, 248 (1990).

Journal 1990 Discusses the right of physicians to refrain from participating in the withdrawal or removal of life-sustaining treatment. Concludes that federal and state legislation is needed to protect the right of conscience of medical personnel in this context. Quotes Opinion 2.20. Note, *I Have A Conscience, Too: The Plight of Medical Personnel Confronting the Right to Die*, 65 Notre Dame L. Rev. 699, 706 (1990).

Journal 1990 Discusses advance medical directives including living wills and durable powers of attorney. Considers the importance of these instruments in patient self-determination. Concludes by examining the physician's role in implementing patient preferences. Cites Opinion 2.20. Orentlicher, *Advance Medical Directives*, 263 J.A.M.A. 2365 (1990).

Journal 1990 Discusses the moral dilemma in deciding whether to withdraw artificial nutrition and hydration from a patient and the appropriate role of the judiciary. States that part of the reason for judicial activism in this private area is because legislatures have not adequately expressed public policy. Concludes that judicial decisions do not represent the moral viewpoint of society and that moral pronouncements should not be made in the courtroom. Quotes Preamble, Principles I, II, III, IV, V, VI, and VII, and Opinion 2.20. Peccarelli, *A Moral Dilemma: The Role of Judicial Intervention in Withholding or Withdrawing Nutrition and Hydration*, 23 John Marshall L. Rev. 537, 539, 540, 541 (1990).

Journal 1990 Explores how recent advances in medical science and technology have resulted in changing views concerning withdrawing and withholding of life support. Concludes that morality plays a key role in dealing with this issue and that physicians should rely upon fundamental principles of medicine for guidance. Quotes Opinion 2.20. Sprung, *Changing Attitudes and Practices in Forgoing Life-Sustaining Treatments*, 263 J.A.M.A. 2211, 2213 (1990).

Journal 1990 Looks into the appropriateness of terminating life-prolonging treatment for patients lacking decision making abilities. Considers relevant legal authorities and issues, including the *Cruzan* case. Concludes that physicians do not risk serious liability for withdrawing life support. References Opinion 2.20. Weir & Gostin, *Decisions to Abate Life-Sustaining Treatment for Nonautonomous Patients: Ethical Standards and Legal Liability for Physicians After Cruzan*, 264 J.A.M.A. 1846, 1849, 1850 (1990).

Journal 1989 Challenges the notion that removal of artificial nutrition from permanently unconscious patients constitutes active euthanasia. Observes that the administration of artificial nutrition constitutes a form of medical treatment that should be administered in accordance with the interests of the patient and humane standards of care. Concludes by observing that the traditional judicial approach, which permits withdrawal of artificial nutrition, is entirely consistent with accepted medical legal and ethical doctrines. Cites Opinion 2.18 (1986) [now Opinion 2.20]. Cantor, *The Permanently Unconscious Patient, Non-Feeding and Euthanasia*, XV Am. J. Law & Med. 381, 385 (1989).

Journal 1989 Examines and criticizes the legal advice that was rendered by hospital counsel in the context of the Samuel Linares case which occurred at Rush-Presbyterian-St. Luke's Medical Center in Chicago, Illinois. There, a minor child's father disconnected his irreversibly comatose son's ventilator while warding off hospital personnel with a handgun. Focusing on such issues as whether foregoing ventilator assistance constitutes murder or child abuse and neglect, concludes that ultraconservative legal advice led to moral paralysis, thereby precipitating the tragic and unnecessary action of the child's father. References Opinion 2.20. Nelson & Cranford, Legal Advice, *Moral Paralysis and the Death of Samuel Linares*, 17 Law, Med. & Health Care 316, 319 (1989).

Journal 1989 Analyzes and evaluates changing attitudes regarding physicians' duties toward hopelessly ill patients. Observes that, while new policies have developed, there is a significant gap between development and implementation of those policies. Urges that this gap be closed and that an overall doctrine of flexible care be developed. References Opinion 2.20. Wanzer, Federman, Adelstein, Cassel, Cassem, Cranford, Hook, Lo, Moertel, Safar, Stone, & Van Eys, *The Physician's Responsibility Toward Hopelessly Ill Patients: A Second Look*, 320 New Eng. J. Med. 844, 844 (1989).

Journal 1988 Considers and challenges certain presumed implications of the definition of death as brain death. Points to the importance of the distinction between death of the person as contrasted with death of the body. Significant emphasis involves the moral impact of such considerations as determination of brain death and the presence or absence of family consent to withdrawal of treatment in cases involving persistent vegetative patients. References Opinion 2.18 (1986) [now Opinion 2.20]. Brody, *Ethical Questions Raised by the Persistent Vegetative Patient*, 18 Hastings Center Rep. 33, 34 (Feb./March 1988).

Journal 1988 Explores the revitalization of the hospice concept and the various structural models available for providing care to the terminally ill. Examines the cost effectiveness of hospice care and discusses various ethical and legal problems that arise in the context of providing hospice care, including withholding or withdrawing life-prolonging medical treatment. References Opinion 2.18 (1986) [now Opinion 2.20]. Comment, *The Hospice Movement: A Renewed View of the Death Process*, 4 J. Contemp. Health L. & Pol'y 295, 312 (1988).

Journal 1988 Focuses on the issue of removal of life-sustaining medical treatment from incompetent patients whose wishes are unknown. The importance of "quality of life" considerations as an aspect of surrogate decision making in this context is emphasized. Guidelines for adoption and implementation of a "capacity for interpersonal relationships" standard are offered. References Opinion 2.18 (1986) [now Opinion 2.20]. Quinn, *The Best Interests of Incompetent Patients: The Capacity for Interpersonal Relationships as a Standard for Decision Making*, 76 Cal. L. Rev. 897, 906 (1988).

Journal 1988 Discusses the legal and moral aspects of the adult patient's right to refuse artificial hydration and nutrition. In particular, examines the meaning and scope of the phrase "artificial feeding," the distinction between ordinary and extraordinary care, and the impact of medical condition and competency on the patient's right to refuse treatment. Concludes that the value of patient autonomy is not the controlling factor in such cases, but only one factor that must be balanced against the nature and probable results of the proposed treatment. Quotes Opinion 2.18 (1986) [now Opinion 2.20]. Snyder, *Artificial Feeding and the Right to Die: The Legal Issues*, 9 J. Legal Med. 349, 351, 352, 357 (1988).

Journal 1988 Discusses numerous judicial decisions in which the courts have focused, among other things, on the withdrawal of artificial feeding from incompetent adult patients. Quoting from the relevant 1986 Opinion of the AMA Council on Ethical and Judicial Affairs and other medical ethical pronouncements, notes an emerging consensus in favor of withdrawal of artificial feeding under appropriate circumstances. Practical suggestions are offered to care givers and relevant policy implications and other unresolved issues are addressed. Quotes from Opinion 2.18

(1986) [now Opinion 2.20]. Steinbrook & Lo, *Artificial Feeding—Solid Ground, Not a Slippery Slope*, 318 New Eng. J. Med. 286, 288 (1988).

Journal 1988 Examines the use of anencephalic infants as organ donors for neonates requiring transplants, and presents a rationale for such use. Discusses moral justification for limited respirator use in prolonging anencephalic infants as organ donors, problems in determining brain death, and the need for additional research relative to anencephalic newborns. Ethical justifications for withdrawal of artificial life support from adult patients who are permanently comatose are offered, by way of analogy, for the purpose of demonstrating the ethical and medical propriety of attaching volunteered, select anencephalic infants to respirators in an effort to obtain scarce organs. Cites Opinion 2.18 (1986) [now Opinion 2.20]. Walters & Ashwal, *Organ Prolongation in Anencephalic Infants: Ethical and Medical Issues*, 18 Hastings Center Rep. 19, 21 (Oct./Nov. 1988).

Journal 1987 Focuses on the issue of withholding nutrition and hydration from comatose patients with emphasis on the questions of what constitutes medical treatment and when it may properly be withheld. Briefly discusses the often cited cases that have addressed these issues, noting the importance of the position of the American Medical Association regarding withholding or withdrawing life-prolonging medical treatment. References Opinion 2.18 (1986) [now Opinion 2.20]. Comment, *Hold On Courts: May a Comatose Patient Be Denied Food and Water*, 31 St. Louis Univ. L. J. 749, 750 (1987).

Journal 1987 Examines the historical and current state of the law relative to family involvement in health care decision making for incompetent patients. Evaluates applicable decision making with emphasis on the role of the courts, physicians, and family members. Following comprehensive analysis of existing common law, notes a trend toward granting families greater autonomy in making decisions for incompetent adult patients. Supports this trend and advocates recognition of a more prominent role for the family in these situations. References Opinion 2.18 (1986) [now Opinion 2.20]. Comment, *The Role of the Family in Medical Decision Making for Incompetent Adult Patients: A Historical Perspective and Case Analysis*, 48 U. Pittsburgh L. Rev. 539, 571, 607, 610-11 (1987).

Journal 1986 Discusses the distinction between the persistent vegetative state and coma, pointing out the confusion of these concepts in various leading "right to die" cases. Addresses philosophical and ethical predicates for withholding treatment noting that, in the final analysis, a balancing of the benefits and burdens of treatment should involve the patient, the family, and the physician. Cites Opinion 2.11 (1981) [now Opinion 2.20]. Berrol, *Considerations for Management of the Persistent Vegetative State*, 67 Arch. Phys. Med. Rehabil. 283, 285 (1986).

Journal 1986 Observes that life-sustaining medical treatment includes artificial nutrition and hydration and that patients have a right to forego such treatment under the Washington State Constitution, applicable common law, and the Washington Natural Death Act. Notes that available judicial standards for surrogate decision making in this context are inadequate, and proposes substantive guidelines for the making of such decisions. References Opinion 2.18 (1986) [now Opinion 2.20]. Comment, *Artificial Nutrition and the Terminally Ill: How Should Washington Decide?*, 61 Wash. L. Rev. 419, 421, 447 (1986).

Journal 1986 Analyzes the law's approach to death by evaluating various legal issues that arise in the context of efforts to define death. Definitions of "cardiopulmonary death," "whole brain death," and "neocortical death" are considered. Against the background of this discussion, it is asserted that "neocortical death" should be viewed as death of the person for all legal purposes. References Opinion 2.18 (1986) [now Opinion 2.20]. Smith, *Legal Recognition of Neocortical Death*, 71 Cornell L. Rev. 850, 860, 876-77 (1986).

Journal 1985 Focuses on the issue of withholding medical care and treatment from infants for whom there is little reasonable expectation of normal development. Urges that parents rather than other persons should assume principal decision making responsibility. Recognizing that the state must have some role in this significant medical legal process, a framework for limited state intervention is offered. References Opinion 2.18 (1986) [now Opinion 2.20]. Haddon, *Baby Doe Cases: Compromise and Moral Dilemma*, 34 Emory L. J. 545, 556 (1985).

Journal 1984 Evaluates two divergent approaches to the legal treatment of withdrawing nourishment. One line of thinking, illustrated by the judicial opinion in *Barber v. California*, 147 Cal. App. 3d 1006, 195 Cal. Rptr. 484 (1983), applies a rule of wide deference to the physician's judgment in such cases. This approach is rejected in favor of the reasoning of the appellate court in *In re Conroy*, 190 N.J. Super. 453, 464 A.2d 303 (1983), which focuses instead on the patient's rights to privacy and to treatment as the primary factors in resolving the issue of withdrawing nourishment. (The New Jersey Supreme Court later reversed this decision. *Matter of Conroy*, 98 N.J. 321, 486 A.2d 1209 (1985)). Quotes Opinion 2.11 (1982) [now Opinion 2.20]. Horan & Grant, *The Legal Aspects of Withdrawing Nourishment, 5 J. Legal Med. 595, 626 (1984)*.

2.21   The previous Opinion 2.21, **Withholding or Withdrawing Life-Prolonging Medical Treatment—Patients' Preferences,** was deleted in 1994 and combined with Opinion 2.20.

2.21   Euthanasia

Euthanasia is the administration of a lethal agent by another person to a patient for the purpose of relieving the patient's intolerable and incurable suffering.

It is understandable, though tragic, that some patients in extreme duress—such as those suffering from a terminal, painful, debilitating illness—may come to decide that death is preferable to life. However, permitting physicians to engage in euthanasia would ultimately cause more harm than good. Euthanasia is fundamentally incompatible with the physician's role as healer, would be difficult or impossible to control, and would pose serious societal risks.

The involvement of physicians in euthanasia heightens the significance of its ethical prohibition. The physician who performs euthanasia assumes unique responsibility for the act of ending the patient's life. Euthanasia could also readily be extended to incompetent patients and other vulnerable populations.

Instead of engaging in euthanasia, physicians must aggressively respond to the needs of patients at the end of life. Patients should not be abandoned once it is determined that a cure is impossible. Patients near the end of life must continue to receive emotional support, comfort care, adequate pain control, respect for patient autonomy, and good communication. (I, IV)

Issued June 1994 based on the report, "Decisions Near the End of Life," adopted June 1991. (JAMA. 1992; 267: 2229-2233).

Updated June 1996.

9th Cir. 1996 Suit was brought by several physicians and not-for-profit corporation which provides information, assistance, and counseling to competent terminally ill adult patients contemplating suicide, asserting that a state statute making it a crime to aid anyone in attempting to commit suicide unconstitutionally prevents terminally ill patients from exercising their protected liberty interests. Appeals court, en banc, held that the choice of how and when to die is a liberty interest and that the statute violates the due process rights of competent, terminally ill adults who wish to hasten their deaths by obtaining medication prescribed by their physicians. Stating that physician-assisted suicide runs counter to medical ethics, the dissent cited Opinions 2.20, 2.21, and 2.211 and quoted Opinion 2.211. *Compassion in Dying v. Washington, 79 F.3d 790, 840, 855 replacing, 49 F.3d 586 (9th Cir. 1995)*.

Journal 1997 Considers the legal and ethical issues involved with physician-assisted suicide and euthanasia. Explores recent legal developments in the courts. Opines that Texas should allow physician-assisted suicide, at least for the terminally ill. Asserts that banning such a practice is unconstitutional. Quotes Opinion 2.211. References Opinion 2.21. Comment, *Physician-Assisted Suicide: Should Texas Be Different?, 33 Hous. L. Rev. 1475, 1480, 1488 (1997)*.

Journal 1997 Discusses goals of care included in advance directives and whether they can be used to predict specific interventions and results. Offers insights provided by survey of physicians at Massachusetts General Hospital. Cites Opinions 2.20 and 2.21. Fischer, Alpert, Stoeckle, & Emanuel, *Can Goals of Care Be Used to Predict Intervention Preferences in an Advance Directive?*, 157 Arch. Intern. Med. 801, 807 (1997).

Journal 1996 Examines the issue of physician-assisted suicide. Observes that it is important not only to consider whether some form of physician-assisted suicide should enjoy legal and ethical support in our society, but whether physicians should be involved. Concludes that physicians, as a profession, probably are not the proper individuals to perform this function. Cites Opinions 2.21 and 2.211. Clark, *Autonomy and Death*, 71 Tul. L. Rev. 45, 89 (1996).

Journal 1996 Explores the issue of legalizing physician-assisted suicide. Opines that the current state of technology increases life expectancy but with a concomitant decrease in dignity and autonomy surrounding one's death. Notes that the elderly are committing suicide at an increasing rate. Cites Opinions 2.20, 2.21, and 2.211. Morgan & Sutherland, *Last Rights? Confronting Physician-Assisted Suicide in Law and Society: Legal Liturgies on Physician-Assisted Suicide*, 26 Stetson L. Rev. 481, 484 (1996).

Journal 1995 Analyzes the case of *Compassion in Dying v. Washington* in which a federal district court judge held that certain people have a constitutional right to physician-assisted suicide. Criticizes the decision for being too broad in that it would protect active euthanasia by physicians on patients who are physically unable to perform the act themselves. Quotes Opinion 2.21. References Opinion 2.211. Larson, *Prescription For Death: A Second Opinion*, 44 DePaul L. Rev. 461, 472 (1995).

Journal 1995 Provides legal and medical definitions of physician-assisted suicide and euthanasia. Offers relevant historical perspectives and provides comprehensive ethical and legal discussion of these compelling social issues. Highlights important legislative developments, including the Oregon Death with Dignity Act, and analyzes significant judicial opinions. Advocates legal tolerance of physician-assisted suicide and euthanasia. Quotes Principles III, IV, and VI and Opinions 2.21 and 9.12. Cites Opinions 2.20 and 8.11. Stone & Winslade, *Physician-Assisted Suicide and Euthanasia in the United States: Legal and Ethical Observations*, 16 J. Legal Med. 481, 483, 490, 497, 498, 499 (1995).

Journal 1993 Considers how life-sustaining treatments have led to prolonged life under unacceptable circumstances. Discusses situations in which patients would prefer to die rather than to stay alive. Recommends quality assurance programs that promote discussion between physicians and patients regarding life-sustaining treatment problems. Cites Opinions 2.20 and 2.21. Pearlman, Cain, Patrick, Appelbaum-Maizel, Starks, Jecker, & Uhlmann, *Insights Pertaining to Patient Assessments of States Worse than Death*, 4 J. Clinical Ethics 33, 40 (1993).

Journal 1992 Analyzes the arguments for and against active euthanasia, including ethical concerns, the slippery slope argument, and the proper role of the physician. Suggests that active euthanasia may be acceptable when its administration is restricted to physicians. References Opinions 2.20 and 2.21. Brock, *Voluntary Active Euthanasia*, 22 Hastings Center Rep. 10 (March/April 1992).

Journal 1992 Considers the debate surrounding medical futility. Observes that this debate is encouraging reexamination of the nature of patient entitlement to medical care as well as the "ends of medicine." References Opinions 2.20, 2.21, and 2.22. Miles, *Medical Futility*, 20 Law, Med. & Health Care 310, 311, 313 (1992).

Journal 1992 Discusses the right of competent, incurably ill patients to commit suicide. Examines the history of the right an individual has over his or her own body, and how the right to commit suicide has evolved from that concept. Emphasizes the *Cruzan* decision. Concludes that the right of an incurably ill person to commit suicide is a personal issue to be decided outside of the judicial system. References Opinions 2.21 and 2.211. Morgan, Marks, & Harty-Golder, *The Issue of Personal Choice: The Competent Incurable Patient and the Right to Commit Suicide?*, 57 Mo. L. Rev. 1, 44, 45 (1992).

2.211 Physician-Assisted Suicide

Physician-assisted suicide occurs when a physician facilitates a patient's death by providing the necessary means and/or information to enable the patient to perform the life-ending act (e.g., the physician provides sleeping pills and information about the lethal dose, while aware that the patient may commit suicide).

It is understandable, though tragic, that some patients in extreme duress—such as those suffering from a terminal, painful, debilitating illness—may come to decide that death is preferable to life. However, allowing physicians to participate in assisted suicide would cause more harm than good. Physician-assisted suicide is fundamentally incompatible with the physician's role as healer, would be difficult or impossible to control, and would pose serious societal risks.

Instead of participating in assisted suicide, physicians must aggressively respond to the needs of patients at the end of life. Patients should not be abandoned once it is determined that a cure is impossible. Multidisciplinary interventions should be sought including specialty consultation, hospice care, pastoral support, family counseling and other modalities. Patients near the end of life must continue to receive emotional support, comfort care, adequate pain control, respect for patient autonomy, and good communication. (I, IV)

Issued 1994 based on the reports, "Decisions Near the End of Life," adopted June 1991, and "Physician-Assisted Suicide," adopted December 1993 (JAMA. 1992; 267: 2229-2233).

Updated June 1996.

U.S. 1997 Several physicians and terminally ill patients sued the state seeking a declaration that its prohibition against physician-assisted suicide violates the Fourteenth Amendment's Equal Protection Clause. The trial court disagreed, but the Second Circuit reversed, holding that the state accords different treatment to those terminally ill patients who wish to hasten their death by self-administering prescribed drugs and to those patients who wish to do so by directing the removal of life support systems. The Supreme Court reversed holding that the prohibition against assisting suicide does not violate the Equal Protection Clause. The Court concluded that there is a distinction between assisting suicide and withdrawing treatment quoting reports of the AMA Council on Ethical and Judicial Affairs [now Opinions 2.20 and 2.211]. *Vacco v. Quill, 117 S. Ct. 2293, 2298, 138 L. Ed. 2d 834.*

U.S. 1997 Several Washington physicians, terminally ill patients, and a not for profit organization that counsels people considering physician-assisted suicide sued the state seeking to have statutory ban on physician-assisted suicide declared unconstitutional. The trial court agreed and the Ninth Circuit affirmed. The Supreme Court, in reversing the decision, held that prohibition against causing or aiding a suicide does not violate the Due Process Clause. The Court also noted that the prohibition was rationally related to legitimate state interests in protecting the integrity and ethics of the medical profession quoting from Opinion 2.211. *Washington v. Glucksberg, 117 S. Ct. 2258, 2273, 138 L. Ed. 2d 772.*

9th Cir. 1996 Suit was brought by several physicians and not-for-profit corporation which provides information, assistance, and counseling to competent terminally ill adult patients contemplating suicide, asserting that a state statute making it a crime to aid anyone in attempting to commit suicide unconstitutionally prevents terminally ill patients from exercising their protected liberty interests. Appeals court, en banc, held that the choice of how and when to die is a liberty interest and that the statute violates the due process rights of competent, terminally ill adults who wish to hasten their deaths by obtaining medication prescribed by their physicians. Stating that physician-assisted suicide runs counter to medical ethics, the dissent cited Opinions 2.20, 2.21, and 2.211 and quoted Opinion 2.211. *Compassion in Dying v. Washington, 79 F.3d 790, 840, 855 replacing, 49 F.3d 586 (9th Cir. 1995).*

9th Cir. 1995 A not-for-profit corporation organized to assist terminally ill persons in committing suicide and several physicians alleged that a state statute making aiding a suicide attempt a crime violated 42 U.S.C. § 1983 and the Constitution. In upholding the statute, the court quoted Opinion 2.211 as articulating the ethical position of the medical profession against assisted suicide. In turn, the court found upholding the ethical integrity of the medical profession to be one of the many state interests outweighing the alleged liberty interest in medically-assisted suicide. *Compassion in Dying v. Washington, 49 F.3d 586, 592, replaced, 79 F.3d 790 (9th Cir. 1996).*

Fla. 1997 A patient, suffering from acquired immune deficiency syndrome (AIDS), and his physician filed suit for a declaratory judgment that state law prohibiting assisted suicide, violated the privacy clause of the state constitution, as well as the due process and equal protection clauses of the Fourteenth Amendment to the United States Constitution. The trial court concluded that the law was unconstitutional. On appeal the state supreme court, relying on the United States Supreme Court's rulings in *Washington v. Glucksberg, 117 S.Ct. 2258 (1997)* and *Vacco v. Quill, 117 S.Ct. 2293 (1997)*, held that the state's ban was not unconstitutional. In determining that the right to assisted suicide is not included in the state's guarantee of privacy, the court quoted from Opinion 2.211. *Krischer v. McIver, 697 So. 2d 97, 103.*

Journal 1997 Reviews the arguments made in *amicus curiae* briefs submitted to the Supreme Court on the topic of assisted suicide. Focuses on key insights into the debate offered by the various *amici curiae*. Quotes Opinion 2.211. Coleson, *The Glucksberg & Quill Amicus Curiae Briefs: Verbatim Arguments Opposing Assisted Suicide, 13 Issues in Law & Med. 3, 67 (1997)*.

Journal 1997 Considers the legal and ethical issues involved with physician-assisted suicide and euthanasia. Explores recent legal developments in the courts. Opines that Texas should allow physician-assisted suicide, at least for the terminally ill. Asserts that banning such a practice is unconstitutional. Quotes Opinion 2.211. References Opinion 2.21. Comment, *Physician-Assisted Suicide: Should Texas Be Different?, 33 Hous. L. Rev. 1475, 1480, 1488 (1997)*.

Journal 1997 Explores a model physician-assisted suicide statute. Explains its history, provisions, and effects. Posits that the Act reaches further than one may suspect. Notes the AMA's position on assisted death and concludes that the Act fails to account for moral tradition. Quotes Opinion 2.211. FitzGibbon & Lai, *The Model Physician-Assisted Suicide Act and the Jurisprudence of Death, 13 Issues in Law & Med. 173, 203-04 (1997)*.

Journal 1997 Considers the right to die. Discusses the extension of the right to refuse treatment to decisions affecting life and death. Explains that courts distinguish between withdrawing life-sustaining treatment and euthanasia or assisted suicide. Emphasizes the importance of quality end-of-life care. Cites Opinion 2.211. Gostin, *Deciding Life and Death in the Courtroom: From Quinlan to Cruzan, Glucksberg, and Vacco—A Brief History and Analysis of Constitutional Protection of the 'Right to Die,' 278 J.A.M.A. 1523, 1525, 1528 (1997)*.

Journal 1997 Examines possible legalization of euthanasia, observing that any form of euthanasia will be a step toward horrible death. Posits that legalizing euthanasia will create unsolvable mortal dangers that conflict with universal values of life. Concludes that physician-assisted suicide would create many victims. Cites Opinion 2.211. McGonnigal, *This is Who Will Die When Doctors Are Allowed To Kill Their Patients, 31 J. Marshall L. Rev. 95, 103 (1997)*.

Journal 1997 Explores the ethical and legal debate over assisted suicide. Examines cases dealing with prohibitions against physician-assisted suicide. Considers the Oregon Death with Dignity Act in light of the ruling in *Lee v. Oregon*. Quotes Opinion 2.211. Note, *Constitutional Aspects of Physician-Assisted Suicide After Lee v. Oregon, XXIII Am. J. Law & Med. 69 (1997)*.

Journal 1997 Discusses the difference between physician-assisted suicide and the withdrawal of life-sustaining medical treatment. Posits that traditional moral arguments cannot justify the distinction. Examines how a right to assisted suicide for terminal patients brings right-to-die laws into alignment with underlying ethical precepts. References Opinion 2.211. Orentlicher, *The Legalization of Physician Assisted Suicide: A Very Modest Revolution, 38 B.C.L. Rev. 443, 459-60 (1997)*.

Journal 1997 Considers the perspectives of medical residents about end-of-life issues. Investigates the differences of opinion held by residents in psychiatry, internal medicine, and emergency medicine. References Opinion 2.211. Roberts, Roberts, Warner, Solomon, Hardee, & McCarty, *Internal Medicine, Psychiatry, and Emergency Medicine Residents' Views of Assisted Death Practices, 157 Arch. Intern. Med. 1603, 1609 (1997)*.

Journal 1996 Proposes a model state statute allowing and controlling physician-assisted suicide. Analyzes the constitutionality of the act and offers public policy justifications for the act's provisions. Concludes that proponents of physician-assisted suicide should provide precise, carefully tailored examples of regulations. Quotes Opinion 2.211. Cites Opinion 2.20. Baron, Bergstresser, Brock, Cole, Dorfman, Johnson, Schnipper, Vorenberg, & Wanzer, *A Model State Act to Authorize and Regulate Physician-Assisted Suicide, 33 Harv. J. on Legis. 1, 2, 7 (1996)*.

Journal 1996 Examines the issue of physician-assisted suicide. Observes that it is important not only to consider whether some form of physician-assisted suicide should enjoy legal and ethical support in our society, but whether physicians should be involved. Concludes that physicians, as a profession, probably are not the proper individuals to perform this function. Cites Opinions 2.21 and 2.211. Clark, *Autonomy and Death*, 71 Tul. L. Rev. 45, 89 (1996).

Journal 1996 Criticizes the circuit court's opinion in *Compassion in Dying*. Suggests that the opinion fails to fully consider the ethical prohibitions against physician-assisted suicide. Concludes that the court's opinion is not based on a complete and accurate presentation of historical views and attitudes about suicide. Quotes Opinion 2.211. Duncan & Lubin, *The Use and Abuse of History in Compassion in Dying*, 20 Harv. J.L. & Pub. Pol'y 175, 183 (1996).

Journal 1996 Examines ethical and legal issues involved in physician-assisted suicide. Asserts that the judiciary is not the proper forum for establishing guidelines regarding these issues. Concludes that individual state legislative enactments are the proper vehicles for delineating appropriate guidelines. Quotes Opinion 2.211. Kass & Lund, *Physician-Assisted Suicide, Medical Ethics and the Future of the Medical Profession*, 35 Duq. L. Rev. 395, 404 (1996).

Journal 1996 Discusses the historical development of the right to die. Considers patient autonomy and paternalism and the role physicians play in end-of-life decisions. Explains the issue in the context of federal cases. Examines the true extent of a protected right to die. Cites Opinion 2.211. Kelly, *The "Right to Die" in America: The Ninth Circuit's Decision in Compassion in Dying v. The State of Washington*, 29 J. Health & Hosp. L. 246, 255 (1996).

Journal 1996 Explores the issue of legalizing physician-assisted suicide. Opines that the current state of technology increases life expectancy but with a concomitant decrease in dignity and autonomy surrounding one's death. Notes that the elderly are committing suicide at an increasing rate. Cites Opinions 2.20, 2.21, and 2.211. Morgan & Sutherland, *Last Rights? Confronting Physician-Assisted Suicide in Law and Society: Legal Liturgies on Physician-Assisted Suicide*, 26 Stetson L. Rev. 481, 484 (1996).

Journal 1996 Considers the right to death with dignity. Suggests that the AMA's position undermines mitigation of suffering and the individuals' right to self-determination. Concludes that restrictions on the right to death with dignity may be constitutionally impermissible. Quotes Opinion 2.211. Cites Opinion 2.20. Note, *Who Decides if There is "Triumph in the Ultimate Agony"? Constitutional Theory and the Emerging Right to Die With Dignity*, 37 Wm. & Mary L. Rev. 827, 829 (1996).

Journal 1996 Explores ethical problems accompanying the power to prolong and preserve life past points previously achievable. Questions whether physician-assisted suicide is a proper and ethically desirable course of treatment. Discusses recent developments and arguments surrounding physician-assisted suicide. References Opinion 2.211. Thomasma, *When Physicians Choose to Participate in the Death of Their Patients: Ethics and Physician-Assisted Suicide*, 24 J. Law, Med. & Ethics 183, 184, 195 (1996).

Journal 1995 Argues that assistance in suicide is an inappropriate societal response to a request for suicide. Suggests that people seeking suicide need life-affirming treatment, not aid in dying. Concludes that the United States Constitution does not require society to stand by while a person seeks suicide. Cites Opinion 2.211. Bopp & Coleson, *The Constitutional Case Against Permitting Physician-Assisted Suicide for Competent Adults With "Terminal Conditions,"* 11 Issues in Law & Med. 239, 250 (1995).

Journal 1995 Examines four essential principles of bioethics: patient autonomy; nonmaleficence; beneficence; and justice. Describes the application of these principles in clinical settings according to bioethical norms and AMA opinions. Concludes that such an approach promotes compassionate medical caregiving and that laws should reflect these values. Quotes Opinions 2.01 and 8.18. References Opinion 2.211. Cohen, *Toward a Bioethics of Compassion*, 28 Ind. L. Rev. 667, 673, 681-82, 683 (1995).

Journal 1995 Analyzes the case of *Compassion in Dying v. Washington* in which a federal district court judge held that certain people have a constitutional right to physician-assisted suicide. Criticizes the decision for being too broad in that it would protect active euthanasia by physicians on patients who are physically unable to perform the act themselves. Quotes Opinion 2.21. References Opinion 2.211. Larson, *Prescription For Death: A Second Opinion*, 44 DePaul L. Rev. 461, 472 (1995).

Journal 1994 Considers the debate over assisted suicide. Argues that assisted suicide is not an implicit right under the fourteenth amendment's liberty guarantee. Examines the difficulty in establishing under what conditions assisted suicide would be protected. Suggests that giving physicians the authority to determine the appropriateness of assisted suicide furthers no legitimate state interest. Cites Opinion 2.06. References Opinion 2.211. Marzen, *"Out, Out Brief Candle": Constitutionally Prescribed Suicide for the Terminally Ill*, 21 Hastings Const. L.Q. 799, 821 (1994).

Journal 1992 Discusses the right of competent, incurably ill patients to commit suicide. Examines the history of the right an individual has over his or her own body, and how the right to commit suicide has evolved from that concept. Emphasizes the *Cruzan* decision. Concludes that the right of an incurably ill person to commit suicide is a personal issue to be decided outside of the judicial system. References Opinions 2.21 and 2.211. Morgan, Marks, & Harty-Golder, *The Issue of Personal Choice: The Competent Incurable Patient and the Right to Commit Suicide?*, 57 Mo. L. Rev. 1, 44, 45 (1992).

Journal 1992 Discusses the historical, legal, and social arguments both for and against assisted suicide and voluntary active euthanasia. Examines Washington's aid-in-dying initiative. Concludes that only physician-assisted suicide should be legalized. References Opinion 2.211. Note, *Aid-in-Dying: Should We Decriminalize Physician-Assisted Suicide and Physician-Committed Euthanasia?*, XVIII Am. J. Law & Med. 369, 370 (1992).

2.215 Treatment Decisions for Seriously Ill Newborns

The primary consideration for decisions regarding life-sustaining treatment for seriously ill newborns should be what is best for the newborn. Factors that should be weighed are: (1) the chance that therapy will succeed, (2) the risks involved with treatment and nontreatment, (3) the degree to which the therapy, if successful, will extend life, (4) the pain and discomfort associated with the therapy, and (5) the anticipated quality of life for the newborn with and without treatment.

Care must be taken to evaluate the newborn's expected quality of life from the child's perspective. Life-sustaining treatment may be withheld or withdrawn from a newborn when the pain and suffering expected to be endured by the child will overwhelm any potential for joy during his or her life. When an infant suffers extreme neurological damage, and is consequently not capable of experiencing either suffering or joy a decision may be made to withhold or withdraw life-sustaining treatment. When life-sustaining treatment is withheld or withdrawn, comfort care must not be discontinued.

When an infant's prognosis is largely uncertain, as is often the case with extremely premature newborns, all life-sustaining and life-enhancing treatment should be initiated. Decisions about life-sustaining treatment should be made once the prognosis becomes more certain. It is not necessary to attain absolute or near absolute prognostic certainty before life-sustaining treatment is withdrawn, since this goal is often unattainable and risks unnecessarily prolonging the infant's suffering.

Physicians must provide full information to parents of seriously ill newborns regarding the nature of treatments, therapeutic options and expected prognosis with and without therapy, so that parents can make informed decisions for their children about life-sustaining treatment. Counseling services and an opportunity to talk with persons who have had to make similar decisions should be available to parents. Ethics committees or infant-review committees should also be utilized to facilitate parental decision making. These committees should help mediate resolutions of conflicts that may arise among parents, physicians and others involved in the care of the infant. These committees should also be responsible for referring cases to the appropriate public agencies when it is concluded that the parents' decision is not a decision that could reasonably be judged to be in the best interests of the infant. (I, III, IV, V)

Issued June 1994 based on the report, "Treatment Decisions for Seriously Ill Newborns," adopted June 1992.

2.22 Do-Not-Resuscitate Orders

Efforts should be made to resuscitate patients who suffer cardiac or respiratory arrest except when circumstances indicate that cardiopulmonary resuscitation (CPR) would be inappropriate or not in accord with the desires or best interests of the patient.

Patients at risk of cardiac or respiratory failure should be encouraged to express in advance their preferences regarding the use of CPR and this should be documented in the patient's medical record. These discussions should include a description of the procedures encompassed by CPR and, when possible, should occur in an outpatient setting when general treatment preferences are discussed, or as early as possible during hospitalization. The physician has an ethical obligation to honor the resuscitation preferences expressed by the patient. Physicians should not permit their personal value judgments about quality of life to obstruct the implementation of a patient's preferences regarding the use of CPR.

If a patient is incapable of rendering a decision regarding the use of CPR, a decision may be made by a surrogate decision maker, based upon the previously expressed preferences of the patient or, if such preferences are unknown, in accordance with the patient's best interests.

If, in the judgment of the attending physician, it would be inappropriate to pursue CPR, the attending physician may enter a do-not-resuscitate (DNR) order into the patient's record. Resuscitative efforts should be considered inappropriate by the attending physician only if they cannot be expected either to restore cardiac or respiratory function to the patient or to meet established ethical criteria, as defined in the Principles of Medical Ethics and Opinions 2.03 and 2.095. When there is adequate time to do so, the physician must first inform the patient, or the incompetent patient's surrogate, of the content of the DNR order, as well as the basis for its implementation. The physician also should be prepared to discuss appropriate alternatives, such as obtaining a second opinion (e.g., consulting a bioethics committee) or arranging for transfer of care to another physician.

DNR orders, as well as the basis for their implementation, should be entered by the attending physician in the patient's medical record.

DNR orders only preclude resuscitative efforts in the event of cardiopulmonary arrest and should not influence other therapeutic interventions that may be appropriate for the patient. (I, IV)

Issued March 1992 based on the report, "Guidelines for the Appropriate Use of Do-Not-Resuscitate Orders," adopted December 1990 (JAMA. 1991; 265: 1868-1871).

Updated June 1994.

Journal 1997 Examines case law pertaining to medical futility disputes. Reviews hospital policies regarding futility and notes a variety of definitions and guidelines. Concludes that, absent a clear consensus, physicians should not act solely to decide questions of futility. References Opinions 2.035 and 2.22. Johnson, Gibbons, Goldner, Wiener, & Eton, *Legal and Institutional Policy Responses to Medical Futility*, 30 J. Health & Hosp. L. 21, 26, 31, 35, 36 (1997).

Journal 1997 Explores the meaning of cardiopulmonary resuscitation and legal issues involving DNR orders. Considers problems created by DNR orders in operating rooms in light of patients' rights. Concludes that hospitals must adopt clear policies for their surgical teams to follow. Quotes Opinion 8.08. References Opinion 2.22. Lonchyna, *To Resuscitate or Not . . . In the Operating Room: The Need for Hospital Policies for Surgeons Regarding DNR Orders*, 6 Annals Health L. 209, 215, 217 (1997).

Journal 1997 Considers individuals' right to die and the value of a wrongful living tort. Proposes that courts should reject any cause of action for wrongful living in situations where patient advance directives are not honored by physicians. References Opinion 2.22. Milani, *Better Off Dead Than Disabled?: Should Courts Recognize A "Wrongful Living" Cause of Action When Doctors Fail to Honor Patients' Advance Directives?*, 54 Wash. & Lee L. Rev. 149, 151-52 (1997).

Journal 1994 Considers how greater patient autonomy has led to situations in which medical care may be viewed as futile. Examines cases in which physicians' medical judgments conflict with requests for medical treatment by patients or families. Suggests that the law has intruded too far into this area of medicine. Quotes Opinion 2.035. Cites Opinions 2.03, 2.095, 2.17, 2.19, 2.20, and 2.22. Cultice, *Medical Futility: When Is Enough, Enough?*, 27 J. Health & Hosp. Law 225, 230, 256 (1994).

Journal 1993 Examines the question of when medical treatment is futile. Discusses physician, patient, and societal concerns about futility. Concludes that futility decisions should be left to physicians. Cites Opinion 2.22. Bennett, *When Is Medical Treatment "Futile"?*, 9 Issues in Law & Med. 35, 39 (1993).

Journal 1993 Considers how patient self-determination may be affected by cardiopulmonary resuscitation and Do-Not-Resuscitate policies. Proposes a traditional informed consent model for medical decision making in this context. Opposes a "futility" exception to informed consent as being violative of a physician's fiduciary duties to patients. Cites Opinion 8.07 (1986) [now Opinion 8.08]. References Opinion 2.22. Boozang, *Death Wish: Resuscitating Self-Determination for the Critically Ill*, 35 Ariz. L. Rev. 23, 24, 28, 52 (1993).

Journal 1993 Discusses the problem of physicians withholding needed medical treatment from HIV-infected infants. Explores the medical aspects of infant HIV infection. Considers ethical and legal issues involving nontreatment. Concludes that current law should be expanded to eliminate this discrimination. Quotes Opinions 2.09, 2.17, 2.20, 2.22, 4.04, and 8.03. Crossley, *Of Diagnoses and Discrimination: Discriminatory Nontreatment of Infants With HIV Infection*, 93 Columbia L. Rev. 1581, 1620, 1621 (1993).

Journal 1993 Discusses the relationship between a physician's professional conscience and end of life decision making. Considers the issue of futile medical treatment—and a physician's responsibility to provide such treatment. Examines case law concerning a patient's right to demand treatment and a physician's obligation to provide it. Proposes a model for resolving physician-patient conflicts in this context. References Opinions 2.20 and 2.22. Daar, *A Clash at the Bedside: Patient Autonomy v. A Physician's Professional Conscience*, 44 Hastings L. J. 1241, 1257, 1268, 1286 (1993).

Journal 1993 Discusses the ethical implications of the American Heart Association's (AHA) Guidelines for Cardiopulmonary Resuscitation and Emergency Cardiac Care. Discusses the AHA's acknowledgment of medical futility, but questions whether its views adequately reflect current ethical perceptions. Proposes ways in which the guidelines should be reformed. References Opinion 2.22. Jecker & Schneiderman, *An Ethical Analysis of the Use of "Futility" in the 1992 American Heart Association Guidelines for Cardiopulmonary Resuscitation and Emergency Cardiac Care*, 153 Arch. Intern. Med. 2195, 2197 (1993).

Journal 1993 Examines the American Heart Association's guidelines for withholding cardiopulmonary resuscitation in emergency medical service systems and criticizes them for being too strict. Argues that a mechanism should be created to facilitate prehospital DNR orders and ensure that they are followed. References Opinion 2.22. McIntyre, *Loosening Criteria for Withholding Prehospital Cardiopulmonary Resuscitation*, 153 Arch. Intern. Med. 2189, 2190 (1993).

Journal 1992 Examines several issues regarding persistent vegetative state (PVS) patients, including whether PVS patients are really dead, whether nutrition and hydration should be withheld, whether life-sustaining treatments are futile or medically inappropriate, and whether ordinary standards for decision making should be applied to PVS patients. Concludes that life-sustaining therapy may be withheld or continued, but that withdrawal of nutrition and hydration, as well as active euthanasia, present more difficult questions. References Opinions 2.20 and 2.22. Brody, *Special Ethical Issues in the Management of PVS Patients*, 20 Law, Med. & Health Care 104, 109 (1992).

Journal 1992 Discusses "Do-Not-Resuscitate" (DNR) orders in light of the Patient Self-Determination Act. Considers occasions when it may be inappropriate to follow such orders. Proposes a policy of required reconsideration of DNR orders in hospitals when a patient enters a treatment setting in which discreet, time-limited therapies are offered that may precipitate cardiac arrest. References Opinion 2.22. Cohen & Cohen, *Required Reconsideration of "Do-Not-Resuscitate" Orders in the Operating Room and Certain Other Treatment Settings*, 20 Law, Med. & Health Care 354, 356 (1992).

Journal 1992 Examines ethical issues surrounding cardiopulmonary resuscitation and emergency cardiac care. Discusses advance directives and proxy decision making, medical futility, resource allocation, and Do-Not-Resuscitate orders. Concludes with a discussion of legal considerations. References Opinions 2.20 and 2.22. Comment, *Ethical Considerations in Resuscitation*, 268 J.A.M.A. 2282, 2283, 2287 (1992).

Journal 1992 Considers the debate surrounding medical futility. Observes that this debate is encouraging reexamination of the nature of patient entitlement to medical care as well as the "ends of medicine." References Opinions 2.20, 2.21, and 2.22. Miles, *Medical Futility*, 20 Law, Med. & Health Care 310, 311, 313 (1992).

Journal 1992 Examines the significance of natural death acts in light of the *Cruzan* decision. Explains how the "terminal condition" requirement in these statutes may reduce the number of people who fall within the scope of coverage. Also indicates that omission of nutrition and hydration from the list of treatments that may be withdrawn limits patient choices. Concludes with a discussion of practical problems faced by persons executing living wills. Quotes Opinion 2.20. References Opinion 2.22. Note, *State Natural Death Acts: Illusory Protection of Individuals' Life-Sustaining Treatment Decisions*, 29 Harvard J. Legis. 175, 186, 194, 195, 201 (1992).

Journal 1992 Discusses results of a study that evaluated the impact of ethics education on Do-Not-Resuscitate (DNR) practices by house officers. Concludes that educational programs improve care for DNR patients. References Opinion 2.22. Sulmasy, Geller, Faden, & Levine, *The Quality of Mercy: Caring for Patients With "Do Not Resuscitate" Orders*, 267 J.A.M.A. 682 (1992).

Journal 1991 Examines the involvement of the legal system in end-of-life medical decision making. Questions whether the law should intrude into the domain. Concludes that judges should become involved primarily to address the "terms of reconciliation" between physicians and patients. References Opinion 2.22. Flick, *The Due Process of Dying*, 79 Cal. L. Rev. 1121, 1152 (1991).

Journal 1990 Examines cardiopulmonary resuscitation policies in North Carolina nursing homes. Finds that a vast majority of nursing homes have written policies, but that there is substantial variation among them. Concludes that such variations risk limiting or ignoring the personal rights of residents. References Opinions 2.20 and 2.22. Brunetti, Weiss, Studenski, & Clipp, *Cardiopulmonary Resuscitation Policies and Practices: A Statewide Nursing Home Study*, 150 Arch. Intern. Med. 121, 122 (1990).

2.225 Optimal Use of Orders-Not-to-Intervene and Advance Directives

More rigorous efforts in advance care planning are required in order to tailor end-of-life care to the preferences of patients so that they can experience a satisfactory last chapter in their lives. There is need for better availability and tracking of advance directives, and more uniform adoption of form documents that can be honored in all states of the United States. The discouraging evidence of inadequate end-of-life decision making indicates the necessity of several improvement strategies:

(1) Patients and physicians should make use of advisory as well as statutory documents. Advisory documents aim to accurately represent a patient's wishes and are legally binding under law. Statutory documents give physicians immunity from malpractice for following a patient's wishes. If a form is not available that combines the two, an advisory document should be appended to the state statutory form.

(2) Advisory documents should be based on validated worksheets, thus ensuring reasonable confidence that preferences for end-of-life treatment can be fairly and effectively elicited and recorded, and that they are applicable to medical decisions.

(3) Physicians should directly discuss the patient's preferences with the patient and the patient's proxy. These discussions should be held ahead of time whenever possible. The key steps of structuring a core discussion and of signing and recording the document in the medical record should not be delegated to a junior member of the health care team.

(4) Central repositories should be established so that completed advisory documents, state statutory documents, identification of a proxy, and identification of the primary physician, can be obtained efficiently in emergency and urgent circumstances as well as routinely.

(5) Health care facilities should honor, and physicians use, a range of orders on the Doctor's Order Sheet to indicate patient wishes regarding avoidable treatments that might otherwise be given on an emergency basis or by a covering physician with less knowledge of the patient's wishes. Treatment avoidance orders might include, along with a Do Not Resuscitate (DNR) order, some of the following: Full Comfort Care Only (FCCO); Do Not Intubate (DNI); Do Not Defibrillate (DND); Do Not Leave Home (DNLH); Do Not Transfer (DNTransfer); No Intravenous Lines (NIL); No Blood Draws (NBD); No Feeding Tube (NFT); No Vital Signs (NVS); and so forth. One common new order, Do Not Treat (DNT), is specifically not included in this list, since it may unintentionally convey the message that no care should be given and the patient may lose the intense attention due to a dying person; FCCO serves the same purpose without the likely misinterpretation. As with DNR orders, these treatment avoidance orders should be revisited periodically to ensure their continued applicability. Active comfort care orders might include Allow Visitors Extended Hours (AVEH) and Inquire About Comfort (IAC) b.i.d. (twice daily). (I)

Issued June 1998 based on the report, "Optimal Use of Orders-Not-to-Intervene and Advance Directives," adopted June 1996.

2.23 HIV Testing

Human Immunodeficiency Virus (HIV) testing is appropriate and should be encouraged for the diagnosis and treatment of HIV infection or of medical conditions that may be affected by HIV. Treatment may prolong the lives of those with AIDS and prolong the symptom-free period in those with an asymptomatic HIV infection. Wider testing is imperative to ensure that individuals in need of treatment are identified and treated.

Physicians should ensure that HIV testing is conducted in a way that respects patient autonomy and assures patient confidentiality as much as possible.

The physician should secure the patient's informed consent specific for HIV testing before testing is performed. Because of the need for pretest counseling and the potential consequences of an HIV test on an individual's job, housing, insurability, and social relationships, the consent should be specific for HIV testing. Consent for HIV testing cannot be inferred from a general consent to treatment.

When a health care provider is at risk for HIV infection because of the occurrence of puncture injury or mucosal contact with potentially infected bodily fluids, it is acceptable to test the patient for HIV infection even if the patient refuses consent. When testing without consent is performed in accordance with the law, the patient should be given the customary pretest counseling.

The confidentiality of the results of HIV testing must be maintained as much as possible and the limits of a patient's confidentiality should be known to the patient before consent is given.

Exceptions to confidentiality are appropriate when necessary to protect the public health or when necessary to protect individuals, including health care workers, who are endangered by persons infected with HIV. If a physician knows that a seropositive individual is endangering a third party, the physician should, within the constraints of the law: (1) attempt to persuade the infected patient to cease endangering the third party; (2) if persuasion fails, notify authorities; and (3) if the authorities take no action, notify the endangered third party.

In order to limit the public spread of HIV infection, physicians should encourage voluntary testing of patients at risk for infection.

It is unethical to deny treatment to HIV-infected individuals because they are HIV seropositive or because they are unwilling to undergo HIV testing, except in the instance where knowledge of the patient's HIV status is vital to the appropriate treatment of the patient. When a patient refuses to be tested after being informed of the physician's medical opinion, the physician may transfer the patient to a second physician who is willing to manage the patient's care in accordance with the patient's preferences about testing. (I, IV)

Issued March 1992 based on the report, "Ethical Issues Involved in the Growing AIDS Crisis," adopted December 1987 (JAMA. 1988; 259: 1360-1361).

Updated June 1994.

Journal 1996 Discusses conflict between physicians' duty of confidentiality to patients and physicians' obligation to warn third parties of foreseeable injuries. Examines physicians' current legal responsibility to breach confidentiality to prevent the spread of infectious diseases, including AIDS. Identifies guidelines for physicians. Cites Opinions 2.23 and 5.057. Comment, *Taking Tarasoff Where No One Has Gone Before: Looking at "Duty to Warn" Under the AIDS Crisis*, 15 St. Louis U. Pub. L. Rev. 471, 499 (1996).

Journal 1995 Explores the ramifications of enacting statutes that criminalize HIV transmission. Observes that such statutes would pose a disincentive for testing and also infringe upon the patient's right to confidentiality because criminal prosecutions are a matter of public record. Concludes that legislatures must carefully consider such issues when drafting legislation to prevent the spread of HIV. Quotes Opinion 2.23. O'Toole, *HIV-Specific Crime Legislation: Targeting an Epidemic for Criminal Prosecution*, 10 J.L. & Health 183, 195, 199 (1995).

Journal 1990 Explores potential physician tort liability for failure to warn at risk individuals of the danger of being infected by the physician's HIV-positive patient. Analyzes the legal bases for such claims and finds strong precedent for imposing liability. Notes that the Centers for Disease Control promulgated standards dealing with this issue and that courts are likely to look to such standards for guidance. Concludes that there is a legal duty requiring health care professionals to warn those persons foreseeably at risk of being infected by an HIV-positive patient. References Opinion 2.23. Labowitz, *Beyond Tarasoff: AIDS and the Obligation to Breach Confidentiality*, 9 St. Louis Univ. Pub. L. Rev. 495, 514 (1990).

Journal 1990 Considers the tension between confidentiality and the duty to warn in the context of AIDS and HIV. Examines the various ways states have dealt with this issue, exploring applicable statutes and case law. Analyzes current state health programs designed to curb the spread of HIV. Considers the appropriateness of mandatory reporting and partner notification. Proposes legal reforms in this area. References Opinion 2.23. Price, *Between Scylla and Charybdis: Charting a Course to Reconcile the Duty of Confidentiality and the Duty to Warn in the AIDS Context*, 94 Dickinson L. Rev. 435, 477 (1990).

3.00 Opinions on Interprofessional Relations

Nonscientific Practitioners

It is unethical to engage in or to aid and abet in treatment which has no scientific basis and is dangerous, is calculated to deceive the patient by giving false hope, or which may cause the patient to delay in seeking proper care.

Physicians should also be mindful of state laws which prohibit a physician from aiding and abetting an unlicensed person in the practice of medicine, aiding or abetting a person with a limited license in providing services beyond the scope of his or her license, or undertaking the joint medical treatment of patients under the foregoing circumstances.

Physicians are otherwise free to accept or decline to serve anyone who seeks their services, regardless of who has recommended that the individual see the physician. (III, VI)

Issued prior to April 1977.

Updated June 1994 and June 1996.

3d Cir. 1984 Osteopathic physician brought class action against hospital and medical staff alleging violation of antitrust statute after hospital refused to grant staff privileges. In determining that the "per se" rule should be used to determine whether the medical staff had violated restraint of trade section of antitrust statute, the court distinguished in a footnote an earlier case which had employed the "rule of reason" analysis in a boycott case involving physicians and chiropractors. The earlier case had concluded that since there was no per se illegal purpose for Principle 3 (1957) [now Opinion 3.01], a rule of reason analysis was appropriate because defendants were asserting a public service/ethical norm justification for their actions; no such rationale for their discriminatory treatment was raised by defendants in the instant case. *Weiss v. York Hosp.*, 745 F.2d 786, 821 n.61, cert. denied, 470 U.S. 1060 (1985).

6th Cir. 1989 Plaintiff, a chiropractic association, alleged that the American Medical Association and several other professional associations violated antitrust law by conspiring to contain and ultimately eliminate the practice of chiropractic. The court provided an historical overview of the Association's gradual, but incomplete, recognition of chiropractors and limited licensed practitioners referring specifically to Principle 3 (1957) as well as to the Opinions and Reports of the Judicial Council Sec. 3, Para. 8 (1969) and to the Opinions and Reports 3.60 and 3.70 (1977) [now Principles VI and Opinions 3.01 and 3.04]. Based on its reading of these Principles and Opinions, the court reversed the trial court's grant of summary judgment to the Association because there remained a material issue of fact of whether it had continued to illegally boycott chiropractic. *Chiropractic Coop. Ass'n v. AMA*, 867 F.2d 270, 272-75.

7th Cir. 1990 Appellate court affirmed district court ruling that American Medical Association and other national professional associations violated federal antitrust laws by illegal conspiracy against chiropractors. Plaintiff alleged in lower court that Association sought by means of boycott to eliminate chiropractic through application of Principle 3 (1957) [now Opinion 3.01] labeling chiropractors as "unscientific practitioners." The appellate court traced the history of the

Association's position regarding chiropractic including references to Principle 3 and Opinion 3.50 (1977) as revised by Opinion 3.01 (1981). The court found the evidence supported finding of an illegal boycott and that injunctive relief was appropriate. *Wilk v. American Medical Ass'n.*, *895 F.2d 352, 355 n.1, 356-58, 361-63, 364 n.2, 365-66, 368-69, 369 n.4.*

7th Cir. 1983 Defendants in antitrust suit appealed the denial of their directed verdict, claiming that the evidence presented by plaintiff failed to show the existence of a conspiracy to eliminate the practice of chiropractic. The Seventh Circuit affirmed the lower court's decision, noting that the adoption of Principle 3 (1957) [now Opinion 3.01], which condemned professional association with any one practicing a method of healing that was not scientifically based, in concert with other actions, might have allowed a jury to reasonably conclude that the defendant orthopaedic association conspired to discourage medical doctors from associating with chiropractors. *Wilk v. American Medical Ass'n.*, *735 F.2d 217, 219, cert. denied, 467 U.S. 1210 (1984).*

7th Cir. 1983 Plaintiff-chiropractors alleged that American Medical Association and others conspired to induce physicians to forego any professional association with chiropractors, to induce hospitals to deny access to chiropractors, and to induce patients to avoid chiropractors, all in violation of the Sherman Act. Plaintiffs argued that Principle 3 (1957) and a 1966 House of Delegates resolution later included in Opinions and Reports of the Judicial Council Sec. 3, Para. 8 (1969) [now Opinion 3.01] reflected defendants' behavior. In response, defendants asserted that their actions were non-commercial and had been taken in the interest of public health, safety, and welfare in the good faith belief that chiropractic was dangerous to patients. The appellate court found the case inappropriate for application of the "per se" rule applying instead the "rule of reason" focusing on whether the challenged activities were anticompetitive. Further, as to the "rule of reason," the court found the defendants could possibly avoid antitrust liability by showing that the dominant motive in their actions was a genuine concern for patient care. However, the court held that only such "patient care" concerns, and not a generalized "public interest" motive could be used as an antitrust defense. *Wilk v. American Medical Ass'n, 719 F.2d 207, 213-15, 225-27, 233, cert. denied, 467 U.S. 1210 (1984).*

N.D. Ill. 1987 Plaintiffs, licensed chiropractors, sued defendant medical associations for violation of antitrust laws. With regard to defendant American Medical Association, plaintiffs alleged that through Principle 3 (1957) [now Opinion 3.01], the Association had successfully precluded physicians from associating professionally with chiropractors. The Association asserted that with the 1980 revision of its Principles, which eliminated the offending portions of Principle 3, any alleged boycott activity directed toward chiropractors had ceased. The court found, however, that plaintiffs did in fact suffer professional rejections and lost opportunities due to lingering effects of the boycott, traceable to the Association's actions. The court also noted that the revised stance of the Association on the legitimacy of chiropractic as reflected in Opinion 3.01 fell short of being an affirmative statement that physicians could professionally associate with chiropractors without fear of reprisal. *Wilk v. American Medical Ass'n., 671 F. Supp 1465, 1470, 1473, 1474, 1475, aff'd, 895 F.2d 352 (7th Cir. 1990).*

N.D. Ill. 1986 In case involving antitrust challenge to rule promulgated by American College of Surgeons, the court concluded that the rule was a "facially legitimate ethical canon" and therefore it would apply the "rule of reason" in deciding the case. The court also rejected defendant's argument that the modified "rule of reason" test in Wilk v. AMA, 719 F.2d 207 (7th Cir. 1983), cert. denied, 467 U.S. 1210 (1984), allowing a defense based upon a "patient care motive" exception to otherwise illegal restraint, should be applicable in this case. The court found that the Wilk exception was limited to Principle 3 (1957) [now Opinion 3.01] pertaining to the importance of scientific method in patient care. *Koefoot v. American College of Surgeons, 652 F. Supp. 882, 889, 890, 891.*

E.D. Mich. 1986 Plaintiff-chiropractors claimed violation of the Sherman Antitrust Act alleging that the American Medical Association conspired with others to injure them professionally and financially. In support of their claim, plaintiffs cited Principle 3 (1957) and the Opinions and Reports of the Judicial Council Sec. 3, Para. 8 (1969) [now Principles VI and Opinions 3.01 and 3.04]. The court, noting the 1977 change in the Association's position regarding chiropractic, reflected in the Opinions and Reports of the Judicial Council 3.60 and 3.70 (1977) [now Opinion 3.04] held that plaintiffs failed to demonstrate evidence of an overt act by the Association within the statutory limitations period. Summary judgment entered for Association. *Chiropractic Coop. Ass'n v. AMA, 1986-2 Trade Cas. (CCH) ¶ 67,294, aff'd in part and rev'd in part, 867 F.2d 270 (6th Cir. 1989).*

E.D. Mich. 1985 In an antitrust case brought by plaintiff-chiropractic association against the American Medical Association, plaintiffs presented the court with a motion in limine asking that the court strike defendant's affirmative defense of a good faith concern with public health and patient care. Plaintiffs argued that the defense was "unprecedented, in conflict with existing law and dramatically wrong." Plaintiffs referred to Principle 3 (1957) [now Principle VI and Opinions 3.01 and 3.04] as the source of the AMA's antitrust violations. The court denied plaintiffs' motion to strike, stating that under the "rule of reason" test, the Association had the right to present evidence that its actions furthered the public interest and patient care. *Chiropractic Coop. Ass'n v. AMA*, 617 F. Supp. 264, 266, aff'd in part and rev'd in part, 867 F.2d 270 (6th Cir. 1989).

D.N.M. 1987 In an antitrust action against major health insurance provider and state medical society, group of chiropractors alleged that a conspiracy existed in which the insurer refused to provide health cost reimbursement coverage for chiropractic services. Plaintiffs urged court to apply a "per se" analysis, rather than the "rule of reason" analysis to determine the legality of defendants' restrictive practices. The court declined to apply the "per se" test. In part, court's conclusion was based on view that concerns of defendant-physicians about relationship with chiropractors because of ethical restrictions imposed by Principle 3 (1957) [now Principle VI and Opinions 3.01 and 3.04] deserved more consideration than the "per se" test would afford. *Johnson v. Blue Cross/Blue Shield*, 677 F. Supp. 1112, 1118.

Ariz. 1965 Physician appealed denial of medical license which was based on alleged violations of local medical society rules and Principles 3, 5, and 10 (1957) [now Principles III and VII, and Opinions 3.01, 8.11, and 9.06]. Alleged violations included treating a patient without first obtaining a prior treating physician's permission, inadequate patient care, performing operations without hospital privileges, and signing the medical record of a deceased patient who had been treated by interns. The court held that the evidence failed to show any clear violation of the Principles and that a local medical society had no right to prescribe a code of ethics for state licensing purposes. *Arizona State Bd. of Medical Examiners v. Clark*, 97 Ariz. 205, 398 P.2d 908, 914-915, 915 n.3.

N.J. 1963 Plaintiff, an osteopath fully licensed to practice medicine and surgery by the state, sought to apply for staff privileges at defendant-hospital, a private, not for profit, general hospital. Defendant refused application based on a bylaw requiring staff members to be graduates of medical schools approved by the American Medical Association and members of the county medical society. In plaintiff's action challenging refusal of the application, the court held that the hospital's power to pass upon staff applications was a fiduciary power, and that plaintiff's application was to be considered on its own merit without regard to the bylaw provision. In its opinion, the court noted the historic opposition of the American Medical Association to osteopathy. The court also referred to a position adopted by the Association in 1961, later reflected in Opinions and Reports of the Judicial Council Sec. 3, Para. 7 (1965) [now Opinion 3.01], allowing for association with osteopaths who follow "scientific principles." *Greisman v. Newcomb Hosp.*, 40 N.J. 389, 192 A.2d 817, 819.

N.J. Super. 1960 Plaintiff, a graduate of a school of osteopathy and licensed to practice medicine and surgery in New Jersey, sought to compel the defendant medical society to admit him to full membership. Defendant claimed as an affirmative defense that to admit plaintiff would violate Principle 3 (1957) [now Principle VI and Opinion 3.01] because plaintiff possessed a degree in osteopathy rather than an M.D. The court noted that the defendant society had virtually monopolistic control of medical practice in the state and that exclusion from membership caused substantial injury. In view of this, the court ordered the defendant society to admit plaintiff to its membership. To bar membership of a licensed graduate of an approved school of osteopathy would, the court held, violate public policy. *Falcone v. Middlesex County Medical Soc'y*, 62 N.J. Super. 184, 162 A.2d 324, 328-329, aff'd, 34 N.J. 582, 170 A.2d 791 (1961).

Journal 1996 Explores the incorporation of holistic health care into modern medical practice. Observes that the AMA previously condemned association with chiropractors as unethical. Concludes that alternative health care methods need to be further integrated into patient treatment plans where warranted. Quotes Principle 3 (1956) [amended and now Opinion 3.01]. Cohen, *Holistic Health Care: Including Alternative and Complementary Medicine in Insurance and Regulatory Schemes*, 38 Ariz. L. Rev. 83, 92 (1996).

3.02 Nurses

The primary bond between the practices of medicine and nursing is mutual ethical concern for patients. One of the duties in providing reasonable care is fulfilled by a nurse who carries out the orders of the attending physician. Where orders appear to the nurse to be in error or contrary to customary medical and nursing practice, the physician has an ethical obligation to hear the nurse's concern and explain those orders to the nurse involved. The ethical physician should neither expect nor insist that nurses follow orders contrary to standards of good medical and nursing practice. In emergencies, when prompt action is necessary and the physician is not immediately available, a nurse may be justified in acting contrary to the physician's standing orders for the safety of the patient. Such occurrences should not be considered to be a breakdown in professional relations. (IV, V)

Issued June 1983.

Updated June 1994.

3.03   **Opinion 3.03, Optometry,** was deleted in June 1994.

3.03   **Allied Health Professionals**

Physicians often practice in concert with allied health professionals such as, but not limited to, optometrists, nurse anesthetists, nurse midwives, and physician assistants in the course of delivering appropriate medical care to their patients. In doing so, physicians should be guided by the following principles:
(1) It is ethical for a physician to work in consultation with or employ allied health professionals, as long as they are appropriately trained and duly licensed to perform the activities being requested.
(2) Physicians have an ethical obligation to the patients for whom they are responsible to insure that medical and surgical conditions are appropriately evaluated and treated.
(3) Physicians may teach in recognized schools for the allied health professionals for the purpose of improving the quality of their education. The scope of teaching may embrace subjects which are within the legitimate scope of the allied health profession and which are designed to prepare students to engage in the practice of the profession within the limits prescribed by law.
(4) It is inappropriate to substitute the services of an allied health professional for those of a physician when the allied health professional is not appropriately trained and duly licensed to provide the medical services being requested. (I, V, VII)

Issued December 1997.

3.04   **Referral of Patients**

A physician may refer a patient for diagnostic or therapeutic services to another physician, limited practitioner, or any other provider of health care services permitted by law to furnish such services, whenever he or she believes that this may benefit the patient. As in the case of referrals to physician-specialists, referrals to limited practitioners should be based on their individual competence and ability to perform the services needed by the patient. A physician should not so refer a patient unless the physician is confident that the services provided on referral will be performed competently and in accordance with accepted scientific standards and legal requirements. (V, VI)

Issued prior to April 1977.

6th Cir. 1989 Plaintiff, a chiropractic association, alleged that the American Medical Association and several other professional associations violated antitrust law by conspiring to contain and ultimately eliminate the practice of chiropractic. The court provided an historical overview of the Association's gradual, but incomplete, recognition of chiropractors and "limited licensed practitioners" referring specifically to Principle 3 (1957) as well as to the Opinions and Reports of the Judicial Council Sec. 3, Para. 8 (1969) and to the Opinions and Reports 3.60 and 3.70 (1977) [now Principles VI and Opinions 3.01 and 3.04]. Based on its reading of these Principles and Opinions, the court reversed the trial court's grant of summary judgment to the Association because there remained a material issue of fact of whether it had continued to illegally boycott chiropractic. *Chiropractic Coop. Ass'n v. AMA*, 867 F.2d 270, 272-75.

E.D. Mich. 1986 Plaintiff-chiropractors claimed violation of the Sherman Antitrust Act alleging that the American Medical Association conspired with others to injure them professionally and financially. In support of their claim, plaintiffs cited Principle 3 (1957) and the Opinions and Reports of the Judicial Council Sec. 3, Para. 8 (1969) [now Principles VI and Opinions 3.01 and 3.04]. The court, noting the 1977 change in the Association's position regarding chiropractic reflected in the Opinions and Reports of the Judicial Council 3.60 and 3.70 (1977) [now Opinion 3.04] held that plaintiffs failed to demonstrate evidence of an overt act by the Association within the statutory limitations period. Summary judgment entered for Association. *Chiropractic Coop. Ass'n v. AMA*, 1986-2 Trade Cas. (CCH) ¶ 67,294, aff'd in part and rev'd in part, 867 F.2d 270 (6th Cir. 1989).

E.D. Mich. 1985 In an antitrust case brought by plaintiff-chiropractic association against the American Medical Association, plaintiffs presented the court with a motion in limine asking that the court strike defendant's affirmative defense of a good faith concern with public health and patient care. Plaintiffs argued that the defense was "unprecedented, in conflict with existing law and dramatically wrong." Plaintiffs referred to Principle 3 (1957) [now Principle VI and Opinions 3.01 and 3.04] as the source of the AMA's antitrust violations. The court denied plaintiffs' motion to strike, stating that under the "rule of reason" test, the Association had the right to present evidence that its actions furthered the public interest and patient care. *Chiropractic Coop. Ass'n v. AMA*, 617 F. Supp. 264, 266, aff'd in part and rev'd in part, 867 F.2d 270 (6th Cir. 1989).

D.N.M. 1987 In an antitrust action against major health insurance provider and state medical society, group of chiropractors alleged that a conspiracy existed in which the insurer refused to provide health cost reimbursement coverage for chiropractic services. Plaintiffs urged court to apply a "per se" analysis, rather than the "rule of reason" analysis to determine the legality of defendants' restrictive practices. The court declined to apply the "per se" test. In part, court's conclusion was based on view that concerns of defendant-physicians about relationship with chiropractors because of ethical restrictions imposed by Principle 3 (1957) [now Principle VI and Opinions 3.01 and 3.04] deserved more consideration than the "per se" test would afford. *Johnson v. Blue Cross/Blue Shield*, 677 F. Supp. 1112, 1118.

S.D. Ohio 1995 Physician accused of soliciting bribes in return for referring patients to Medicaid provider moved to dismiss the indictment which alleged mail fraud and violations of Medicaid antikickback statute. In denying physician's motion to dismiss indictment, the court noted that physician's fiduciary duty under Opinion 3.04 supported an intangible rights mail fraud charge. *United States v. Neufeld*, 908 F. Supp. 491, 500.

Journal 1994 Focuses on physicians' legal and ethical duties to pregnant women to provide medical information relevant to patient choice regarding abortion and to make referrals for services that physicians are unable or unwilling to perform. Argues that physicians' own moral views on abortion do not excuse obligations to facilitate choice for patients. Concludes that medical educators, professional associations, women's groups, and state legislatures should address these issues. Cites Opinions 3.04 and 8.04. Law, *Silent No More: Physicians' Legal and Ethical Obligations to Patients Seeking Abortions*, 21 N.Y.U. Rev. L. & Soc. Change 279, 289, 290, 300 (1994).

Journal 1993 Considers the problem of exclusion of chiropractors by health maintenance organizations (HMOs) and the effect it has on access to care. Focuses on how antitrust laws might be used to prevent this exclusion by discussing two theories under which it might be illegal. Concludes that chiropractors challenging their exclusion from HMOs may establish an antitrust claim under the theories of "structural conspiracy" and "tacit collusion" if certain criteria are met. Quotes Opinion 3.04. Note, *HMO Exclusion of Chiropractors*, 66 So. Cal. L. Rev. 807, 823 (1993).

3.041 Chiropractic

It is ethical for a physician to associate professionally with chiropractors provided that the physician believes that such association is in the best interests of his or her patient. A physician may refer a patient for diagnostic or therapeutic services to a chiropractor permitted by law to furnish such services whenever the physician believes that this may benefit his or her patient. Physicians may also ethically teach in recognized schools of chiropractic. (V, VI)

Issued March 1992.

3.05   **Opinion 3.05, Specialists,** was deleted in June 1994.

3.06 Sports Medicine

Physicians should assist athletes to make informed decisions about their participation in amateur and professional contact sports which entail risks of bodily injury.

The professional responsibility of the physician who serves in a medical capacity at an athletic contest or sporting event is to protect the health and safety of the contestants. The desire of spectators, promoters of the event or even the injured athlete that he or she not be removed from the contest should not be controlling. The physician's judgment should be governed only by medical considerations. (I, VII)

Issued June 1983.

Updated June 1994.

Journal 1993 Discusses an athlete's rights to assume serious health risks by playing a sport, despite a physical abnormality or medical condition. Considers the team physician's conflicting duties toward the patient/player and the team. Proposes that medical societies establish guidelines to assist team physicians in making participation recommendations and to aid courts in setting relevant standards. Emphasizes an athlete's duty to use reasonable care to protect his or her health. Concludes that physicians or athletes should bear legal responsibility if either violates their obligations in this context. Cites Opinion 3.06. Mitten, *Team Physicians and Competitive Athletes: Allocating Legal Responsibility for Athletic Injuries*, 55 U. Pitt. L. Rev. 129, 140 (1993).

3.07   **Opinion 3.07, Teaching,** was deleted in June 1994.

3.08   Sexual Harassment and Exploitation Between Medical Supervisors and Trainees

Sexual harassment may be defined as sexual advances, requests for sexual favors, and other verbal or physical conduct of a sexual nature when (1) such conduct interferes with an individual's work or academic performance or creates an intimidating, hostile, or offensive work or academic environment or (2) accepting or rejecting such conduct affects or may be perceived to affect employment decisions or academic evaluations concerning the individual. Sexual harassment is unethical.

Sexual relationships between medical supervisors and their medical trainees raise concerns because of inherent inequalities in the status and power that medical supervisors wield in relation to medical trainees and may adversely affect patient care. Sexual relationships between a medical trainee and a supervisor even when consensual are not acceptable regardless of the degree of supervision in any given situation. The supervisory role should be eliminated if the parties involved wish to pursue their relationship. (II, IV, VII)

Issued March 1992 based on the report, "Sexual Harassment and Exploitation Between Medical Supervisors and Trainees," adopted June 1989.

Updated June 1994.

4.00 Opinions on Hospital Relations

4.01 Admission Fee

Charging a separate and distinct fee for the incidental, administrative, non-medical service the physician performs in securing the admission of a patient to a hospital is unethical. Physicians should derive their income from medical services rendered, in keeping with the traditions of the American Medical Association. (IV)

Issued prior to April 1977.

Updated June 1994.

4.02 Assessments, Compulsory

It is improper to condition medical staff membership or privileges on compulsory assessments for any purpose. However, self-imposed assessments by vote of the medical staff are acceptable. (IV)

Issued prior to April 1977.

Updated June 1994.

4.03 Billing for House Staff and Student Services

When a physician assumes responsibility for the services rendered to a patient by a resident or student, the physician may ethically bill the patient for services which were performed under the physician's direct personal observation, direction and supervision. (II)

Issued prior to April 1977.

Updated June 1994.

4.04 Economic Incentives and Levels of Care

The primary obligation of the hospital medical staff is to safeguard the quality of care provided within the institution. The medical staff has the responsibility to perform essential functions on behalf of the hospital in accordance with licensing laws and accreditation requirements. Treatment or hospitalization that is willfully excessive or inadequate constitutes unethical practice. The organized medical staff has an obligation to avoid wasteful practices and unnecessary treatment that may cause the hospital needless expense. In a situation where the economic interests of the hospital are in conflict with patient welfare, patient welfare takes priority. (I, II, IV, V, VI)

Issued June 1986.

Journal 1996 Considers the change from traditional medical care systems to managed care, noting the conflicts of interest this creates between physicians' ethical obligations and financial concerns. Discusses these issues in the context of managed behavioral health care. Suggests community-based care and social supports as a solution. Quotes Opinion 2.03 and 4.04. Petrila, *Ethics, Money, and the Problem of Coercion in Managed Behavioral Health Care*, 40 St. Louis U. L. J. 359, 377 (1996).

Journal 1994 Observes that health care reform proposals present significant challenges to the role and ethics of attending physicians. Emphasizes that reform proposals must set forth the role envisioned for physicians and must articulate an acceptable ethical framework within which physicians may fulfill that role. Quotes Opinions 4.04, 9.121, and 9.122. Cites Opinions 2.03, 2.09, 5.01, and 8.03. Wolf, *Health Care Reform and the Future of Physician Ethics*, 24 Hastings Center Rep. 28, 32, 40 (March/April 1994).

Journal 1993 Discusses the problem of physicians withholding needed medical treatment from HIV-infected infants. Explores the medical aspects of infant HIV infection. Considers ethical and legal issues involving nontreatment. Concludes that current law should be expanded to eliminate this discrimination. Quotes Opinions 2.09, 2.17, 2.20, 2.22, 4.04, and 8.03. Crossley, *Of Diagnoses and Discrimination: Discriminatory Nontreatment of Infants With HIV Infection*, 93 Columbia L. Rev. 1581, 1620, 1621 (1993).

Journal 1992 Examines the major health care rationing issues facing the United States including increasing costs and decreasing access. Considers the reasons for the rising cost of medical care as well as possible solutions. Explores the concept of the standard of care and considers whether it should be changed. Concludes that the standard of care should not be changed and that rationing should be a separate enterprise undertaken pursuant to explicit criteria. Quotes Opinions 2.03, 2.09, and 4.04. Hirshfeld, *Should Ethical and Legal Standards for Physicians Be Changed to Accommodate New Models for Rationing Health Care?*, 140 Univ. Pa. L. Rev. 1809, 1816 (1992).

Journal 1990 Discusses efforts of third party payors to control health care expenditures for beneficiaries. Focuses on use of financial incentives to encourage providers to minimize the amount of care provided. Also discusses monitoring of requests for payment to determine necessity of care provided. Raises questions regarding impact of cost control mechanisms on quality of care, observing that available evidence is equivocal. Evaluates importance of disclosure to beneficiaries of use of financial incentives to limit care as well as other cost control mechanisms. Concludes that financial incentives and other cost control techniques should be disclosed and that the rationale for such disclosure is compelling. Quotes Opinions 2.03, 2.09, and 8.03. Cites Opinions 2.19, 4.04, and 4.06. Hirshfeld, *Should Third Party Payors of Health Care Services Disclose Cost Control Mechanisms to Potential Beneficiaries?*, 14 Seton Hall Legis. J. 115, 130, 131, 144, 145, 146 (1990).

4.05 Organized Medical Staff

The organized medical staff performs essential hospital functions even though it may often consist primarily of independent practicing physicians who are not hospital employees. As a practical matter, however, the organized medical staff may enjoy a dual status. In addition to functioning as a division of the hospital, members of the organized medical staff may choose to act as a group for the purpose of communicating and dealing with the governing board and others with respect to matters that concern the interest of the organized medical staff and its members. This is ethical so long as there is no adverse interference with patient care or violation of applicable laws. (IV, VI)

Issued July 1983.

Updated June 1994.

4.06   Physician-Hospital Contractual Relations

There are various financial or contractual arrangements that physicians and hospitals may enter into and find mutually satisfactory. A physician may, for example, be a hospital employee, a hospital-associated medical specialist, or an independent practitioner with staff privileges. The form of the contractual or financial arrangement between physicians and hospitals depends on the facts and circumstances of each situation. A physician may be employed by a hospital for a fixed annual amount, for a certain amount per hour, or pursuant to other similar arrangements that are related to the professional services, skill, education, expertise, or time involved. (VI)

Issued March 1981.

Updated June 1994.

Journal 1990 Discusses efforts of third party payors to control health care expenditures for beneficiaries. Focuses on use of financial incentives to encourage providers to minimize the amount of care provided. Also discusses monitoring of requests for payment to determine necessity of care provided. Raises questions regarding impact of cost control mechanisms on quality of care, observing that available evidence is equivocal. Evaluates importance of disclosure to beneficiaries of use of financial incentives to limit care as well as other cost control mechanisms. Concludes that financial incentives and other cost control techniques should be disclosed and that the rationale for such disclosure is compelling. Quotes Opinions 2.03, 2.09, and 8.03. Cites Opinions 2.19, 4.04, and 4.06. Hirshfeld, *Should Third Party Payors of Health Care Services Disclose Cost Control Mechanisms to Potential Beneficiaries?*, 14 Seton Hall Legis. J. 115, 130, 131, 144, 145, 146 (1990).

4.07   Staff Privileges

The mutual objective of both the governing board and the medical staff is to improve the quality and efficiency of patient care in the hospital. Decisions regarding hospital privileges should be based upon the training, experience, and demonstrated competence of candidates, taking into consideration the availability of facilities and the overall medical needs of the community, the hospital, and especially patients. Privileges should not be based on numbers of patients admitted to the facility or the economic or insurance status of the patient. Personal friendships, antagonisms, jurisdictional disputes, or fear of competition should not play a role in making these decisions. Physicians who are involved in the granting, denying, or termination of hospital privileges have an ethical responsibility to be guided primarily by concern for the welfare and best interests of patients in discharging this responsibility. (IV, VI, VII)

Issued July 1983.

Updated June 1994.

Journal 1990 Presents current issues, policies, legislation, and judicial decisions regarding impaired physicians. Considers confidentiality problems that arise in the disciplinary process. Concludes by proposing enhanced confidentiality requirements in disciplinary proceedings and nationwide adoption of a uniform law in this area. Quotes Opinion 4.07. References Principle IV. Walzer, *Impaired Physicians: An Overview and Update of the Legal Issues*, 11 J. Legal Med. 131, 174, 192 (1990).

5.00 Opinions on Confidentiality, Advertising, and Communications Media Relations

5.01 Advertising and Managed Care Organizations

A physician may provide medical services to members of a prepaid medical care plan or to members of a health maintenance organization which seeks members or subscribers through advertising. Physicians practicing in prepaid plans or managed care organizations are subject to the same ethical principles as are other physicians. Advertising which would lead prospective members or subscribers to believe that the services of a named physician who has a reputation for outstanding skill would be routinely available to all members or subscribers, if in fact this is not so, is deceptive. However, the publication by name of the roster of physicians who provide services to members, the type of practice in which each is engaged, biographical and other relevant information is not a deceptive practice. (II, VI)

Issued prior to April 1977.

Updated June 1996.

Journal 1994 Observes that health care reform proposals present significant challenges to the role and ethics of attending physicians. Emphasizes that reform proposals must set forth the role envisioned for physicians and must articulate an acceptable ethical framework within which physicians may fulfill that role. Quotes Opinions 4.04, 9.121, and 9.122. Cites Opinions 2.03, 2.09, 5.01, and 8.03. Wolf, *Health Care Reform and the Future of Physician Ethics*, 24 *Hastings Center Rep.* 28, 32, 40 (March/April 1994).

5.02 Advertising and Publicity

There are no restrictions on advertising by physicians except those that can be specifically justified to protect the public from deceptive practices. A physician may publicize him- or herself as a physician through any commercial publicity or other form of public communication (including any newspaper, magazine, telephone directory, radio, television, direct mail, or other advertising) provided that the communication shall not be misleading because of the omission of necessary material information, shall not contain any false or misleading statement, or shall not otherwise operate to deceive.

Because the public can sometimes be deceived by the use of medical terms or illustrations that are difficult to understand, physicians should design the form of communication to communicate the information contained therein to the public in a readily comprehensible manner. Aggressive, high pressure advertising and publicity should be avoided if they create unjustified medical expectations or are accompanied by deceptive claims. The key issue, however, is whether advertising or publicity, regardless of format or content, is true and not materially misleading.

The communication may include: (a) the educational background of the physician; (b) the basis on which fees are determined (including charges for specific services); (c) available credit or other methods of payment; and (d) any other nondeceptive information.

Nothing in this opinion is intended to discourage or to limit advertising and representations which are not false or deceptive within the meaning of Section 5 of the Federal Trade Commission Act. At the same time, however, physicians are advised that certain types of communications have a significant potential for deception and should therefore receive special attention. For example, testimonials of patients as to the physician's skill or the quality of the physician's professional services tend to be deceptive when they do not reflect the results that patients with conditions comparable to the testimoniant's condition generally receive.

Objective claims regarding experience, competence and the quality of physicians and the services they provide may be made only if they are factually supportable. Similarly, generalized statements of satisfaction with a physician's services may be made if they are representative of the experiences of that physician's patients.

Because physicians have an ethical obligation to share medical advances, it is unlikely that a physician will have a truly exclusive or unique skill or remedy. Claims that imply such a skill or remedy therefore can be deceptive. Statements that a physician has an exclusive or unique skill or remedy in a particular geographic area, if true, however, are permissible. Similarly, a statement that a physician has cured or successfully treated a large number of cases involving a particular serious ailment is deceptive if it implies a certainty of result and creates unjustified and misleading expectations in prospective patients.

Consistent with federal regulatory standards which apply to commercial advertising, a physician who is considering the placement of an advertisement or publicity release, whether in print, radio or television, should determine in advance that the communication or message is explicitly and implicitly truthful and not misleading. These standards require the advertiser to have a reasonable basis for claims before they are used in advertising. The reasonable basis must be established by those facts known to the advertiser, and those which a reasonable, prudent advertiser should have discovered. Inclusion of the physician's name in advertising may help to assure that these guidelines are being met. (II)

Issued prior to April 1977.

Updated June 1996.

U.S. 1977 Disciplinary sanctions were imposed by state bar against attorneys who violated state rule prohibiting advertising. After state court upheld sanctions, attorneys appealed to Supreme Court arguing that state rule violated federal antitrust laws and was unconstitutional. State bar argued that rule prohibiting advertising was justified to prevent adverse impact on the legal profession. In questioning this assertion, the Court referred to the position of the American Medical Association announced in 235 JAMA 2328 (1976) and included in Opinions and Reports of the Judicial Council 6.00 (1977) [now Opinion 5.02], that the medical profession permits advertising by physicians. The Court held that the state may regulate some aspects of advertising, but that a blanket prohibition against advertising by attorneys was unconstitutional as a violation of the first amendment. *Bates v. State Bar of Ariz., 433 U.S. 350, 369-70 n.20.*

1st Cir. 1966 Physician sued electric shaver manufacturer for libel on basis of its use of reprints of an article quoting a study favorably mentioning manufacturer which allegedly falsely indicated that physician was one of the co-authors of the research study. Plaintiff asserted that he had agreed to participate in the research only if his name was not used in advertising claims since this would be a violation of "established rules of ethics of the American Medical Association," Opinions and Reports of the Judicial Council Sec. 5, Para. 29 (1965) [now Opinion 5.02]. These facts were considered sufficient to submit to the jury. *Sperry Rand Corp. v. Hill, 356 F.2d 181, 184, cert. denied, 384 U.S. 973 (1966).*

2d Cir. 1980 Federal Trade Commission ordered American Medical Association and others to cease, with some exceptions, imposing restraints on advertising and "contract practice" by physicians, as well as on business relations between physicians and laypersons. Commission found restraints violated 15 U.S.C. Sec. 45 (a) (1). See 94 F.T.C. 701 (1979). Association petitioned for judicial review of Commission's order. Court reviewed order, noting specific ethical pronouncements of Association which Commission found improper, including the following: restrictions upon advertising and solicitation, Principle 5 (1957) and Opinions and Reports of the Judicial Council Sec. 5, Para. 11 (1971) [now Opinion 5.02]; restrictions on "contract practice", Principle 6 (1957) and Opinions and Reports of the Judicial Council Sec. 6, Paras. 3, 4, and 5 (1971) [now Opinion 8.05]; and restrictions on business organizations and relations with laypersons, Opinions and Reports of the Judicial Council, Sec.6, Paras. 14 and 15 (1971). The court rejected the Association's argument that its ethical rules did not provide impetus for local and state medical societies to act against physicians violating its rules. Further, the court rejected the Association's position that liability should be precluded because of revisions in the Opinions in 1977 and the Principles in 1980. Specifically, the court found that removal of the ban on patient solicitation and changes reflected in Principles II and IV (1980) did not render Commission's order moot. The order was therefore enforced with modifications. Dissenting judge, referring to 1980 revisions in Principles and to Opinions and Reports of the Judicial Council 4.05 and 6.00 (1977) [now Opinions 5.02 and 8.05], concluded order should not be enforced on grounds of mootness. *American Medical Ass'n v. FTC, 638 F.2d 443, 446, 446 n.1, 448, 449, 449 n.5, 450, 451, 455-57, aff'd, 455 U.S. 676 (1982).*

D.C. Cir. 1980 Professional associations, including American Medical Association, filed for judicial review of a Federal Trade Commission rule limiting the ability of states and professional associations to restrict advertising of eye exams as well as ophthalmic goods and services. Since the United States Supreme Court had found certain restrictions on lawyer advertising unconstitutional while the case was pending, the court remanded the case for further consideration by the Commission. In its analysis of advertising in the eye care profession, the court quoted Principle 5 (1957) and the Opinions and Reports of the Judicial Council Sec. 10, Para. 4 (1971) which prohibited solicitation and advertising. However, the court also noted the intervening changes in the American Medical Association's position regarding advertising, quoting the Opinions and Reports of the Judicial Council 6.00 (1977) [now Opinion 5.02] which permitted nondeceptive advertising. *American Optometric Ass'n v. F.T.C., 626 F.2d 896, 900-01, 913, 914, 914 n.11.*

E.D. Va. 1976 Health planning agency, which sought to compile directory of services and fees of community physicians, and consumer group interested in obtaining such information, challenged state statute which prohibited direct or indirect advertisement by physicians. In holding that the statute violated first amendment rights, court noted that to protect the public from being misled as to medical quality, directory was designed in conformity with American Medical Association advertising guidelines. Court quoted Judicial Council position published in 235 JAMA 2328 (1976), later included in Opinions and Reports of the Judicial Council 6.00 (1977) [now Opinion 5.02] to support analysis. *Health Sys. Agency v. Virginia State Bd. of Medicine, 424 F. Supp. 267, 274, 275 n.11, 276 Appendix B.*

Cal. App. 1968 Plaintiff-physician sought dissolution of a medical partnership with defendant's decedent, and also sought a larger percentage of the partnership receipts based upon an alleged oral agreement. Defendant crossclaimed to enjoin plaintiff from taking physical control of the partnership offices and patient records. The trial court enjoined plaintiff from treating previous patients, requiring that he return all medical records and pay defendant all fees received from patients he had treated during the time of dispute. The appellate court reversed insofar as the injunction prohibited plaintiff from treating the patient who desired to continue to receive his services or prevented access to medical records essential for this purpose, citing Opinions and Reports of the Judicial Council Sec. 7, Para. 16, Sec. 5, Para. 21, and Sec. 9 (1966) [now Opinions 6.08, 5.02, and 5.05] to support view that patients may not be regarded as the subject of ownership. *Jones v. Fakehany, 261 Cal. App. 2d 298, 67 Cal. Rptr. 810, 815, 816 n.1.*

Fla. App. 1968 Physician sued to enjoin county medical association and telephone company from eliminating medical specialty headings in classified section of directory pursuant to guidelines issued by American Medical Association's Judicial Council in June, 1966 [now Opinion 5.02]. The court held that where medical association had no statutory authority to dictate directory listings, association's restrictions interfered with individual physicians' right to contract and deprived them of due process. *Dade County Medical Ass'n v. Samartino, 213 So. 2d 627, 629, n.2, 631.*

Mich. Att'y Gen. 1978 Opinion was requested from state attorney general as to constitutionality of blanket statutory prohibition of advertising by physicians and as to legality of expulsion of a member of a professional society for advertising that is otherwise proper. In finding the statutory restrictions unconstitutional, the opinion refers to the Judicial Council's advertising statement at 235 JAMA 2328 (1976) included as Opinion 6.00 (1977) [now Opinion 5.02]. *Michigan Att'y. Gen. Opinion N. 5024, 1977-78 Att'y Gen. Op. 299, 303.*

N.Y. Sup. 1965 Physician sued publishing company to bar insertion of advertisement for baby and child care products in physician's book, seeking declaration that book contract was void to the extent that it allowed inclusion of such an advertisement. Physician asserted that the advertisement was contrary to public policy, citing Opinions and Reports of the Judicial Council Sec. 5, Para. 29 (1965) [now Opinion 5.02] which stated that a doctor should not lend his name to any product. In rejecting the physician's claim, the court was willing to give careful consideration to the American Medical Association's view but concluded that it did not, in itself, constitute an expression of public policy. *Spock v. Pocket Books, Inc., 48 Misc. 2d 812, 266 N.Y.S.2d 77, 79.*

Journal 1990 Provides an overview of the recent developments in the area of physician advertising. Considers arguments for and against specialty advertising. Analyzes current trends in limiting and restricting physician advertisement. Evaluates the effect of those trends. Proposes alternative solutions to the practical and ethical problems raised. Quotes Opinion 5.02. Olson, *Physician Specialty Advertising: The Tendency to Deceive?, 11 J. Legal Med. 351, 354 (1990).*

Journal 1984 Discusses the AMA policy on physician advertising and identifies several factors that may affect the decision to advertise. Among the important factors are variations in prominence of physician advertising from region to region and state to state, local attitudes of patients and physicians toward physician advertising, and acceptable forms of physician advertising. Quotes Opinion 5.01 (1984) [now Opinion 5.02]. Porter, *Physician Advertising—What is Legal? What is Ethical? What is Acceptable?, 80 Ohio State Med. J. 437, 437, 439 (1984).*

5.025 Physician Advisory or Referral Services by Telecommunication

Telecommunication advisory services, by way of phone, fax or computer, distinct from an existing patient-physician relationship can be a helpful source of medical information for the public. Often, people are not sure where to turn for information of a general medical nature or do not have easy access to other sources of information. Individuals also may be embarrassed about directly bringing up certain questions with their physicians. Although telecommunication advisory services can provide only limited medical services, they can be a useful complement to more comprehensive services, if used properly.

Any telecommunication advisory service should employ certain safeguards to prevent misuse. For example, the physician responding to the call should not make a clinical diagnosis. Diagnosis by telecommunication is done without the benefit of a physician examination or even a face-to-face meeting with the caller. Critical medical data may be unavailable to the physician. Physicians who respond to callers should therefore act within the limitations of telecommunication services and ensure that callers understand the limitations of the services. Under no circumstances should medications be prescribed.

Physicians who respond to the calls should elicit all necessary information from the callers. When callers are charged by the minute, they may try to hurry their calls to limit their costs. As a result, important information may not be disclosed to the physician. Physicians should also ensure that callers do not incur large bills inadvertently or without understanding the billing system.

Physician referral services can also offer important information to the public. Referral services are often provided by medical societies, hospitals and for-profit entities. To ensure that the service bases its recommendation on medically legitimate considerations rather than the likelihood of being paid by the physician, when the service charges physicians a fee to participate, physicians should not pay the service per referral. Also, callers should be told how the list is created. For example, callers should be informed whether the list includes physicians who pay a flat fee to be listed, members of a particular hospital staff or medical society, or physicians who meet some general quality-based criteria.

While these safeguards are described as applying primarily to telephone services, they should be considered equally applicable to any other communication media, such as radio or television, in which the physician and patient do not meet face-to-face. (I, IV, VI)

Issued June 1994.

Updated June 1996.

5.03   **The previous Opinion 5.03, Communications Media: Press Relations,** issued prior to April 1977, was deleted in June 1996 and combined with Opinion 5.04.

5.04   Communications Media: Standards of Professional Responsibility

Physicians are ethically and legally required to protect the personal privacy and other legal rights of patients. When information concerning a specific patient is requested by the media, the physician must obtain the consent of the patient or an authorized representative before releasing such information. The physician may release only the authorized information or that which is public knowledge. The patient-physician relationship and its confidential nature must be maintained.

With these considerations in mind, the physician may assist the representatives of the media in every way possible. When the patient or authorized representative consents to the release of information, physicians should cooperate with the press to insure that medical news is available more promptly and more accurately than would be possible without their assistance. Inasmuch as a diagnosis may be made only by a physician and may depend upon X-ray and laboratory studies, no statement regarding diagnosis should be made except by or on behalf of the attending physician. For the same reason, prognosis will be given only by the attending physician or at the attending physician's direction.

Statements regarding the circumstances surrounding shootings, knifings, and poisonings are properly police matters, and questions whether they were accidental should be referred to the appropriate authorities.

Certain news that is part of the public record, such as deaths, may be made available without the consent of the patient or authorized representative. (IV)

Issued prior to April 1977

Updated June 1994.

Journal 1995 Addresses presidential disability, its past impact on American government, and possible solutions to potential problems. Suggests guidelines for implementation of the Twenty-Fifth Amendment. Examines the effectiveness of a medical commission in determining presidential disability. Proposes enhancement of the role of the President's physician. Quotes Opinion 8.03. Cites Opinions 5.04 and 5.05. Abrams, *The Vulnerable President and the Twenty-Fifth Amendment, with Observations on Guidelines, a Health Commission, and the Role of the President's Physician, 30 Wake Forest L. Rev. 453, 466, 471 (1995).*

Journal 1984 Discusses the broad content of medical records, noting that they are being demanded for use in a variety of contexts. Observes that available ethical and legal guidelines are insufficient to aid physicians in addressing issues of patient privacy and confidentiality. Concludes that there is need for legislation in order to provide suitable guidance to physicians who fulfill an important role in protecting patient privacy. Cites 1981 Opinions 5.03, 5.04, 5.05 [now Opinion 5.06], 5.06 [now Opinion 5.07], 5.07 [now Opinion 5.08], and 5.08 [now Opinion 5.09]. Gellman, *Prescribing Privacy: The Uncertain Role of the Physician in the Protection of Patient Privacy, 62 No. Carolina L. Rev. 255, 271 (1984).*

5.05   Confidentiality

The information disclosed to a physician during the course of the relationship between physician and patient is confidential to the greatest possible degree. The patient should feel free to make a full disclosure of information to the physician in order that the physician may most effectively provide needed services. The patient should be able to make this disclosure with the knowledge that the physician will respect the confidential nature of the communication. The physician should not reveal confidential communications or information without the express consent of the patient, unless required to do so by law.

The obligation to safeguard patient confidences is subject to certain exceptions which are ethically and legally justified because of overriding social considerations. Where a patient threatens to inflict serious bodily harm to another person or to him or herself and there is a reasonable probability that the patient may carry out the threat, the physician should take reasonable precautions for the protection of the intended victim, including notification of law enforcement authorities. Also, communicable diseases, gun shot and knife wounds should be reported as required by applicable statutes or ordinances. (IV)

Issued December 1983.

Updated June 1994.

E.D. Ark. 1992 Plaintiff sought an injunction to prevent defendant's attorneys from contacting patient's non-party treating physicians and interviewing them privately without the patient's consent. Quoting Opinion 5.05, the court stated that patients have a right not to have privileged information disclosed by their physician without express authorization. While the privilege may be partially waived where the patient's medical condition is put in issue by the filing of a lawsuit, patients still retain the right to insist that disclosure be made pursuant to formal discovery methods, absent express consent to ex parte contact. *Harlan v. Lewis, 141 F.R.D. 107, 109 n.5.*

D. Kan. 1991 With apparent reliance on Principle IV and Opinion 5.05, plaintiff claimed that other than in discovery or judicial proceedings, the physician-patient privilege is absolute and precludes ex parte communications with defense counsel. While recognizing the confidential nature of the physician-patient relationship, the court held that the ethical standards promulgated by the AMA are not binding law and that, where a litigant-patient has placed his or her medical status in issue, the physician is released from the constraints imposed by the physician-patient relationship for the purposes of the litigation. *Bryant v. Hilst, 136 F.R.D. 487, 490.*

E.D. Pa. 1992 Patient sued state mental institution and psychiatrist for violation of her right to privacy under the Fourteenth Amendment. Defendants had disclosed to law enforcement personnel and to plaintiff's supervisor threats made by plaintiff during the course of her treatment. While recognizing a strong public policy against breaches of confidentiality, the court held that the state's interest in protecting its citizens from serious bodily harm was overriding. The court noted that the limits placed on patient-therapist confidentiality by Opinion 5.05 (1989) are in accordance with the judicially recognized duty that a mental health professional take reasonable steps to prevent harm to others threatened by his or her patient. *Ms. B. v. Montgomery County Emergency Service, Inc., 799 F. Supp. 534, 539 cert denied, 114 S.Ct. 174 (1993).*

M.D. Pa. 1987 Plaintiff in a medical malpractice action sought to preclude his treating physicians from serving as defendant's expert witnesses at trial. The court held that defense counsel's failure to provide prior notice of ex parte communication with plaintiff's treating physicians barred their use as defense experts. Referring to Petrillo v. Syntex Laboratories, Inc., 148 Ill. App. 3d 581, 499 N.E.2d 952 (1986), the court noted that the court there favorably cited Principle IV and Opinions 5.05, 5.06, and 5.07 (1984) in support of a public policy protecting confidentiality between physician and patient and against ex parte discussion. *Manion v. N.P.W. Medical Center of N.E. Pa., Inc., 676 F. Supp. 585, 591.*

Ala. 1973 Physician revealed patient information to the patient's employer, contrary to instructions of patient. Patient sued for breach of fiduciary duty. Citing Principle 9 (1957) [now Principle IV and Opinion 5.05] as well as cases from other states, the court held that even in the absence of a testimonial privilege statute, as a matter of public policy, a physician has a fiduciary duty not to make extrajudicial disclosures of patient information acquired in the course of treatment unless the public interest or the private interest of the patient demands otherwise. In holding that the physician had breached his contract with patient, the court found the Principles together with state licensing requirements sufficient to establish the public policy of confidentiality. *Horne v. Patton, 291 Ala. 701, 287 So. 2d 824, 829, 832.*

Alaska 1977 Physician-school board member failed to fully comply with state's conflict of interest law by refusing to reveal the names of patients from whom he had received over $100 in income. The physician claimed a legal privilege or ethical duty not to disclose the information under Principle 9 (1957) [now Principle IV and Opinion 5.05] and, alternatively, that the conflict of interest law unconstitutionally invaded a patient's right to privacy. The court held that disclosure was not barred by a legal privilege or ethical mandate, but that the conflict of interest law unconstitutionally invaded patient privacy due to the absence of protective regulations. In ruling on the ethical duty issue, the court noted that under Alaska law, a physician's license may be revoked for violating the Principles. However, the court found this licensing provision irrelevant to the privileged relationship exception in the conflict of interest law. The court found that otherwise the privilege exception in the statute could be changed by the American Medical Association, a private organization, simply by amending the Principles. *Falcon v. Alaska Pub. Offices Comm'n, 570 P.2d 469, 474 n.13.*

Ariz. App. 1989 In a medical malpractice action, defense counsel interviewed several of plaintiff's treating physicians ex parte and notified plaintiff of this in preparation for a medical liability review panel hearing. Plaintiff moved to bar all testimony by those physicians and to disqualify defense counsel from representing defendants. The appellate court noted a physician's obligation of confidentiality pursuant to Principle IV and Opinion 5.05 and held that "defense counsel in a medical malpractice action may not engage in non-consensual ex parte communications with plaintiff's treating physicians." *Duquette v. Superior Court, 161 Ariz. 269, 778 P.2d 634, 641.*

Cal. 1994 Plaintiff alleged that treating physician and medical group violated her statutory and constitutional right to privacy by engaging in ex parte communications with original physician's insurance company during discovery in a medical malpractice action against her original physician. The court concluded that state law clearly exempts the defendants from liability and that plaintiff failed to allege a sufficiently serious invasion of privacy to warrant relief. The dissent quoted Opinion 5.05 to emphasize the fiduciary nature of the physician-patient relationship. *Heller v. Norcal Mutual Ins. Co.*, 8 Cal. 4th 30, 876 P.2d 999, 32 Cal. Rptr. 2d 200, 220, cert. denied, 115 S. Ct. 669, 130 L. Ed. 2d 602 (1994).

Cal. 1976 Parents sued psychotherapists to recover for murder of daughter by psychiatric patient, alleging that failure to warn victim of patient's violent threat was a proximate cause of her death. In considering whether such a revelation would have been a violation of professional ethics, the Court noted that Principle 9 (1957) [now Principle IV and Opinion 5.05] recognized that the confidential nature of a physician-patient communication must yield when disclosure is necessary to protect an individual or community as a whole. The court concluded that, in the circumstances of this case, disclosure would not have violated medical ethics and held that psychotherapists are under a duty to warn when they determine or should determine that a patient poses a serious danger of violence to someone else. *Tarasoff v. Regents of Univ. of Cal.*, 17 Cal. 3d 425, 551 P.2d 334, 347, 131 Cal. Rptr. 14, 27.

Cal. 1970 Psychiatrist-witness in civil assault case applied for writ of habeas corpus after being held in contempt of court for refusing to produce patient's psychiatric records. Patient, plaintiff in the assault action, neither expressly claimed nor waived the statutory psychotherapist-patient privilege. The court held that the litigant-patient exception to the statutory psychotherapist-patient privilege does not unconstitutionally infringe rights of privacy of either psychotherapists or their patients. The court noted that in such a context a psychiatrist does not violate Principle 9 (1957) [now Principle IV and Opinion 5.05] since the Principle allows for legally compelled disclosure. *In re Lifschutz*, 2 Cal. 3d 415, 467 P.2d 557, 565-66 n.9, 85 Cal. Rptr. 829, 837-38 n.9.

Cal. App. 1982 Defendant was convicted of lewd act with a child and child molestation or annoyance, after licensed clinical psychologist reported defendant's admission of sexual conduct to authorities. The court held that the psychologist's testimony was properly admitted since a statute requiring the reporting of actual or suspected child abuse expressly made the psychotherapist-patient privilege inapplicable. The court quoted Principle 9 (1957) [now Principle IV and Opinions 2.02 and 5.05] in concluding the disclosure was not a breach of professional ethics. *People v. Stritzinger*, 126 Cal. App. 3d 135, 186 Cal. Rptr. 750, 752 rev'd, 34 Cal. 3d 505, 668 P.2d 738, 194 Cal. Rptr. 431 (1983).

Cal. App. 1968 Plaintiff-physician sought dissolution of a medical partnership with defendant's decedent, and also sought a larger percentage of the partnership receipts based upon an alleged oral agreement. Defendant crossclaimed to enjoin plaintiff from taking physical control of the partnership offices and patient records. The trial court enjoined plaintiff from treating previous patients, requiring that he return all medical records and pay defendant all fees received from patients he had treated during the time of dispute. The appellate court reversed insofar as the injunction prohibited the plaintiff from treating patient who desired to continue to receive his services or prevented access to medical records essential for this purpose, citing Opinions and Reports of the Judicial Council Sec. 7, Para. 16, Sec. 5, Para. 21, and Sec. 9 (1966) [now Opinions 6.08, 5.02, and 5.05] to support view that patients may not be regarded as the subject of ownership. *Jones v. Fakehany*, 261 Cal. App. 2d 298, 67 Cal. Rptr. 810, 815, 816 n.1.

Colo. 1989 Spouse of police officer killed by released psychiatric patient sued state mental hospital and psychiatrist for negligence. Patient had blamed police for his misfortunes during repeated involuntary commitments for paranoid schizophrenia, and psychiatrist knew that patient would have access to a gun after release. The court held that a psychiatrist owed a duty of care in determining whether patient had propensity for violence and posed unreasonable risk of serious bodily harm to others. In so holding, the court cited Principle 9 (1957) [now Principle IV and Opinion 5.05], in support of the view that there are situations in which the need to protect an individual or the community from the threat of harm from a patient may outweigh the strong policy in favor of non-disclosure of patient confidences. *Perreira v. State*, 768 P.2d 1198, 1210 n.7.

D.C. App. 1985 Patient sued plastic surgeon for breach of confidential physician-patient relationship following surgeon's use of before and after photographs of her plastic surgery in a department store presentation. In considering whether such a breach was an actionable tort, the court made reference to an earlier case quoting Principles Ch. II, Sec. 2 (1947) [erroneously cited in the earlier case as Ch. II, Sec. 1 (1943); [now Principle IV and Opinion 5.05], as evidence of the strong public policy which exists in favor of maintaining a patient's confidences. *Vassiliades v. Garfinckel's, Brooks Bros.*, 492 A.2d 580, 590, 591.

Fla. App. 1995 The court considered the issue of the effect of § 455.241(2) of the Florida Statutes on right of defense in a medical malpractice action to engage in ex parte communications with plaintiff's non-party treating physician. The court held that a 1988 amendment to § 455.241(2) negated the applicability of the statute to medical malpractice cases. The dissent, citing Petrillo v. Syntex Laboratories, Inc., 148 Ill. App. 3d 581, 499 N.E.2d 952 (1986), quoted Principles II and IV and Opinions 5.05, 5.06, and 5.08 as strong public policy support for its position that ex parte communications should be barred altogether. *Castillo-Plaza v. Green*, 655 So. 2d 197, 206 n.4.

Ill. 1997 Trial court held various statutory sections, including those permitting unlimited disclosure of a patient's medical records, unconstitutional. On appeal, state supreme court affirmed. Regarding provisions mandating consent to the disclosure of medical records, the court noted, with reference to Principle IV and Opinion 5.05, the crucial importance of confidentiality in the physician-patient relationship. *Best v. Taylor Machine Works*, 179 Ill. 2d 367, 689 N.E. 2d 1057, 1099.

Ill. App. 1987 In appeal of malpractice action, an issue was whether expert testimony of plaintiff's treating physician, based upon discussions with the defense counsel without patient's consent, was admissible. The court held that ex parte communications between a plaintiff's treating physician and legal adversary violated public policy. In determining the existence of such a policy favoring the sanctity of the doctor-patient relationship, the court noted Petrillo v. Syntex Laboratories, Inc., 148 Ill. App. 3d 581, 499 N.E.2d 952 (1st Dist. 1986) and its reference to the Principles and Opinions, namely Principle IV and Opinion 5.05 (1984), which establish an ethical obligation to keep physician-patient communications confidential, generally requiring a patient's consent before information is released. *Yates v. El-Deiry*, 160 Ill. App. 3d 198, 513 N.E.2d 519, 522.

Ill. App. 1986 Defense attorney in product liability suit was held in contempt of court for conducting ex parte discussions with plaintiff-patient's treating physician without patient's consent and contrary to authorized methods of discovery. The court held that the strong public policy favoring physician-patient confidentiality articulated in Principles II and IV and Opinions 5.05, 5.06, 5.07, and 5.08 (1984) justified a rule against such ex parte discussions. Further, the court held that the public has the right to rely on physicians to faithfully execute their ethical obligations. *Petrillo v. Syntex Laboratories, Inc.*, 148 Ill. App. 3d 581, 499 N.E.2d 952, 957, 958, 959, cert. denied, 483 U.S. 1007 (1987).

Ill. App. 1979 Patient filed suit against physician for breach of contract and breach of confidential relationship after physician's employee disclosed patient's name to police. Patient alleged that implied contract arose out of a statutory physician-patient privilege, and provisions of the Canons of Medical Ethics, with apparent reference to Principle 9 (1957) [now Principle IV and Opinion 5.05]. The court held that disclosure of patient's name alone by a physician or the physician's agents is insufficient to state a cause of action in contract and does not violate the physician-patient privilege. *Geisberger v. Willuhn*, 72 Ill. App. 3d 435, 390 N.E.2d 945, 946, 948.

Ind. App. 1996 A patient filed suit against a mental health counseling center for disclosing to a third party death threats made by the patient during therapy. The patient claimed this was a breach of the standard of care owed to her. The trial court found that the counseling center was not statutorily prohibited from disclosing death threats the patient made. On appeal, the court affirmed the decision. It noted, with apparent reference to Principle IV and Opinion 5.05, that physicians may disclose confidential information to ensure the safety of the public or of individuals. In clarifying its holding, the court observed that while free and frank communication should be promoted to aid proper diagnosis and treatment, public policy supports disclosure of confidential information when appropriate. *Rocca v. Southern Hills Counseling Center, Inc.*, 671 N.E. 2d 913, 916.

Md. Att'y Gen. 1977 Opinion addresses the obligation of a psychiatrist to report child abuse information obtained from a parent-patient. Referring to state statutes and to Principle 9 (1957) [now Principle IV and Opinions 2.02 and 5.05] the opinion concludes that the question of whether to disclose suspected child abuse is a matter left to the individual psychiatrist's professional and moral judgment. *Maryland Att'y. Gen. Opinion*, 62 Op. Att'y Gen. Md. 157, 160.

Mass. 1984 Employee sued employer for libel and invasion of privacy following disclosure of medical facts about employee to other employees. In part, claim involved disclosure of opinion about employee's mental state to his supervisor by physician retained by employer. Citing

Principle 9 (1957) [now Principle IV and Opinions 5.05 and 5.09], the court held that a physician retained by an employer may disclose to the employer information concerning an employee if receipt of the information is reasonably necessary to serve a substantial and valid business interest of the employer. *Bratt v. Int'l Business Mach. Corp., 392 Mass. 508, 467 N.E.2d 126, 137 n.23.*

Minn. 1976 Plaintiff-patient in malpractice action appealed trial court's order to provide authorization for private, informal interview between defense counsel and patient's treating physician. In holding that formal pretrial discovery provided the exclusive procedure by which defendant could obtain medical testimony, the court noted, without deciding the issue, that a physician who discloses confidential patient information in a private interview may be subject to tort liability for breach of patient's right to privacy or professional discipline for unprofessional conduct, citing Principle 9 (1957) [now Principle IV and Opinion 5.05]. *Wenninger v. Muesing, 240 N.W.2d 333, 337 n.3.*

Mo. 1993 Patient sued physicians alleging a breach of fiduciary duty of confidentiality for participating in an unauthorized ex parte discussion with defendant's attorney. While recognizing this duty, the court held that, where the plaintiff's medical condition is in issue, this constitutes a waiver of both the testimonial privilege and the physician's fiduciary duty in so far as the information is related to the medical issues. Quoting Opinion 5.05 and citing Principle IV, the court stated that courts may apply ethical principles to frame the specific limits of the legal duty of confidentiality. *Brandt v. Medical Defense Assoc., 856 S.W.2d 667, 671 n.1.*

Mo. 1989 In a personal injury suit, plaintiff challenged trial court's authority to compel plaintiff to authorize ex parte meetings between defendant insurance company and plaintiff's treating physician. Applying a balancing test between preserving the physician-patient confidential and fiduciary relationship, the physician-patient testimonial privilege, and the quest for truth in civil litigation, the court held that such information could be obtained through the methods of formal discovery. The court quoted Principle IV and Opinion 5.05 (1984) as statements of the policy underlying medical confidentiality and a basis for a patient's affirmative right to rely on the confidential nature of disclosures to a treating physician. *State ex. rel. Woytus v. Ryan, 776 S.W.2d 389, 392-93.*

Mo. App. 1985 In a prohibition proceeding arising from a medical malpractice action, defense attorneys sought order compelling plaintiff to authorize a private interview between defense attorneys and physician who treated plaintiff for injuries allegedly caused by defendant-physician. The appellate court, after discussing Principle IV and Opinion 5.05 (1984), held that the defense attorneys had the right to seek an ex parte interview with the treating physician, subject to the willingness of the physician to grant the interview. Furthermore, the court noted that Opinion 5.05 prevents a physician from revealing a patient's confidences only where there is a lack of consent from the patient and found that consent did exist here in the form of a medical authorization executed by plaintiff during pendency of the malpractice action. *State ex rel. Stufflebam v. Appelquist, 694 S.W.2d 882, 886, 888 n.7, overruled by State ex. rel. Woytus v. Ryan, 776 S.W.2d 389 (Mo. 1989).*

N.J. 1985 Plaintiff provided authorization for release of decedent's medical records from former treating physicians but refused to consent to depositions or interviews between defense counsel and physicians. The court noted physicians' ethical duty to avoid unauthorized disclosure, as stated in Principle 9 (1957) [now Principle IV and Opinion 5.05], but recognized that a patient's right to confidentiality was not absolute. After balancing the competing interests involved, the court held that defense counsel had a right to seek ex parte interviews of decedent's other treating physicians regarding litigation matters, provided procedural safeguards were met including clear statements that participation in such an interview is voluntary on the part of a physician. *Stempler v. Speidell, 100 N.J. 368, 495 A.2d 857, 860, cert. denied, 483 U.S. 1007 (1987).*

N.J. 1979 In wrongful death action against a psychiatrist whose patient murdered plaintiff's decedent, the court concluded, in accord with Principle 9 (1957) [now Principle IV], that a psychiatrist may owe a duty to warn potential victims of possible danger from psychiatrist's patient despite the general emphasis on confidentiality. The court also noted the Preamble and Principles 1 and 3 (1957) [now revised Preamble, Principle I and Opinion 5.05] in discussing the psychiatrist-patient relationship. *McIntosh v. Milano, 168 N.J. Super. 466, 403 A.2d 500, 510, 512-13.*

N.J. 1962 Parents sued pediatrician for unauthorized disclosure to life insurer of deceased infant's congenital heart defect. The court quoted Principle 9 (1957) [now Principle IV and Opinion 5.05] as an articulation of a physician's legal duty to his or her patient subject to exceptions of compelling social or patient interests. The court held that the parents had lost their limited right to nondisclosure by filing an insurance claim. *Hague v. Williams*, 37 N.J. 328, 181 A.2d 345, 347.

N.J. Super. 1991 Physician's estate sued hospital alleging that it violated state law against discrimination by restricting the physician's surgery privileges and requiring him to inform patients of his HIV-infected status before performing invasive procedures. The defendant hospital was also alleged to have breached its duty to maintain confidentiality of his seropositive diagnosis. The court held that the hospital had not discriminated against the physician since the hospital had relied on ethical and professional standards, including a report of the Council on Ethical and Judicial Affairs of the AMA dealing with the issue of AIDS [now Opinions 9.13 and 9.131]. However, the hospital was held to have breached its fiduciary duty to maintain the confidentiality of the physician's medical records. Referring to McIntosh v. Milano, 168 N.J. Super. 466, 403 A.2d 500 (1979) which had quoted AMA Principles of Medical Ethics sec. 9 (1957) [now Principle IV and Opinion 5.05] in applying the "duty to warn" exception, the court noted that the disclosure in this case went far beyond the medical personnel directly involved in the treatment of the physician and those patients entitled to informed consent. *Estate of Behringer v. Medical Ctr.*, 249 N.J. Super. 597, 614, 633, 592 A.2d 1251, 1259, 1268.

N.J. Super. 1988 Several portions of state Department of Corrections regulations concerning exceptions to privileged communications between psychologist and inmates were invalidated by appellate court because they permitted disclosure of confidences that did not present clear and imminent danger to the inmate or others, or failed to identify any intended victim. Court made general reference (with erroneous quotation) to Principle 9 (1957) [now Principle IV and Opinion 5.05]. *In re Rules Adoption*, 224 N.J. Super. 252, 540 A.2d 212, 215.

N.J. Super. 1987 Defendant in a personal injury suit sought to offer testimony from plaintiff's treating physician regarding plaintiff's prognosis. The court denied plaintiff's motion to exclude that evidence, despite the ethical obligation of physicians to uphold patients' communications as confidential under Principle 9 (1957) [now Principle IV and Opinion 5.05]. The court's decision was based on New Jersey case law permitting disclosure of a patient's medical condition to someone having a legitimate interest "where the physical condition of the patient is made an element of a claim." *Kurdek v. West Orange Bd. of Educ.*, 222 N.J. Super. 218, 536 A.2d 332, 335.

N.J. Super. 1967 In a suit for separate maintenance, communications between plaintiff-wife and her psychiatrist were not protected from disclosure during depositions, despite Principle 9 (1957) [now Principle IV and Opinion 5.05] which prohibited physicians from disclosing patient confidences except where "necessary to protect the welfare of the individual or of the community." The court concluded that the patient had only a limited right of nondisclosure, subject to exceptions created by "supervening interest of society" and that the institution of litigation by the patient constituted a vitiation of that right. *Ritt v. Ritt*, 98 N.J. Super. 590, 238 A.2d 196, 199, rev'd, 52 N.J. 177, 244 A.2d 497 (1968).

N.Y. Sup. 1977 Plaintiff, a psychiatric patient, sued her psychiatrist and the psychiatrist's spouse for violating several state statutes and her privacy rights by publishing a book about the intimate details of plaintiff's psychotherapy. The court found for plaintiff, basing its decision in part upon Principle 9 (1957) [now Principle IV and Opinion 5.05] which requires a physician to uphold the confidences of a patient. *Doe v. Roe*, 93 Misc. 2d 201, 400 N.Y.S.2d 668, 674.

N.Y. Surr. 1977 In a discovery proceeding, respondent-psychiatrist, who had treated some patients of deceased psychiatrist subsequent to his death, allegedly misappropriated decedent's patient records. Estate petitioned court for return of records and damages for injury to value of decedent's practice. Respondent sought dismissal of claim arguing that estate could not sell patient records. The court rejected respondent's request. In so ruling, the court noted that under Principle 9 (1957) [now Principle IV and Opinion 5.05] prohibiting physicians from revealing patient confidences, various guidelines had been issued regarding sale of a medical practice [now Opinion 7.04]. Whether respondent's actions had interfered with the estate's efforts to dispose of decedent's practice in keeping with these guidelines presented the court with factual issues for later resolution. *Estate of Finkle*, 90 Misc. 2d 550, 395 N.Y.S.2d 343, 346.

N.C. 1990 Plaintiff in a malpractice case was granted an order prohibiting ex parte conferences between defendant's attorney and non-party treating physicians. The court noted that both the Principles of Medical Ethics and Current Opinions affirm the physician's duty to protect patient confidentiality, in apparent reference to Principle IV and Opinion 5.05. In consideration of (1) the patient's right to privacy, (2) physician-patient confidentiality, (3) the adequacy of formal discovery procedures, and (4) the dilemma in which non-party treating physicians are placed by conferences are unnecessary. Quotes Principle IV and Opinion 5.05. Kassel, *Counterpoint . . . Defense Counsel's Ex Parte Communication with Plaintiff's Doctors: A Bad One-Sided Deal*, 9 S.C. Law. 42, 43 (Sept./Oct. 1997).

Journal 1997 Considers Connecticut AIDS statute, which relates to testing and confidentiality of patient medical information. Discusses statutory construction of provisions of this law by the Connecticut Supreme Court in *Doe v. Marselle*. Quotes Opinion 5.05. Note, *A Case Study of New Textualism in State Courts: Doe v. Marselle and the Confidentiality of HIV-Related Information*, 30 Conn. L. Rev. 295, 297 (1997).

Journal 1997 Considers whether the physician-patient privilege should be extended to protect communications to alternative health practitioners. Suggests that these practitioners treat and diagnose patients within the meaning of the privilege. Advocates an extension of the privilege to recognize the importance of confidentiality. Quotes Opinion 5.05. Note, *Healer-Patient Privilege: Extending the Physician-Patient Privilege to Alternative Health Practitioners in California*, 48 Hastings L. J. 633, 657 (1997).

Journal 1996 Explains the benefits of high-tech access to patient information by pharmacists. Considers related issues of patient confidentiality. Advocates a pharmacist-patient privilege. Quotes Opinion 5.05. Berger, *Patient Confidentiality in a High Tech World*, 5 J. Pharmacy & L., 139, 141 (1996).

Journal 1996 Suggests that attorneys representing HIV-infected and sexually active adolescents face an ethical conflict between their duty of client confidentiality and the duty to protect third parties. Notes that attorneys failing to warn third parties may face liability. Concludes that clients should be informed of potential limitations on the right to confidentiality. Quotes Opinion 5.05. Katner, *The Ethical Dilemma Awaiting Counsel Who Represent Adolescents with HIV/AIDS: Criminal Law and Tort Suits Pressure Counsel to Breach the Confidentiality of the Clients' Medical Status*, 70 Tul. L. Rev. 2311, 2341 (1996).

Journal 1996 Discusses sexual abuse litigation in which accusers have recovered memories of molestation in psychotherapy sessions. Observes that, to successfully defend against such claims, it is necessary for the accused to have access to the clinical record. Posits that confidentiality problems can be eliminated with *in camera* record inspections. References Principle IV and Opinion 5.05. Loftus, Paddock, & Guernsey, *Patient-Psychotherapist Privilege: Access to Clinical Records in the Tangled Web of Repressed Memory Litigation*, 30 U. Rich L. Rev. 109, 127 (1996).

Journal 1996 Reviews two Washington state supreme court decisions in which subsequent treating physicians testified against their patients and on behalf of defendant physicians in malpractice litigation. Observes that these decisions erode the physician-patient privilege. Posits that the decisions are inconsistent with current medical ethics and proposes a statutory enactment as a solution. Quotes Opinion 5.05. Cites Principle 9 (1957) [now Principle IV]. Oppenheim, *Physicians as Experts Against Their Own Patients? What Happened to the Privilege?*, 63 Def. Couns. J. 254, 257, 261 (1996).

Journal 1996 Considers prearraignment forensic evaluations. Notes the prohibition against use of such evaluations. Examines underlying ethical precepts. Observes that principles of beneficence are misapplied to forensic psychiatry in this context. Advocates a new ethical framework. Quotes Preamble. References Principle IV and Opinion 5.05. Ornish, Mills, & Ornish, *Prearraignment Forensic Evaluations: Toward a New Policy*, 24 Bull. Am. Acad. Psychiatry Law 453, 454, 469 (1996).

Journal 1996 Examines the psychiatrist-patient duty of confidentiality. Notes that Principles of Medical Ethics prohibit the disclosure of patient confidences and medical records. Observes that exceptions to this prohibition exist when required by law or to protect the community. Quotes Principle 9 (1957) [now Principle IV and Opinion 5.05]. Sadoff, *Ethical Obligations for the Psychiatrist: Confidentiality, Privilege, and Privacy in Psychiatric Treatment*, 29 Loy. L.A. L. Rev. 1709, 1710, 1711 (1996).

Journal 1995 Addresses presidential disability, its past impact on American government, and possible solutions to potential problems. Suggests guidelines for implementation of the Twenty-Fifth Amendment. Examines the effectiveness of a medical commission in determining presidential disability. Proposes enhancement of the role of the President's physician. Quotes Opinion 8.03. Cites Opinions 5.04 and 5.05. Abrams, *The Vulnerable President and the Twenty-Fifth Amendment, with Observations on Guidelines, a Health Commission, and the Role of the President's Physician*, 30 Wake Forest L. Rev. 453, 466, 471 (1995).

Journal 1995 Discusses the belief of health care providers that they have an ethical obligation to warn the partners of HIV-positive patients. Provides an overview of the ethical and legal principles concerning confidentiality and the duty to warn. Examines both the scope of a Massachusetts statute that prevents providers from releasing HIV test results of patients and possible defenses that providers may assert. Quotes Principle IV and Opinion 5.05. Friedland, *HIV Confidentiality and the Right to Warn—The Health Care Provider's Dilemma*, 80 Mass. L. Rev. 3, 4 (March 1995).

Journal 1995 Considers how the use of health care identification cards and medical record databases would threaten privacy rights. Evaluates both the existing law that applies to medical record privacy and proposals to protect such privacy under health reform. Concludes that federal legislation should be enacted to protect health care record privacy and prevent misuse of health care identification cards. Quotes Opinion 5.05. Minor, *Identity Cards and Databases in Health Care: The Need for Federal Privacy Protections*, 28 Colum. J.L. & Soc. Probs. 253, 279 (1995).

Journal 1995 Examines the impact of health care reform on physician-patient relationships. Observes that patients' primary relationships may be with their insurers (HMOs) rather than their physicians. Discusses how reform may threaten the physician's fiduciary duty of loyalty by forcing physicians to make rationing decisions and giving physicians financial incentives to limit use of health care resources. Considers how these potentially harmful effects may be mitigated. Quotes Fundamental Elements (5). Cites Opinion 5.05. Orentlicher, *Health Care Reform and the Patient-Physician Relationship*, 5 Health Matrix 141, 143, 148 (1995).

Journal 1995 Analyzes the secular approach to the duty to treat HIV-infected individuals and the duty to warn those who are sexual partners of, or who share needles with, people infected with HIV. Observes that the secular approach leaves these issues unresolved; but indicates that Jewish law compels physicians both to treat and to warn. Quotes Opinions 5.05 and 9.131. Shorr, *AIDS, Judaism, and the Limits of the Secular Society*, 20 Second Opinion 23, 24, 27 (1995).

Journal 1994 Considers whether an exception should be made to physician-patient confidentiality that would allow a physician to reveal parental medical history to a child. Discusses whether parents should be required to divulge their medical history to their children. Concludes that such an exception would not completely erode physician-patient confidentiality. Quotes Principles IV, Fundamental Elements (4), and Opinion 5.05. Cites Principle I and Fundamental Elements (1). Friedland, *Physician-Patient Confidentiality: Time to Re-Examine a Venerable Concept in Light of Contemporary Society and Advances in Medicine*, 15 J. Legal Med. 249, 257, 264, 276 (1994).

Journal 1994 Explores the ethical issues involved in a multidisciplinary team working with children in legal proceedings. Focuses on the relationships between professionals and the conflicts that arise regarding disclosure of confidential information and forced disclosure of non-privileged information. Examines theories supporting protection of client information. Quotes Principles III, IV, Fundamental Elements (4) and Opinions 1.02 (1992) and 5.07 (1992) [now Opinion 5.05]. Cites Opinions 2.02. Glynn, *Multidisciplinary Representation of Children: Conflicts Over Disclosures of Client Communications*, 27 J. Marshall L. Rev. 617, 625, 626, 630-32, 637, 639, 643 (1994).

Journal 1994 Compares Texas law with Illinois law on the issue of ex parte communications between defense counsel and the patient/plaintiff's physician in civil litigation. Argues that preservation of the physician-patient relationship requires prohibition of such contact. Quotes Principles II and IV and Opinion 5.05. Comment, *From the Land of Lincoln a Healing Rule: Proposed Texas Rule of Civil Procedure Prohibiting Ex Parte Contact Between Defense Counsel and a Plaintiff's Treating Physician*, 25 Tex. Tech L. Rev. 1081, 1081, 1082 (1994).

Journal 1994 Considers how computerized medical records might threaten patient confidentiality. Examines existing legal protections and their shortcomings. Explores proposed legislation for computerized records and the potential need for new legal standards in this area. Cites Opinion 5.05. Field, *Overview: Computerized Medical Records Create New Legal and Business Confidentiality Problems*, 11 HealthSpan 3, 4 (1994).

Journal 1993 Discusses family privacy rights and a physician's ethical responsibility to report violence. Considers the meaning of justice, self respect, and the fundamental principles of physician ethics. Concludes that physicians have an ethical duty to intervene in domestic violence so long as such intervention does not breach confidentiality or violate patient autonomy. Quotes Principle IV and Opinion 5.05. References Opinions 8.14 and 9.131. Jecker, *Privacy Beliefs and the Violent Family: Extending the Ethical Argument for Physician Intervention*, 269 J.A.M.A. 776, 778, 779 (1993).

Journal 1993 Evaluates the legal issues surrounding AIDS and HIV. Examines various aspects of the law that would be relevant to a medical or health care lawyer. Quotes Opinion 5.05. Skiver & Hickey, *AIDS: Legal Issues 1992, 19 Ohio No. Univ. L. Rev. 839, 860 (1993).*

Journal 1991 Discusses current law protecting confidential genetic information obtained in the workplace. Presents several mechanisms designed to safeguard this information. Analyzes the legal grounds upon which various parties may access this information. Proposes a model law. References Opinion 5.05. Andrews & Jaeger, *Confidentiality of Genetic Information in the Workplace, XVII Am. J. Law & Med. 75, 78 (1991).*

Journal 1991 Examines the problem of AIDS in this country and the risk of HIV transmission via sexual assault. Discusses attendant problems for the criminal justice system and possible mandatory testing of offenders. Considers the constitutionality of such a scheme. Analyzes state laws requiring HIV testing for sex offenders. Concludes that such laws are necessary to preserve the rights of victims of sexual assault. Quotes Opinion 5.05. McGuire, *AIDS and the Sexual Offender: The Epidemic Now Poses New Threats to the Victim and the Criminal Justice System, 96 Dickinson L. Rev. 95, 109, 110 (1991).*

Journal 1991 Considers the issue of the physician-patient privilege and the restriction of ex parte interviews. Focuses on the case *Crist v. Moffatt,* where a court permitted ex parte interview of a plaintiff's physician only after the plaintiff signed a written authorization. Concludes that *Crist* was correctly decided, but warns against expanding the decision to the point of unduly restricting discovery. Quotes Opinion 5.05. Note, *Restricting Ex Parte Interviews With Nonparty Treating Physicians: Crist v. Moffatt, 69 No. Carolina L. Rev. 1381, 1391, 1392 (1991).*

Journal 1991 Discusses confidentiality with respect to a patient's HIV status. Examines laws regulating the dissemination of AIDS information. Notes how confidentiality may be lost in the hospital setting and emphasizes importance of heightened attention to this issue by institutional health care providers. Quotes Opinion 5.05. Obade, *Whisper Down the Lane: AIDS, Privacy, and the Hospital "Grapevine," 2 J. Clinical Ethics 133, 133 (1991).*

Journal 1990 Discusses the legal and ethical considerations associated with genetic research, including recombinant DNA technology. Explores issues raised by the application of this technology in the clinical setting. Offers case examples illustrating these issues. Quotes Opinion 5.05. Elsas, *A Clinical Approach to Legal and Ethical Problems in Human Genetics, 39 Emory L.J. 811, 816, 820 (1990).*

Journal 1990 Advocates physician liability for failure to warn third parties of the potential risk of being infected with HIV from the physician's patient. Discusses a physician's common law duty to warn third parties in other situations and applies that duty in the AIDS context. Explores the possibility of physician liability for breach of confidentiality. Concludes that there should be no liability for disclosure because public health concerns outweigh an individual patient's right to confidentiality. References Opinion 5.05. Note, *AIDS: Establishing a Physician's Duty to Warn, 21 Rutgers L.J. 645, 652 (1990).*

Journal 1989 Discusses the history of the physician-patient privilege up through changes implemented under the Ohio Tort Reform Act of 1987. Aspects of the physician-patient privilege that are most significantly affected by this Tort Reform Act are highlighted, with recommendations for further refinement of the privilege in Ohio. Quotes Principles II and IV and Opinion 5.05. Note, *The Ohio Physician-Patient Privilege: Modified, Revised, and Defined, 49 Ohio St. L. J. 1147, 1167 (1989).*

5.055 Confidential Care for Minors

Physicians who treat minors have an ethical duty to promote the autonomy of minor patients by involving them in the medical decision making process to a degree commensurate with their abilities.

When minors request confidential services, physicians should encourage them to involve their parents. This includes making efforts to obtain the minor's reasons for not involving their parents and correcting misconceptions that may be motivating their objections.

Where the law does not require otherwise, physicians should permit a competent minor to consent to medical care and should not notify parents without the patient's consent. Depending on the seriousness of the decision, competence may be evaluated by physicians for most minors. When necessary, experts in adolescent medicine or child psychological development should be consulted. Use of the courts for competence determinations should be made only as a last resort.

When an immature minor requests contraceptive services, pregnancy-related care (including pregnancy testing, prenatal and postnatal care, and delivery services), or treatment for sexually transmitted disease, drug and alcohol abuse, or mental illness, physicians must recognize that requiring parental involvement may be counterproductive to the health of the patient. Physicians should encourage parental involvement in these situations. However, if the minor continues to object, his or her wishes ordinarily should be respected. If the physician is uncomfortable with providing services without parental involvement, and alternative confidential services are available, the minor may be referred to those services. In cases when the physician believes that without parental involvement and guidance, the minor will face a serious health threat, and there is reason to believe that the parents will be helpful and understanding, disclosing the problem to the parents is ethically justified. When the physician does breach confidentiality to the parents, he or she must discuss the reasons for the breach with the minor prior to the disclosure.

For minors who are mature enough to be unaccompanied by their parents for their examination, confidentiality of information disclosed during an exam, interview, or in counseling should be maintained. Such information may be disclosed to parents when the patient consents to disclosure. Confidentiality may be justifiably breached in situations for which confidentiality for adults may be breached, according to Opinion 5.05. In addition, confidentiality for immature minors may be ethically breached when necessary to enable the parent(s) to make an informed decision about treatment for the minor or when such a breach is necessary to avert serious harm to the minor. (IV)

Issued June 1994 based on the report, "Confidential Care for Minors," adopted June 1992.

Updated June 1996.

5.057 Confidentiality of HIV Status on Autopsy Reports

Physicians should maintain the confidentiality of HIV status on autopsy reports to the greatest extent possible.

Physicians who perform autopsies or who have access to autopsy information regarding a patient's HIV status should be familiar with state law governing: (1) the reporting of HIV and AIDS to public health authorities; (2) obligations to inform third parties who may be at risk for HIV infection through contact with an HIV-infected decedent; (3) other parties to whom reporting may be required (e.g., funeral directors, health care personnel involved in the care of the patient); and (4) the extent of confidentiality of autopsy records.

HIV status which appears on autopsy records performed under the authority of a hospital are part of the decedent's medical record and should be held confidential. The physician should comply with state laws regarding disclosure to public health authorities and at-risk third parties, and, where such laws are absent, fulfill ethical obligations to notify endangered third parties (e.g., identified sexual or needle-sharing partners). This includes reporting to organ or tissue procurement agencies if any parts of the decedent's body were taken for use in transplantation.

HIV status which appears on autopsy records performed by a medical examiner in the case of suspicious, accidental, or unexplained death should be kept confidential where autopsy records are not accessible to the public. The physician should comply with state laws regarding disclosure to public health authorities and at-risk third parties, and, where such laws are absent, fulfill ethical obligations to notify endangered third parties (e.g., sexual and needle-sharing partners). This includes reporting to organ or tissue procurement agencies if any parts of the decedent's body were taken for use in transplantation.

In cases where autopsies are done under the auspices of the medical examiner's office and state law mandates that the autopsy information be accessible to the public, then physicians should comply with state law. However, in these instances, HIV status should only be recorded when the HIV status of the decedent would be relevant to determining the patient's cause-of-death. In addition, although a patient's HIV status may be learned from public records in some jurisdictions, it is still unethical for a physician to make a public disclosure of an individual patient's HIV status independent of the legal requirements governing the filing or processing of autopsy records. The physician should comply with state laws regarding disclosure to public health authorities and at-risk third parties, and, where such laws are absent, fulfill ethical obligations to notify endangered third parties (e.g., sexual and needle-sharing partners). This includes reporting to organ or tissue procurement agencies if any parts of the decedent's body were taken for use in transplantation. (IV)

Issued June 1994 based on the report, "Confidentiality of HIV Status on Autopsy Reports," adopted June 1992 (*Arch Pathol Lab Med.* 1992; 116: 1120-1123).

Journal 1997 Compares past ethical opinions to current opinions and notes the differences. Comments on the forces that have changed medical ethics through the years. Notes differing theories on the future course of medical ethics. Quotes Fundamental Elements (Preamble) and Opinions 5.05, 5.057, 7.01, 8.12, 9.12, and 9.131. Cites Fundamental Elements (5) and Opinions 8.115 and 8.13. Buchanan, *Medical Ethics at the Millennium: A Brief Retrospective,* 26 *Colo. Law. 141, 142, 143, 144, 145* (1997).

Journal 1996 Discusses conflict between physicians' duty of confidentiality to patients and physicians' obligation to warn third parties of foreseeable injuries. Examines physicians' current legal responsibility to breach confidentiality to prevent the spread of infectious diseases, including AIDS. Identifies guidelines for physicians. Cites Opinions 2.23 and 5.057. Comment, *Taking Tarasoff Where No One Has Gone Before: Looking at "Duty to Warn" Under the AIDS Crisis,* 15 *St. Louis U. Pub. L. Rev. 471, 499* (1996).

5.06   Confidentiality: Physician-Attorney Relation

The patient's history, diagnosis, treatment, and prognosis may be discussed with the patient's attorney with the consent of the patient or the patient's lawful representative.

A physician may testify in court or before a worker's compensation board or the like in any personal injury or related case. (IV)

Issued prior to April 1977.

M.D. Pa. 1987 Plaintiff in a medical malpractice action sought to preclude his treating physicians from serving as defendant's expert witnesses at trial. The court held that defense counsel's failure to provide prior notice of ex parte communication with plaintiff's treating physicians barred their use as defense experts. Referring to Petrillo v. Syntex Laboratories, Inc., 148 Ill. App. 3d 581, 499 N.E.2d 952 (1986), the court noted that the court there favorably cited Principle IV and Opinions 5.05, 5.06, and 5.07 (1984) in support of a public policy protecting confidentiality between physician and patient and against ex parte discussion. *Manion v. N.P.W. Medical Center of N.E. Pa., Inc., 676 F. Supp. 585, 591.*

Fla. App. 1995 The court considered the issue of the effect of § 455.241(2) of the Florida Statutes on right of defense in a medical malpractice action to engage in ex parte communications with plaintiff's non-party treating physician. The court held that a 1988 amendment to § 455.241(2) negated the applicability of the statute to medical malpractice cases. The dissent, citing Petrillo v. Syntex Laboratories, Inc., 148 Ill. App. 3d 581, 499 N.E.2d 952 (1986), quoted Principles II and IV and Opinions 5.05, 5.06, and 5.08 as strong public policy support for its position that ex parte communications should be barred altogether. *Castillo-Plaza v. Green, 655 So. 2d 197, 206 n.4.*

Ill. App. 1986 Defense attorney in product liability suit was held in contempt of court for conducting ex parte discussions with plaintiff-patient's treating physician without patient's consent and contrary to authorized methods of discovery. The court held that the strong public policy favoring physician-patient confidentiality articulated in Principles II and IV and Opinions 5.05, 5.06, 5.07, and 5.08 (1984) justified a rule against such ex parte discussions. Further, the court held that the public has the right to rely on physicians to faithfully execute their ethical obligations. *Petrillo v. Syntex Laboratories, Inc., 148 Ill. App. 3d 581, 499 N.E.2d 952, 957, 958, 959 cert. denied, 483 U.S. 1007 (1987).*

Journal 1997 Considers how breast cancer has given rise to numerous medical malpractice lawsuits. Discusses trial techniques and strategies for litigating these types of claims. Quotes Opinions 5.05 and 5.06. Hillerich, Ellerin, & Frieder, *Selecting and Presenting a Failure to Diagnose Breast Cancer Case, 20 Am. J. Trial Advoc. 253, 271 (1996-97).*

Journal 1991 Discusses the case of *Crist v. Moffat*, which prohibits ex parte communications with a plaintiff's treating physician in North Carolina. Examines the physician-patient privilege and looks at various jurisdictions that permit and forbid ex parte communications. Concludes that *Crist* is a reaffirmation of North Carolina's commitment to protecting the physician-patient relationship. Quotes Principle IV and Opinion 5.06. Comment, *Shielding the Plaintiff and Physician: The Prohibition of Ex Parte Contacts With a Plaintiff's Treating Physician, 13 Campbell L. Rev. 233, 243, 248 (1991).*

Journal 1984 Discusses the broad content of medical records, noting that they are being demanded for use in a variety of contexts. Observes that available ethical and legal guidelines are insufficient to aid physicians in addressing issues of patient privacy and confidentiality. Concludes that there is need for legislation in order to provide suitable guidance to physicians who fulfill an important role in protecting patient privacy. Cites 1981 Opinions 5.03, 5.04, 5.05 [now Opinion 5.06], 5.06 [now Opinion 5.07], 5.07 [now Opinion 5.08], and 5.08 [now Opinion 5.09]. Gellman, *Prescribing Privacy: The Uncertain Role of the Physician in the Protection of Patient Privacy, 62 No. Carolina L. Rev. 255, 271 (1984).*

5.07   Confidentiality: Computers

The utmost effort and care must be taken to protect the confidentiality of all medical records, including computerized medical records.

The guidelines below are offered to assist physicians and computer service organizations in maintaining the confidentiality of information in medical records when that information is stored in computerized data bases:

(1) Confidential medical information should be entered into the computer-based patient record only by authorized personnel. Additions to the record should be time and date stamped, and the person making the additions should be identified in the record.

(2) The patient and physician should be advised about the existence of computerized data bases in which medical information concerning the patient is stored. Such information should be communicated to the physician and patient prior to the physician's release of the medical information to the entity or entities maintaining the computer data bases. All individuals and organizations with some form of access to the computerized data bases, and the level of access permitted, should be specifically identified in advance. Full disclosure of this information to the patient is necessary in obtaining informed consent to treatment. Patient data should be assigned a security level appropriate for the data's degree of sensitivity, which should be used to control who has access to the information.

(3) The physician and patient should be notified of the distribution of all reports reflecting identifiable patient data prior to distribution of the reports by the computer facility. There should be approval by the patient and notification of the physician prior to the release of patient-identifiable clinical and administrative data to individuals or organizations external to the medical care environment. Such information should not be released without the express permission of the patient.

(4) The dissemination of confidential medical data should be limited to only those individuals or agencies with a bona fide use for the data. Only the data necessary for the bona fide use should be released. Patient identifiers should be omitted when appropriate. Release of confidential medical information from the data base should be confined to the specific purpose for which the information is requested and limited to the specific time frame requested. All such organizations or individuals should be advised that authorized release of data to them does not authorize their further release of the data to additional individuals or organizations, or subsequent use of the data for other purposes.

(5) Procedures for adding to or changing data on the computerized data base should indicate individuals authorized to make changes, time periods in which changes take place, and those individuals who will be informed about changes in the data from the medical records.

(6) Procedures for purging the computerized data base of archaic or inaccurate data should be established and the patient and physician should be notified before and after the data has been purged. There should be no mixing of a physician's computerized patient records with those of other computer service bureau clients. In addition, procedures should be developed to protect against inadvertent mixing of individual reports or segments thereof.

(7) The computerized medical data base should be on-line to the computer terminal only when authorized computer programs requiring the medical data are being used. Individuals and organizations external to the clinical facility should not be provided on-line access to a computerized data base containing identifiable data from medical records concerning patients. Access to the computerized data base should be controlled through security measures

such as passwords, encryption (encoding) of information, and scannable badges or other user identification.

(8) Back-up systems and other mechanisms should be in place to prevent data loss and downtime as a result of hardware or software failure.

(9) Security:

(a) Stringent security procedures should be in place to prevent unauthorized access to computer-based patient records. Personnel audit procedures should be developed to establish a record in the event of unauthorized disclosure of medical data. Terminated or former employees in the data processing environment should have no access to data from the medical records concerning patients.

(b) Upon termination of computer services for a physician, those computer files maintained for the physician should be physically turned over to the physician. They may be destroyed (erased) only if it is established that the physician has another copy (in some form). In the event of file erasure, the computer service bureau should verify in writing to the physician that the erasure has taken place. (IV)

Issued prior to April 1977.

Updated June 1994.

M.D. Pa. 1987 Plaintiff in a medical malpractice action sought to preclude his treating physicians from serving as defendant's expert witnesses at trial. The court held that defense counsel's failure to provide prior notice of ex parte communication with plaintiff's treating physicians barred their use as defense experts. Referring to Petrillo v. Syntex Laboratories, Inc., 148 Ill. App. 3d 581, 499 N.E.2d 952 (1986), the court noted that the court there favorably cited Principle IV and Opinions 5.05, 5.06, and 5.07 (1984) in support of a public policy protecting confidentiality between physician and patient and against ex parte discussion. *Manion v. N.P.W. Medical Center of N.E. Pa., Inc.*, 676 F.Supp. 585, 591.

Ill. App. 1986 Defense attorney in product liability suit was held in contempt of court for conducting ex parte discussions with plaintiff-patient's treating physician without patient's consent and contrary to authorized methods of discovery. The court held that the strong public policy favoring physician-patient confidentiality articulated in Principles II and IV and Opinions 5.05, 5.06, 5.07, and 5.08 (1984) justified a rule against such ex parte discussions. Further, the court held that the public has the right to rely on physicians to faithfully execute their ethical obligations. *Petrillo v. Syntex Laboratories, Inc.*, 148 Ill. App. 3d 581, 499 N.E.2d 952, 957, 958, 959, cert. denied 483 U.S. 1007 (1987).

Pa. Super. 1988 Plaintiff-patient sued her physician for breach of confidentiality when physician conferred with defense counsel in plaintiff's malpractice suit against the hospital (physician's employer). In its majority opinion, the court cited Principle IV, commenting that it gave very little guidance to physicians but nonetheless was not violated by the physician. The court also noted Opinion 5.07 (1986) finding that the plaintiff's suit minimized her expectations of confidentiality. The dissent, however, interpreted these same provisions, along with Opinion 5.05 (1986), as protecting plaintiff's expectations of confidentiality. *Moses v. McWilliams*, 379 Pa. Super. 150, 549 A.2d 950, 956, 962 (dissent) appeal denied 521 Pa. 630, 558 A.2d 532 (1989).

Journal 1997 Examines the benefits of unconstrained access to personal medical information. Discusses drawbacks to full disclosure and absolute confidentiality of medical information. Advocates increased awareness of how medical data are used. Proposes guidelines for the best approach to regulation of health care data. Cites Opinion 5.07. Schwartz, *Privacy and the Economics of Personal Health Care Information*, 76 Tex. L. Rev. 1, 59 (1997).

Journal 1997 Considers new data-collection technology enabling collection, storage, and dissemination of data, including medical records information. Discusses the confidentiality problems triggered by increased utilization of computers in health care delivery. Quotes Opinion 5.07. Woodward, *Medical Record Confidentiality and Data Collection: Current Dilemmas*, 25 J. Law, Med. & Ethics 88, 90, 95 (1997).

Journal 1995 Examines federal legislative proposals intended to protect confidentiality of computerized medical records. Notes flaws in these proposals. Concludes that proposed legislation will significantly undermine confidentiality. Cites Opinion 5.07. References Principle IV. Hoge, *Proposed Federal Legislation Jeopardizes Patient Privacy*, 23 Bull. Am. Acad. Psychiatry Law 495, 498, 500 (1995).

Journal 1993 Discusses the issues surrounding the confidentiality of electronic and computerized medical records. Examines the factors that conflict with desirable security measures, such as cost and accessibility. Concludes that any legal standard addressing this problem should balance the need to protect patient confidentiality with the practical constraints limiting ideal security. References Principle IV and Opinion 5.07. Waller & Fulton, *The Electronic Chart; Keeping it Confidential and Secure*, 26 J. Health & Hosp. L. 104, 105 (April 1993).

Journal 1984 Discusses the broad content of medical records, noting that they are being demanded for use in a variety of contexts. Observes that available ethical and legal guidelines are insufficient to aid physicians in addressing issues of patient privacy and confidentiality. Concludes that there is need for legislation in order to provide suitable guidance to physicians who fulfill an important role in protecting patient privacy. Cites 1981 Opinions 5.03, 5.04, 5.05 [now Opinion 5.06], 5.06 [now Opinion 5.07], 5.07 [now Opinion 5.08], and 5.08 [now Opinion 5.09]. Gellman, *Prescribing Privacy: The Uncertain Role of the Physician in the Protection of Patient Privacy*, 62 No. Carolina L. Rev. 255, 271 (1984).

5.075 Confidentiality: Disclosure of Records to Data Collection Companies

Data collection from computerized or other patient records for marketing purposes raises serious ethical concerns. In some cases, firms have sought to amass information on physicians' prescribing practices on behalf of pharmaceutical houses for marketing purposes. Often, physicians are offered incentives such as computer hardware and software packages in return for agreeing to such an arrangement. They may be told that data-collecting software does not capture patients' names.

These arrangements may violate principles of informed consent and patient confidentiality. Patients divulge information to their physicians only for purposes of diagnosis and treatment. If other uses are to be made of the information, patients must give their permission after being fully informed about the purpose of such disclosures. If permission is not obtained, physicians violate patient confidentiality by sharing specific and intimate information from patients' records with commercial interests.

Arrangements of this kind may also violate Opinion 8.061 on gifts to physicians from industry.

Finally, these arrangements may harm the integrity of the patient-physician relationship. The trust that is fundamental to this relationship is based on the principle that the physicians are the agents first and foremost of their patients. (I, II, IV)

Issued June 1994.

5.08 Confidentiality: Insurance Company Representative

History, diagnosis, prognosis, and the like acquired during the patient-physician relationship may be disclosed to an insurance company representative only if the patient or a lawful representative has consented to the disclosure. A physician's responsibilities to patients are not limited to the actual practice of medicine. They also include the performance of some services ancillary to the practice of medicine. These services might include certification that the patient was under the physician's care and comment on the diagnosis and therapy in the particular case. See also Opinion 2.135. (IV)

Issued prior to April 1977.

N.D. Ohio 1965 Plaintiff-patient alleged that the defendant-malpractice insurer induced physician to reveal confidential information about plaintiff on pretext that plaintiff filed a malpractice suit. In denying defendant's motion for reconsideration of the court's earlier opinion, the court confirmed its holding that actions of a third party inducing a physician to divulge confidential information may result in liability to the patient. In so holding, the court quoted (with incorrect citation to Ch. II, Sec.1) Principles Ch. I, Sec.2 (1912), [now Principle IV and Opinion 5.08], to emphasize the medical profession's established views regarding confidentiality. *Hammonds v. Aetna Casualty & Sur. Co.*, 243 F. Supp. 793, 803.

Fla. App. 1995 The court considered the issue of the effect of § 455.241(2) of the Florida Statutes on right of defense in a medical malpractice action to engage in ex parte communications with plaintiff's non-party treating physician. The court held that a 1988 amendment to § 455.241(2) negated the applicability of the statute to medical malpractice cases. The dissent, citing Petrillo v. Syntex Laboratories, Inc., 148 Ill. App. 3d 581, 499 N.E.2d 952 (1986), quoted Principles II and IV and Opinions 5.05, 5.06, and 5.08 as strong public policy support for its position that ex parte communications should be barred altogether. *Castillo-Plaza v. Green*, 655 So. 2d 197, 206 n.4.

Ill. App. 1986 Defense attorney in product liability suit was held in contempt of court for conducting ex parte discussions with plaintiff-patient's treating physician without patient's consent and contrary to authorized methods of discovery. The court held that the strong public policy favoring physician-patient confidentiality articulated in Principles II and IV and Opinions 5.05, 5.06, 5.07, and 5.08 (1984) justified a rule against such ex parte discussions. Further, the court held that the public has the right to rely on physicians to faithfully execute their ethical obligations. *Petrillo v. Syntex Laboratories, Inc.*, 148 Ill. App. 3d 581, 499 N.E.2d 952, 957, 958, 959, cert. denied, 483 U.S. 1007 (1987).

Journal 1984 Discusses the broad content of medical records, noting that they are being demanded for use in a variety of contexts. Observes that available ethical and legal guidelines are insufficient to aid physicians in addressing issues of patient privacy and confidentiality. Concludes that there is need for legislation in order to provide suitable guidance to physicians who fulfill an important role in protecting patient privacy. Cites 1981 Opinions 5.03, 5.04, 5.05 [now Opinion 5.06], 5.06 [now Opinion 5.07], 5.07 [now Opinion 5.08], and 5.08 [now Opinion 5.09]. Gellman, *Prescribing Privacy: The Uncertain Role of the Physician in the Protection of Patient Privacy*, 62 No. Carolina L. Rev. 255, 271 (1984).

5.09*   Confidentiality: Physicians in Industry

Where a physician's services are limited to pre-employment physical examinations or examinations to determine if an employee who has been ill or injured is able to return to work, no physician-patient relationship should be considered to exist between the physician and those individuals. However, a physician is obligated to divulge important health information to the patient which the physician discovers as a result of the examination. Nevertheless, the information obtained by the physician as a result of such examinations is confidential and should not be communicated to a third party without the individual's prior written consent, unless it is required by law. If the individual authorized

* This opinion is currently under reconsideration by the Council, and may be amended in the next edition of the Code of Medical Ethics. Contact the Ethics Standards Division of the AMA for the most up-to-date version.

the release of medical information to an employer or a potential employer, the physician should release only that information which is reasonably relevant to the employer's decision regarding that individual's ability to perform the work required by the job.

A physician-patient relationship does exist when a physician renders treatment to an employee, even though the physician is paid by the employer. If the employee's illness or injury is work-related, the release of medical information as to the treatment provided to the employer may be subject to the provisions of worker's compensation laws. The physician must comply with the requirements of such laws, if applicable. However, the physician may not otherwise discuss the employee's health condition with the employer without the employee's consent or, in the event of the employee's incapacity, the family's consent.

Whenever statistical information about employees' health is released, all employee identities should be deleted. (IV)

Issued July 1983.

Updated June 1994 and June 1996.

Mass. 1984 Employee sued employer for libel and invasion of privacy following disclosure of medical facts about employee to other employees. In part, claim involved disclosure of opinion about employee's mental state to his supervisor by physician retained by employer. Citing Principle 9 (1957) [now Principle IV and Opinions 5.05 and 5.09], the court held that a physician retained by an employer may disclose to the employer information concerning an employee if receipt of the information is reasonably necessary to serve a substantial and valid business interest of the employer. *Bratt v. International Business Mach. Corp.*, 392 Mass. 508, 467 N.E.2d 126, 137 n.23.

Journal 1991 Explores ethical problems unique to the field of forensic psychiatry. Presents the results of a survey of members of the American Academy of Psychiatry and the Law (AAPL), asking their opinions regarding proposed ethical guidelines. Concludes that AAPL members are both interested in and sensitive to current ethical issues. Quotes Opinions 1.02 and 5.09. Weinstock, Leong, & Silva, *Opinions by AAPL Forensic Psychiatrists on Controversial Ethical Guidelines: A Survey*, 19 Bull. Am. Acad. Psychiatry Law 237, 238 (1991).

Journal 1984 Discusses the broad content of medical records, noting that they are being demanded for use in a variety of contexts. Observes that available ethical and legal guidelines are insufficient to aid physicians in addressing issues of patient privacy and confidentiality. Concludes that there is need for legislation in order to provide suitable guidance to physicians who fulfill an important role in protecting patient privacy. Cites 1981 Opinions 5.03, 5.04, 5.05 [now Opinion 5.06], 5.06 [now Opinion 5.07], 5.07 [now Opinion 5.08], and 5.08 [now Opinion 5.09]. Gellman, *Prescribing Privacy: The Uncertain Role of the Physician in the Protection of Patient Privacy*, 62 No. Carolina L. Rev. 255, 271 (1984).

6.00 Opinions on Fees and Charges

6.01 Contingent Physician Fees

If a physician's fee for medical service is contingent on the successful outcome of a claim, such as a malpractice or worker's compensation claim, there is the ever-present danger that the physician may become less of a healer and more of an advocate or partisan in the proceedings. Accordingly, a physician's fee for medical services should be based on the value of the service provided by the physician to the patient and not on the uncertain outcome of a contingency that does not in any way relate to the value of the medical service.

A physician's fee should not be made contingent on the successful outcome of medical treatment. Such arrangements are unethical because they imply that successful outcomes from treatment are guaranteed, thus creating unrealistic expectations of medicine and false promises to consumers. (VI)

Issued prior to April 1977.

Updated June 1994.

Cal. App. 1992 Lower court held that a contingent fee agreement between plaintiff and a medical-legal consulting service violated public policy and was void. In reversing, appellate court referred to Polo v. Gotchel 225 N.J. Super. 492, 542 A.2d 947 (1987) and Dupree v. Malpractice Research, Inc., 179 Mich. App. 254, 445 N.W.2d 498 (1989) which had relied on Opinion 8.04 (1984) [now Opinion 6.01] to hold that contingent fee consulting contracts were per se invalid. The court was unpersuaded by the reasoning of these decisions, stating that (1) the contingent fee agreement was with a company, not with a physician, and (2) the term "medical services" in the Opinion refers to patient treatment and not to consulting services provided in conjunction with the services of an attorney. Ojeda v. Sharp Cabrillo Hosp., 8 Cal. App. 4th 1, 12, 13 n.11, 14, 10 Cal. Rptr. 2d 230, 237 n.11, 238.

Mich. App. 1989 Plaintiffs, who settled an underlying medical malpractice suit, sought to invalidate contingent fee contract with expert witness service. Plaintiffs had paid witness and report fees, travel costs, and other expenses in advance according to a fee schedule but objected to a charge of 20 percent of their recovery. The court, citing Opinion 8.04 (1984) [now Opinion 6.01], held that the contingent fee contract for expert witnesses was repugnant to the public policy of preserving the plaintiff's recovery and preventing the exaggeration of favorable testimony and would not be enforced. Further, the court refused to consider defendant's quantum meruit claim, since some fees had been paid in advance, and any further attempt to collect fees would fail to deter such contracts. Dupree v. Malpractice Research, Inc., 179 Mich. App. 254, 445 N.W.2d 498, 501.

N.J. Super. 1987 Contingent fee agreement between plaintiff's attorney in a medical malpractice action and a medical-legal consulting service which linked plaintiff with potential expert witnesses violated public policy and was void. The court cited with approval Opinion 8.04 (1984) [now Opinion 6.01], which states that a physician's fees should not be based upon the outcome of litigation because of the risk that the physician may become more of an advocate than a healer. Polo v. Gotchel, 225 N.J. Super. 429, 542 A.2d 947, 948.

Journal 1991 Looks at the problem of high expert witness fees and lack of access to expert testimony by those who may need it. Considers the possibility of a contingent fee arrangement for expert witnesses. Analyzes the reasoning behind the current ban on such arrangements. Proposes revamping the current system to allow certain types of contingent fee arrangements. Quotes Opinion 8.04 (1984) [now Opinion 6.01]. Note, *Contingent Expert Witness Fees: Access and Legitimacy*, 64 So. Cal. L. Rev. 1363, 1374, 1382 (1991).

Journal 1990 Examines conflicting court decisions that have addressed the appropriateness of medical-legal consulting services and their use of contingent fee arrangements. Considers ethical opinions on this issue. Cautions against engaging the services of consulting groups charging contingent fees. Concludes by discussing the need for a less troublesome solution to the problems plaintiffs face in malpractice and personal injury cases. Quotes Opinion 6.01. Cites Opinions 6.12 (1989) [now Opinion 6.05] and 9.07. Dillon, *Contingent Fees and Medical-Legal Consulting Services: Economical or Unethical?*, 11 J. Legal Med. 93, 101, 111 (1990).

6.02   Fee Splitting

Payment by or to a physician solely for the referral of a patient is fee splitting and is unethical.

A physician may not accept payment of any kind, in any form, from any source, such as a pharmaceutical company or pharmacist, an optical company or the manufacturer of medical appliances and devices, for prescribing or referring a patient to said source.

In each case, the payment violates the requirement to deal honestly with patients and colleagues. The patient relies upon the advice of the physician on matters of referral. All referrals and prescriptions must be based on the skill and quality of the physician to whom the patient has been referred or the quality and efficacy of the drug or product prescribed. (II)

Issued prior to April 1977.

Updated June 1994.

Kan. App. 1985 Members of a medical partnership sought an injunction to enforce a covenant not to compete against defendant-physician, a former partner. Defendant asserted that the covenant was void as against public policy relying on Opinion 9.02 (1984). The court however ruled that the covenant was reasonable as defined by precedent and that it was bound to follow this precedent as opposed to the American Medical Association's position regarding such covenants. Defendant further argued enforcement of the covenant was precluded because the partnership had violated ethical norms, apparently referring to Opinions 6.03 and 6.04 (1984) [now Opinions 6.02 and 6.03] which were part of partnership contract. The court held that defendant was estopped from complaining about the partnership's actions due to his own conduct. *Axtell Clinic v. Cranston*, No. 56,745 (Kan. Ct. App. June 20, 1985) (LEXIS, States Library, Kan. file).

Mass. 1955 Plaintiff-physician was charged under state licensing statute by defendant-board with conspiracy and fee-splitting. Both parties sought a declaratory judgment as to whether the defendant-board had jurisdiction to determine plaintiff's guilt or innocence. In holding that the board was qualified to determine if plaintiff's actions constituted "gross misconduct" under the statute, the court referred to Principles Ch. I, Secs. 1 and 6 (1947) [now Principle II and Opinion 6.02] delineating, in part, limitations on payment for medical services. These provisions, the court said, reflected the medical profession's understanding of its "peculiar obligations." *Forziati v. Board of Registration in Medicine*, 333 Mass. 125, 128 N.E.2d 789, 791.

Journal 1985 Focuses on the importance of patient autonomy in medical decisionmaking. Initially describes how existing doctrines protect the value of autonomy in the context of the physician-patient relationship, then examines various problems in the current protective scheme. Case law is evaluated wherein enhanced protection is afforded to patient autonomy. Concludes by recommending the creation of an independent articulable protected interest in patient autonomy. Quotes Principles II and IV. Cites Opinions 4.04 (1984) [now Opinion 8.08] and 6.03

(1984) [now Opinion 6.02]. Shultz, *From Informed Consent to Patient Choice: A New Protected Interest*, 95 Yale L. J. 219, 275 (1985).

6.03 Fee Splitting: Referrals to Health Care Facilities

Clinics, laboratories, hospitals, or other health care facilities that compensate physicians for referral of patients are engaged in fee splitting which is unethical.

Health care facilities should not compensate a physician who refers patients there for the physician's cognitive services in prescribing, monitoring, or revising the patient's course of treatment. Payment for these cognitive services is acceptable when it comes from patients, who are the beneficiaries of the physician's services, or from the patient's designated third-party payer.

Offering or accepting payment for referring patients to research studies (finder's fees) is also unethical. (II)

Issued prior to April 1977.

Updated June 1994 and June 1996 based on the report, "Finder's Fees: Payment for the Referral of Patients to Clinical Research Studies," adopted December 1994.

Kan. App. 1985 Members of a medical partnership sought an injunction to enforce a covenant not to compete against defendant-physician, a former partner. Defendant asserted that the covenant was void as against public policy relying on Opinion 9.02 (1984). The court however ruled that the covenant was reasonable as defined by precedent and that it was bound to follow this precedent as opposed to the American Medical Association's position regarding such covenants. Defendant further argued enforcement of the covenant was precluded because the partnership had violated ethical norms, apparently referring to Opinions 6.03 and 6.04 (1984) [now Opinions 6.02 and 6.03] which were part of partnership contract. The court held that defendant was estopped from complaining about the partnership's actions due to his own conduct. *Axtell Clinic v. Cranston*, No. 56,745 (Kan. Ct. App. June 20, 1985) (LEXIS, States Library, Kan. file).

6.04 Fee Splitting: Drug or Device Prescription Rebates

A physician may not accept any kind of payment or compensation from a drug company or device manufacturer for prescribing its products. The physician should keep the following considerations in mind:

(1) A physician should only prescribe a drug or device based on reasonable expectations of the effectiveness of the drug or device for the particular patient.

(2) The quantity of the drug prescribed should be no greater than that which is reasonably required for the patient's condition. (II)

Issued March 1980.

Ohio 1980 A physician, charged with violating the state medical licensing statute by distributing controlled substances without a proper license and writing prescriptions for narcotics in the name of one person when they were intended for another, challenged the state medical board's decision to suspend his license and place him on two years probation. Under the statute, a physician could be disciplined for various activities including "violation of any provision of a code of ethics of a national professional organization" such as the American Medical Association. The board found in part that the physician's actions violated Principles 4 and 7 (1957) [now Principles II and III and Opinions 6.04 and 9.04]. The trial court reversed, holding that the board had insufficient evidence for its decision, and the court of appeals affirmed. On appeal, the supreme court held that expert testimony was not required at a hearing before a medical licensing board because they were experts and could determine for themselves whether the Principles had been violated. *Arlen v. State*, 61 Ohio St. 2d 168, 399 N.E.2d 1251, 1252, 1253-54.

Journal 1992 Surveys federal and state antikickback and antireferral statutes pertaining to drug and device marketing activities. Considers the effectiveness of regulatory safe harbors. Reviews the AMA's ethical guidelines concerning gifts to physicians from industry. Quotes Opinion 6.04. References Opinion 8.061. Kirschenbaum & Kuhlik, *Federal and State Laws Affecting Discounts, Rebates, and Other Marketing Practices for Drugs and Devices*, 47 Food & Drug L. J. 533, 560 (1992).

6.05   Fees for Medical Services

A physician should not charge or collect an illegal or excessive fee. For example, an illegal fee occurs when a physician accepts an assignment as full payment for services rendered to a Medicare patient and then bills the patient for an additional amount. A fee is excessive when after a review of the facts a person knowledgeable as to current charges made by physicians would be left with a definite and firm conviction that the fee is in excess of a reasonable fee. Factors to be considered as guides in determining the reasonableness of a fee include the following:

(1) the difficulty and/or uniqueness of the services performed and the time, skill, and experience required;

(2) the fee customarily charged in the locality for similar physician services;

(3) the amount of the charges involved;

(4) the quality of performance;

(5) the experience, reputation, and ability of the physician in performing the kind of services involved. (II)

Issued prior to April 1977.

Updated June 1994.

Journal 1990 Examines conflicting court decisions that have addressed the appropriateness of medical-legal consulting services and their use of contingent fee arrangements. Considers ethical opinions on this issue. Cautions against engaging the services of consulting groups charging contingent fees. Concludes by discussing the need for a less troublesome solution to the problems plaintiffs face in malpractice and personal injury cases. Quotes Opinion 6.01. Cites Opinions 6.12 (1989) [now Opinion 6.05] and 9.07. Dillon, *Contingent Fees and Medical-Legal Consulting Services: Economical or Unethical?*, 11 J. Legal Med. 93, 101, 111 (1990).

6.06   **Opinion 6.06, Fees: Group Practice,** issued in March 1981, was deleted in June 1994.

6.07   Insurance Form Completion Charges

The attending physician should complete without charge the appropriate "simplified" insurance claim form as a part of service to the patient to enable the patient to receive his or her benefits. A charge for more complex or multiple forms may be made in conformity with local custom. (II)

Issued prior to April 1977.

Updated June 1994.

Journal 1992 Discusses the ethical and legal boundaries of medical treatment. Examines occasions when these boundaries are crossed, including sexual and financial improprieties. Concludes that minor boundary violations occur frequently, but warns that if they become too frequent or serious, physicians risk substantial liability. Quotes Opinion 6.06 [sic] 6.07. Simon, *Treatment Boundary Violations: Clinical, Ethical, and Legal Considerations*, 20 *Bull. Am. Acad. Psychiatry Law* 269, 282 (1992).

6.08   Interest Charges and Finance Charges

Although harsh or commercial collection practices are discouraged in the practice of medicine, a physician who has experienced problems with delinquent accounts may properly choose to request that payment be made at the time of treatment or add interest or other reasonable charges to delinquent accounts. The patient must be notified in advance of the interest or other reasonable finance or service charges by such means as the posting of a notice in the physician's waiting room, the distribution of leaflets describing the office billing practices and appropriate notations on the billing statement. The physician must comply with state and federal laws and regulations applicable to the imposition of such charges. Physicians are encouraged to review their accounting/collection policies to ensure that no patient's account is sent to collection without the physician's knowledge. Physicians who choose to add an interest or finance charge to accounts not paid within a reasonable time are encouraged to use compassion and discretion in hardship cases. (II)

Issued prior to April 1977.

Updated June 1994.

Cal. App. 1968 Plaintiff-physician sought dissolution of a medical partnership with defendant's decedent, and also sought a larger percentage of the partnership receipts based upon an alleged oral agreement. Defendant crossclaimed to enjoin plaintiff from taking physical control of the partnership offices and patient records. The trial court enjoined plaintiff from treating previous patients, requiring that he return all medical records and pay defendant all fees received from patients he had treated during the time of dispute. The appellate court reversed insofar as the injunction prohibited the plaintiff from treating patient who desired to continue to receive his services or prevented access to medical records essential for this purpose, citing Opinions and Reports of the Judicial Council Sec. 7, Para. 16, Sec. 5, Para. 21 and Sec. 9 (1966) [now Opinions 6.08, 5.02, and 5.05] to support view that patients may not be regarded as the subject of "ownership". *Jones v. Fakehany*, 261 *Cal. App.* 2d 298, 67 *Cal. Rptr.* 810, 815, 816 n.1.

6.09   Laboratory Bill

When it is not possible for the laboratory bill to be sent directly to the patient, the referring physician's bill to the patient should indicate the actual charges for laboratory services, including the name of the laboratory, as well as any separate charges for the physician's own professional services. (II)

Issued prior to April 1977.

6.10   Services Provided by Multiple Physicians

Each physician engaged in the care of the patient is entitled to compensation commensurate with the value of the service he or she has personally rendered.

No physician should bill or be paid for a service which is not performed; mere referral does not constitute a professional service for which a professional charge should be made or for which a fee may be ethically paid or received.

When services are provided by more than one physician, each physician should submit his or her own bill to the patient and be compensated separately, if possible. A physician should not charge a markup, commission, or profit on the services rendered by others.

It is ethically permissible in certain circumstances, however, for a surgeon to engage other physicians to assist in the performance of a surgical procedure and to pay a reasonable amount for such assistance, provided the nature of the financial arrangement is made known to the patient. This principle applies whether or not the assisting physician is the referring physician. (II)

Issued prior to April 1977.

Updated June 1994.

6.11   Competition

Competition between and among physicians and other health care practitioners on the basis of competitive factors such as quality of services, skill, experience, miscellaneous conveniences offered to patients, credit terms, fees charged, etc., is not only ethical but is encouraged. Ethical medical practice thrives best under free market conditions when prospective patients have adequate information and opportunity to choose freely between and among competing physicians and alternate systems of medical care. (VII)

Issued July 1983.

Ohio App. 1991 Medical corporation sought an injunction to enforce a covenant not to compete against defendant-physician. The lower court granted summary judgment based on a referee's report which concluded that, under Principle VI and Opinions 6.11, 9.02, and 9.06 (1989) restrictive covenants were *per se* unenforceable as a matter of public policy. While recognizing a strong public interest in allowing open access to health care, the appellate court in reversing held that Opinion 9.02, which applied specifically to restrictive covenants, only "discouraged" such covenants. *Ohio Urology, Inc. v. Poll, 72 Ohio. App. 446, 450, 451, 594 N.E.2d 1027, 1030, 1031.*

Journal 1997 Examines noncompetition clauses in the medical field. Reviews policy concerns and historical and common-law analyses of agreements not to compete. Posits that, the more commercialized the medical profession becomes, the more noncompetition clauses infringe upon the physician-patient relationship and patients' rights. Quotes Opinions 9.02 and 9.06. Cites Preamble and Opinion 6.11. Comment, *Noncompetition Clauses in Physician Employment Contracts in Oregon, 76 Or. L. Rev. 195, 204-06 (1997).*

Journal 1993 Discusses the controversies surrounding advertising in medicine and physician self-referral. Proposes adoption of the model of the physician as either professional or honest businessman. Considers the implications of these models with respect to advertising and self-referral. Quotes Opinion 6.11. Brody, *The Physician as Professional and the Physician as Honest Businessman, 119 Arch. Otolaryngol. Head Neck Surg. 495, 496 (1993).*

Journal 1991 Considers the question of whether physicians should provide medical treatment to those who come to them for second opinions. Analyzes important ethical and legal guidelines. Concludes that each physician must individually decide whether to treat these patients. Quotes Opinions 6.11, 9.06, and 9.12. Cites Opinion 9.02. Ile, *Should Physicians Treat Patients Who Seek Second Opinions?*, 266 J.A.M.A. 273, 274 (1991).

6.12 Forgiveness or Waiver of Insurance Copayments

Under the terms of many health insurance policies or programs, patients are made more conscious of the cost of their medical care through copayments. By imposing copayments for office visits and other medical services, insurers hope to discourage unnecessary health care. In some cases, financial hardship may deter patients from seeking necessary care if they would be responsible for a copayment for the care. Physicians commonly forgive or waive copayments to facilitate patient access to needed medical care. When a copayment is a barrier to needed care because of financial hardship, physicians should forgive or waive the copayment.

A number of clinics have advertised their willingness to provide detailed medical evaluations and accept the insurer's payment but waive the copayment for all patients. Cases have been reported in which some of these clinics have conducted excessive and unnecessary medical testing while certifying to insurers that the testing is medically necessary. Such fraudulent activity exacerbates the high cost of health care, violates Opinion 2.19 and is unethical.

Physicians should be aware that forgiveness or waiver of copayments may violate the policies of some insurers, both public and private; other insurers may permit forgiveness or waiver if they are aware of the reasons for the forgiveness or waiver. Routine forgiveness or waiver of copayments may constitute fraud under state and federal law. Physicians should ensure that their policies on copayments are consistent with applicable law and with the requirements of their agreements with insurers. (II)

Issued June 1993.

6.13 Professional Courtesy

Professional courtesy refers to the provision of medical care to physician colleagues or their families free of charge or at a reduced rate. While professional courtesy is a long-standing tradition in the medical profession, it is not an ethical requirement. Physicians should use their own judgment in deciding whether to waive or reduce their fees when treating fellow physicians or their families. Physicians should be aware that accepting insurance payments while waiving patient co-payments may violate Opinion 6.12. (II, IV)

Issued June 1994.

7.00 Opinions on Physician Records

7.01 Records of Physicians: Availability of Information to Other Physicians

The interest of the patient is paramount in the practice of medicine, and everything that can reasonably and lawfully be done to serve that interest must be done by all physicians who have served or are serving the patient. A physician who formerly treated a patient should not refuse for any reason to make records of that patient promptly available on request to another physician presently treating the patient. Proper authorization for the use of records must be granted by the patient. Medical reports should not be withheld because of an unpaid bill for medical services. (IV)

Issued prior to April 1977.

N.Y. Surr. 1968 Patients of a deceased physician filed an action seeking to obtain or copy records maintained by the decedent during his lifetime regarding them. The executor had refused to deliver the records by reason of a provision in the decedent's will directing that his "office records" be destroyed. Quoting Opinions and Reports of the Judicial Council, Sec. 9 Paras. 3, 4, 5, 6, and 7 (1966) [now Opinions 7.01, 7.02, 7.03, and 7.05], the court ruled that, while patient records are the property of the physician, it would be against public policy to permit their destruction. As a result, the court ordered the executor to make the records available to the patients' succeeding physicians at their request. *In re Culbertson's Will, 57 Misc. 2d 391, 292 N.Y.S.2d 806, 808-10.*

S.C. Att'y Gen. 1978 Citing Opinions 5.61, 5.62, and 5.63 (1977) [now Opinions 7.01, 7.02, and 7.03], state attorney general found that patient medical records are the property of the physician or hospital which compiled them and that patients have no ownership rights in them. Further, the opinion concludes that patients have a right to information contained in their records and the right to have records sent to another physician. Patients do not, however, have the right to unlimited direct access to their medical records. *South Carolina Att'y Gen. Op., 1978 S.C. AG LEXIS 806.*

Journal 1997 Compares past ethical opinions to current opinions and notes the differences. Comments on the forces that have changed medical ethics through the years. Notes differing theories on the future course of medical ethics. Quotes Fundamental Elements (Preamble) and Opinions 5.05, 5.057, 7.01, 8.12, 9.12, and 9.131. Cites Fundamental Elements (5) and Opinions 8.115 and 8.13. Buchanan, *Medical Ethics at the Millennium: A Brief Retrospective, 26 Colo. Law. 141, 142, 143, 144, 145 (1997).*

7.02 Records of Physicians: Information and Patients

Notes made in treating a patient are primarily for the physician's own use and constitute his or her personal property. However, on request of the patient a physician should provide a copy or a summary of the record to the patient or to another physician, an attorney, or other person designated by the patient.

Most states have enacted statutes that authorize patient access to medical records. These statutes vary in scope and mechanism for permitting patients to review or copy medical records. Access to mental health records, particularly, may be limited by statute or regulation. A physician should become familiar with the applicable laws, rules, or regulations on patient access to medical records.

The record is a confidential document involving the patient-physician relationship and should not be communicated to a third party without the patient's prior written consent, unless required by law or to protect the welfare of the individual or the community. Medical reports should not be withheld because of an unpaid bill for medical services. Physicians may charge a reasonable fee for copying medical records. (IV)

Issued prior to April 1977.

Updated June 1994.

N.Y. Surr. 1968 Patients of a deceased physician filed an action seeking to obtain or copy records maintained by the decedent during his lifetime regarding them. The executor had refused to deliver the records by reason of a provision in the decedent's will directing that his "office records" be destroyed. Quoting Opinions and Reports of the Judicial Council, Sec. 9 Paras. 3, 4, 5, 6, and 7 (1966) [now Opinions 7.01, 7.02, 7.03, and 7.05], the court ruled that, while patient records are the property of the physician, it would be against public policy to permit their destruction. As a result, the court ordered the executor to make the records available to the patients' succeeding physicians at their request. *In re Culbertson's Will, 57 Misc. 2d 391, 292 N.Y.S.2d 806, 808-10.*

S.C. Att'y Gen. 1978 Citing Opinions 5.61, 5.62, and 5.63 (1977) [now Opinions 7.01, 7.02, and 7.03], state attorney general found that patient medical records are the property of the physician or hospital which compiled them and that patients have no ownership rights in them. Further, the opinion concludes that patients have a right to information contained in their records and the right to have records sent to another physician. Patients do not, however, have the right to unlimited direct access to their medical records. *South Carolina Att'y Gen. Op., 1978 S.C. AG LEXIS 806.*

7.03   Records of Physicians Upon Retirement or Departure From a Group

A patient's records may be necessary to the patient in the future not only for medical care but also for employment, insurance, litigation, or other reasons. When a physician retires or dies, patients should be notified and urged to find a new physician and should be informed that upon authorization, records will be sent to the new physician. Records which may be of value to a patient and which are not forwarded to a new physician should be retained, either by the treating physician, another physician, or such other person lawfully permitted to act as a custodian of the records.

The patients of a physician who leaves a group practice should be notified that the physician is leaving the group. Patients of the physician should also be notified of the physician's new address and offered the opportunity to have their medical records forwarded to the departing physician at his or her new practice. It is unethical to withhold such information upon request of a patient. If the responsibility for notifying patients falls to the departing physician rather than to the group, the group should not interfere with the discharge of these duties by withholding patient lists or other necessary information. (IV)

Issued prior to April 1977.

Updated June 1994 and June 1996.

N.D. Ill. 1996 A corporation which provided hair transplants brought suit against a physician group under contract to provide medical services to the corporation. The complaint alleged that the defendants had breached the contract in bad faith by attempting to start their own company, by hiring staff members away, and by threatening to enforce noncompetition covenants in their contracts should any physicians attempt to remain with the corporation. The court referred to Opinion 9.02 as explicitly discouraging the use of restrictive covenants in contracts with physicians. Additionally, with apparent reference to Opinion 7.03, the court noted that defendants had not sent notices advising patients of the departure of physicians from the corporation, or of the departing physicians' new practice locations. *Cleveland Hair Clinic, Inc. v. Puig, 968 F. Supp. 1227, 1246.*

N.Y. Surr. 1968 Patients of a deceased physician filed an action seeking to obtain or copy records maintained by the decedent during his lifetime regarding them. The executor had refused to deliver the records by reason of a provision in the decedent's will directing that his "office records" be destroyed. Quoting Opinions and Reports of the Judicial Council, Sec. 9 Paras. 3, 4, 5, 6, and 7 (1966) [now Opinions 7.01, 7.02, 7.03, and 7.05], the court ruled that, while patient records are the property of the physician, it would be against public policy to permit their destruction. As a result, the court ordered the executor to make the records available to the patients' succeeding physicians at their request. *In re Culbertson's Will, 57 Misc. 2d 391, 292 N.Y.S.2d 806, 808-10.*

S.C. Att'y Gen. 1978 Citing Opinions 5.61, 5.62, and 5.63 (1977) [now Opinions 7.01, 7.02, and 7.03], state attorney general found that patient medical records are the property of the physician or hospital which compiled them and that patients have no ownership rights in them. Further, the opinion concludes that patients have a right to information contained in their records and the right to have records sent to another physician. Patients do not, however, have the right to unlimited direct access to their medical records. *South Carolina Att'y Gen. Op., 1978 S.C. AG LEXIS 806.*

7.04	**Sale of a Medical Practice**

A physician or the estate of a deceased physician may sell to another physician the elements which comprise his or her practice, such as furniture, fixtures, equipment, office leasehold, and goodwill. In the sale of a medical practice, the purchaser is buying not only furniture and fixtures, but also goodwill, i.e., the opportunity to take over the patients of the seller.

The transfer of records of patients is subject, however, to the following:

(1) All active patients should be notified that the physician (or the estate) is transferring the practice to another physician who will retain custody of their records and that at their written request, within a reasonable time as specified in the notice, the records or copies will be sent to any other physician of their choice. Rather than destroy the records of a deceased physician, it is better that they be transferred to a practicing physician who will retain them subject to requests from patients that they be sent to another physician.

(2) A reasonable charge may be made for the cost of duplicating records. (IV)

Issued July 1983.

N.Y. Surr. 1977 In a discovery proceeding, respondent-psychiatrist, who had treated some patients of deceased psychiatrist subsequent to his death, allegedly misappropriated decedent's patient records. Estate petitioned court for return of records and damages for injury to value of decedent's practice. Respondent sought dismissal of claim arguing that estate could not sell patient records. The court rejected respondent's request. In so ruling, the court noted that under Principle 9 (1957) [now Principle IV and Opinion 5.05] prohibiting physicians from revealing patient confidences, various guidelines had been issued regarding sale of a medical practice [now

Opinion 7.04]. Whether respondent's actions had interfered with the estate's efforts to dispose of decedent's practice in keeping with these guidelines presented the court with factual issues for later resolution. *Estate of Finkle, 90 Misc. 2d 550, 395 N.Y.S.2d 343, 346.*

7.05 Retention of Medical Records

Physicians have an obligation to retain patient records which may reasonably be of value to a patient. The following guidelines are offered to assist physicians in meeting their ethical and legal obligations:

(1) Medical considerations are the primary basis for deciding how long to retain medical records. For example, operative notes and chemotherapy records should always be part of the patient's chart. In deciding whether to keep certain parts of the record, an appropriate criterion is whether a physician would want the information if he or she were seeing the patient for the first time.

(2) If a particular record no longer needs to be kept for medical reasons, the physician should check state laws to see if there is a requirement that records be kept for a minimum length of time. Most states will not have such a provision. If they do, it will be part of the statutory code or state licensing board.

(3) In all cases, medical records should be kept for at least as long as the length of time of the statute of limitations for medical malpractice claims. The statute of limitations may be three or more years, depending on the state law. State medical associations and insurance carriers are the best resources for this information.

(4) Whatever the statute of limitations, a physician should measure time from the last professional contact with the patient.

(5) If a patient is a minor, the statute of limitations for medical malpractice claims may not apply until the patient reaches the age of majority.

(6) Immunization records always must be kept.

(7) The records of any patient covered by Medicare or Medicaid must be kept at least five years.

(8) In order to preserve confidentiality when discarding old records, all documents should be destroyed.

(9) Before discarding old records, patients should be given an opportunity to claim the records or have them sent to another physician, if it is feasible to give them the opportunity.

Issued prior to April 1977.

Updated June 1994.

N.Y. Surr. 1968 Patients of a deceased physician filed an action seeking to obtain or copy records maintained by the decedent during his lifetime regarding them. The executor had refused to deliver the records by reason of a provision in the decedent's will directing that his "office records" be destroyed. Quoting Opinions and Reports of the Judicial Council, Sec. 9 Paras. 3, 4, 5, 6, and 7 (1966) [now Opinions 7.01, 7.02, 7.03, and 7.05], the court ruled that, while patient records are the property of the physician, it would be against public policy to permit their destruction. As a result, the court ordered the executor to make the records available to the patients' succeeding physicians at their request. *In re Culbertson's Will, 57 Misc. 2d 391, 292 N.Y.S.2d 806, 808-10.*

8.00 Opinions on Practice Matters

8.01 Appointment Charges

A physician may charge a patient for a missed appointment or for one not cancelled 24 hours in advance if the patient is fully advised that the physician will make such a charge. (VI)

Issued prior to April 1977.

Updated June 1994.

8.02 The previous Opinion 8.02, Clinics, was deleted in June 1994.

8.02 Ethical Guidelines for Physicians in Management Positions and Other Non-Clinical Roles

Physicians in administrative and other non-clinical roles must put the needs of patients first. At least since the time of Hippocrates, physicians have cultivated the trust of their patients by placing patient welfare before all other concerns. The ethical obligations of physicians are not suspended when a physician assumes a position that does not directly involve patient care. (I, VII)

Issued June 1994 based on the report, "Ethical Guidelines for Medical Consultants," adopted December 1992.

Updated June 1998.

8.03 Conflicts of Interest: Guidelines

Under no circumstances may physicians place their own financial interests above the welfare of their patients. The primary objective of the medical profession is to render service to humanity; reward or financial gain is a subordinate consideration. For a physician unnecessarily to hospitalize a patient, prescribe a drug, or conduct diagnostic tests for the physician's financial benefit is unethical. If a conflict develops between the physician's financial interest and the physician's responsibilities to the patient, the conflict must be resolved to the patient's benefit. (II)

Issued July 1986.

Updated June 1994.

7th Cir. 1984 Plaintiff brought medical malpractice suit against several physicians appointed to the Veterans Administration Department of Medicine and Surgery. The court held that "strict control" test for determining whether defendants ought to be considered employees or independent contractors under the Federal Tort Claims Act was not appropriate because the ethical obligation of a physician to a patient, evidenced by Principle 6 (1957) [now Opinions 8.03 and 8.05], required that independent judgment be exercised, preventing a physician from being "strictly controlled" by the Veterans Administration. *Quilico v. Kaplan, 749 F.2d 480, 483-84.*

10th Cir. 1983 Pursuant to the Federal Tort Claims Act, plaintiff sued the federal government for the negligence of a neurosurgeon, allegedly an employee of a Veteran's Administration hospital. Plaintiff argued that applying the traditional control test to determine a physician's employment status was inappropriate because physicians are bound by Principle 6 (1957) [now Opinions 8.03 and 8.05] requiring them to have "free and complete exercise of [their] medical judgment and skill...." However, the court did not reach the merits of that argument because the contractual agreement between the neurosurgeon and the VA hospital was "outside the parameters of an employer-employee relationship with the government," thus precluding plaintiff's claim. *Lurch v. United States, 719 F.2d 333, 337, cert. denied, 466 U.S. 927. (1984).*

Cal. App. 1967 Physician-stockholders of publicly-owned pharmaceutical corporations and physicians whose medical partnerships owned and operated pharmacies challenged statutory prohibition of physician membership, proprietory interest, and co-ownership of pharmacies. The court quoted Principles Ch. I, Sec. 6 (1947) and a 1960 Judicial Council rule, later included in Opinions and Reports of the Judicial Council Sec. 7, Para. 38 (1965) [now Opinions 8.03, 8.032, and 8.06] in its discussion of the potential conflict of interest created by such ownership. The court held that the statute prohibited physician partnerships from directly owning pharmacies but did not apply to an individual physician or a partnership of physicians who own stock in a corporation which owns and operates a pharamacy. *Magan Medical Clinic v. California State Bd. of Medical Examiners, 249 Cal. App. 2d 124, 57 Cal. Rptr. 256, 262.*

Mich. Att'y Gen. 1977 State attorney general determined that, within limits, it was not illegal for physicians to refer patient specimens to clinical laboratories which they own or in which they have a financial interest. Opinion observes however that, under the Opinions and Reports of the Judicial Council Sec. 7, Paras. 21 and 22 (1972) [now Opinions 8.03 and 8.032] such referrals may be unethical. *Mich. Att'y Gen. Opinion No. 5229, 1977-78 Att'y. Gen. Op. 234.*

Journal 1997 Discusses physician-patient trust in the managed care environment. Explores options for enhancing trustworthiness in this context. Quotes Opinion 8.03. Gray, *Trust and Trustworthy Care in the Managed Care Era, 16 Health Affairs 34, 38, 47-48 (1997).*

Journal 1995 Addresses presidential disability, its past impact on American government, and possible solutions to potential problems. Suggests guidelines for implementation of the Twenty-Fifth Amendment. Examines the effectiveness of a medical commission in determining presidential disability. Proposes enhancement of the role of the President's physician. Quotes Opinion 8.03. Cites Opinions 5.04 and 5.05. Abrams, *The Vulnerable President and the Twenty-Fifth Amendment, with Observations on Guidelines, a Health Commission, and the Role of the President's Physician, 30 Wake Forest L. Rev. 453, 466, 471 (1995).*

Journal 1994 Discusses the issue of whom physicians must serve first—themselves, their patients, insurers, or society. Explores attempts by the legal system to resolve this issue within the framework of risks that may arise in the physician-patient relationship. Focuses on risks arising out of provider economic arrangements and risks arising out of other individual physician characteristics. Quotes Opinions 8.03 and 9.13. Cites Opinion 8.15. Bobinski, *Autonomy and Privacy: Protecting Patients from Their Physicians, 55 U. Pitt. L. Rev. 291, 302, 313 (1994).*

Journal 1994 Observes that health care reform proposals present significant challenges to the role and ethics of attending physicians. Emphasizes that reform proposals must set forth the role envisioned for physicians and must articulate an acceptable ethical framework within which physicians may fulfill that role. Quotes Opinions 4.04, 9.121, and 9.122. Cites Opinions 2.03, 2.09, 5.01, and 8.03. Wolf, *Health Care Reform and the Future of Physician Ethics, 24 Hastings Center Rep. 28, 32, 40 (March/April 1994).*

Journal 1993 Discusses the problem of physicians withholding needed medical treatment from HIV-infected infants. Explores the medical aspects of infant HIV infection. Considers ethical and legal issues involving nontreatment. Concludes that current law should be expanded to eliminate this discrimination. Quotes Opinions 2.09, 2.17, 2.20, 2.22, 4.04, and 8.03. Crossley, *Of Diagnoses and Discrimination: Discriminatory Nontreatment of Infants With HIV Infection, 93 Columbia L. Rev. 1581, 1620, 1621 (1993).*

Journal 1992 Considers the responsibility of HIV-infected health care workers to protect patients from infection. Examines several issues related to this subject including mandatory testing, disclosure to co-workers and supervisors, and the degree to which the practice of an HIV-infected health care worker should be modified. Focuses on whether there is a duty to disclose HIV-positive status to patients. Concludes that courts likely will impose such a requirement when there is a substantial risk of HIV transmission. Quotes Opinions 8.03 (1989) [now Opinion 8.032], and 8.07 (1989) [now Opinion 8.03]. References Opinion 9.131. Lieberman & Derse, *HIV-Positive Health Care Workers and the Obligation to Disclose: Do Patients Have a Right to Know?*, 13 J. Legal Med. 333, 353, 354 (1992).

Journal 1990 Discusses the federal Medicare and Medicaid Anti-Fraud and Abuse statute and physician investment and referral. Explains how this law limits the ability of physicians to adapt investment and referral strategies to an increasingly competitive health care marketplace. Proposes giving regulatory power over physician investments back to the states, which are more able to recognize and exempt beneficial arrangements from otherwise restrictive statutory schemes. Cites Opinion 8.03. Comment, *Regulating Physician Investment and Referral Behavior in the Competitive Health Care Marketplace of the '90s—An Argument for Decentralization*, 65 Wash. L. Rev. 657, 658 (1990).

Journal 1990 Examines various cost control mechanisms utilized by prepaid health plans and other managed care programs and considers the impact of such mechanisms on clinical decision-making. Various reports, commentaries, and studies are evaluated with respect to the impact, if any, of financial incentives on the quality of patient care. Emphasis is placed on the possible existence of conflicts of interest on the part of health care providers in this context and discussion of legal and ethical duties and responsibilities is offered. Quotes Opinions 8.03 [now Opinions 8.03 and 8.032] and 8.13. Hirshfeld, *Defining Full and Fair Disclosure in Managed Care Contracts*, 60 The Citation 67, 70 (1990).

Journal 1990 Discusses efforts of third party payors to control health care expenditures for beneficiaries. Focuses on use of financial incentives to encourage providers to minimize the amount of care provided. Also discusses monitoring of requests for payment to determine necessity of care provided. Raises questions regarding impact of cost control mechanisms on quality of care, observing that available evidence is equivocal. Evaluates importance of disclosure to beneficiaries of use of financial incentives to limit care as well as other cost control mechanisms. Concludes that financial incentives and other cost control techniques should be disclosed and that the rationale for such disclosure is compelling. Quotes Opinions 2.03, 2.09, and 8.03 [now Opinions 8.03 and 8.032]. Cites Opinions 2.19, 4.04, and 4.06. Hirshfeld, *Should Third Party Payors of Health Care Services Disclose Cost Control Mechanisms to Potential Beneficiaries?*, 14 Seton Hall Legis. J. 115, 130, 131, 144, 145, 146 (1990).

Journal 1989 Analyzes the Medicare and Medicaid Patient and Program Protection Act of 1987 and discusses the complexity of fraud and abuse issues that confront hospitals and health care providers who undertake financially attractive business arrangements. Concludes that the 1987 Act, along with its implementing regulations, can offer meaningful guidance in an area of uncertainty for the health care industry. Quotes Opinion 4.05 (1986) [now Opinion 8.03]. Comment, *Curing the Health Care Industry: Government Response to Medicare Fraud and Abuse*, 5 J. Contemp. Health L. & Pol'y 175, 189 (1989).

Journal 1985 Focuses on the importance of patient autonomy in medical decisionmaking. Initially describes how existing doctrines protect the value of autonomy in the context of the physician-patient relationship, then examines various problems in the current protective scheme. Case law is evaluated wherein enhanced protection is afforded to patient autonomy. Concludes by recommending the creation of an independent articulable protected interest in patient autonomy. Quotes Principles II and IV. Cites Opinions 4.04 (1984) [now Opinions 8.03 and 8.032] and 6.03 (1984) [now Opinion 6.02]. Shultz, *From Informed Consent to Patient Choice: A New Protected Interest*, 95 Yale L. J. 219, 275 (1985).

8.031 Conflicts of Interest: Biomedical Research

Avoidance of real or perceived conflicts of interest in clinical research is imperative if the medical community is to ensure objectivity and maintain individual and institutional integrity. All medical centers should develop specific guidelines for their clinical staff on conflicts of interest. These guidelines should include the following rules: (1) once a clinical investigator becomes involved in a research project for a company or knows that he or she might become involved, she or he, as an individual cannot ethically buy or sell the company's stock until the involvement ends and the results of the research are published or otherwise disseminated to the public; (2) any remuneration received by the researcher from the company whose product is being studied must be commensurate with the efforts of the researcher on behalf of the company; (3) clinical investigators should disclose any material ties to companies whose products they are investigating. They should disclose their financial ties, participation in educational activities supported by the companies, participation in other research projects funded by the companies, consulting arrangements, and any other ties. The disclosures should be made in writing to the medical center where the research is conducted, organizations that are funding the research, and journals that publish the results of the research.

In addition, medical centers should form review committees to examine disclosures by clinical staff about financial associations with commercial corporations. (II, IV)

Issued March 1992 based on the report, "Conflicts of Interest in Biomedical Research," adopted December 1989 (JAMA. 1990; 263: 2790-2793).

Journal 1996 Explores biotechnology advances made possible through cooperation between universities and industries. Observes that clinical investigators involved in company research are ethically prohibited from buying or selling company stock, until results are published. Concludes that cooperation in the biotechnology field will benefit society. Cites Opinion 8.031. Comment, *Alliances for the Future: Cultivating a Cooperative Environment for Biotech Success*, 11 *Berkeley Tech. L. J. 311, 344 (1996)*.

Journal 1991 Considers whether patients should be permitted or required to pay for research in which they participate. Concludes that patient-funded research may be useful, so long as the potential for individual harm and abuse can be minimized. References Opinion 8.031. Morreim, *Patient-Funded Research: Paying the Piper or Protecting the Patient?*, 13 *IRB* 1,2 (May/June 1991).

Journal 1991 Discusses the ethical issues involved when physicians and scientists enroll patients in drug company-sponsored clinical trials in exchange for reimbursement. Focuses on the two major ethical issues raised—informed consent and potential conflicts of interest. Concludes that financial arrangements between drug companies and scientists give the appearance and the opportunity for conflict of interest; thus physicians should be required to disclose funding sources to patients. References Opinion 8.031. Shimm & Spece, *Conflict of Interest and Informed Consent in Industry—Sponsored Clinical Trials*, 12 *J. Legal Med. 477, 481, 507, 510 (1991)*.

8.032 Conflicts of Interest: Health Facility Ownership by a Physician

Physician ownership interests in commercial ventures can provide important benefits in patient care. Physicians are free to enter lawful contractual relationships, including the acquisition of ownership interests in health facilities, products, or equipment. However, when physicians refer patients to facilities in which they have an ownership interest, a potential conflict of interest exists. In general, physicians should not refer patients to a health care facility which is outside their office practice and at which they do not directly provide care or services when they have an investment interest in that facility. The requirement that the physician *directly* provide the care or services should be interpreted as commonly understood. The physician needs to have personal involvement with the provision of care on site.

There may be situations in which a needed facility would not be built if referring physicians were prohibited from investing in the facility. Physicians may invest in and refer to an outside facility, whether or not they provide direct care or services at the facility, if there is a demonstrated need in the community for the facility and alternative financing is not available. Need might exist when there is no facility of reasonable quality in the community or when use of existing facilities is onerous for patients. Self-referral based on demonstrated need cannot be justified simply if the facility would offer some marginal improvement over the quality of services in the community. The potential benefits of the facility should be substantial. The use of existing facilities may be considered onerous when patients face undue delays in receiving services, delays that compromise the patient's care or affect the curability or reversibility of the patient's condition. The requirement that alternative financing not be available carries a burden of proof. The builder would have to undertake efforts to secure funding from banks, other financial institutions, and venture capitalists before turning to self-referring physicians.

Where there is a true demonstrated need in the community for the facility, the following requirements should also be met: (1) physicians should disclose their investment interest to their patients when making a referral, provide a list of effective alternative facilities if they are available, inform their patients that they have free choice to obtain the medical services elsewhere, and assure their patients that they will not be treated differently if they do not choose the physician-owned facility; (2) individuals not in a position to refer patients to the facility should be given a bona fide opportunity to invest in the facility on the same terms that are offered to referring physicians; (3) the opportunity to invest and the terms of investment should not be related to the past or expected volume of referrals or other business generated by the physician investor or owner; (4) there should be no requirement that a physician investor make referrals to the entity or otherwise generate business as a condition for remaining an investor; (5) the return on the physician's investment should be tied to the physician's equity in the facility rather than to the volume of referrals; (6) the entity should not loan funds or guarantee a loan for physicians in a position to refer to the entity; (7) investment contracts should not include "noncompetition clauses" that prevent physicians from investing in other facilities; (8) the physician's ownership interest should be disclosed to third party payers upon request; (9) an internal utilization review program should be established to ensure that investing physicians do not exploit their patients in any way, as by inappropriate or unnecessary utilization; (10) when a physician's commercial interest conflicts to the detriment of the patient, the physician should make alternative arrangements for the care of the patient. (II, III, IV)

Issued prior to April 1977.

Updated March 1992 based on the report, "Conflicts of Interest: Physician Ownership of Medical Facilities," adopted December 1991 (JAMA. 1992; 267: 2366-2369).

Updated June 1994.

C.D. Ill. 1992 A contractual agreement between a clinic and hospital providing undisclosed financial incentives for referrals constituted a "business" aspect of the medical profession and was not exempt from state's Consumer Fraud Act. Reference is made to Council on Ethical Judicial Affairs, Conflicts of Interest—Physician Ownership of Medical Facilities, 267 JAMA 2366 (1992) [now Opinion 8.032], which mandates that a physician disclose his financial interest to his patient when making a referral. *Gadson v. Newman, 807 F. Supp. 1412, 1416.*

E.D. N.Y. 1975 Medical laboratories sought injunction against city's award of exclusive contracts for Medicaid services. The court granted a preliminary injunction and held that the laboratories had a substantial probability of success on the merits of the claim that Medicaid recipients would be deprived of statutory right of free choice of providers. In balancing the equities, the court also noted that the contracts would create an ethical dilemma for physicians who are required to provide patients with free choice of ancillary services under Opinions and Reports of the Judicial Council Sec. 1, Paras. 6 and 14 (1971) [now Opinions 8.032, 8.06, and 9.06]. *Bay Ridge Diagnostic Laboratory, Inc. v. Dumpson, 400 F. Supp. 1104, 1109-10.*

E.D. Va. 1995 Claimants sustained personal injuries when ships collided. In an admiralty action, court had to determine the extent of probable injuries sustained by the claimants. The court observed that a treating physician had referred one of the claimants for tests to a facility in which the physician had a substantial ownership interest. In finding that these tests and procedures were unnecessary and unreasonable, the court quoted Opinion 8.032. *In re Capt. Wool, Inc., 1995 U.S. Dist. LEXIS 20128.*

Cal. App. 1967 Physician-stockholders of publicly-owned pharmaceutical corporations and physicians whose medical partnerships owned and operated pharmacies challenged statutory prohibition of physician membership, proprietory interest, and co-ownership of pharmacies. The court quoted Principles Ch. I, Sec. 6 (1947) and a 1960 Judicial Council rule, later included in Opinions and Reports of the Judicial Council Sec. 7, Para. 38 (1965) [now Opinions 8.03, 8.032 and 8.06] in its discussion of the potential conflict of interest created by such ownership. The court held that the statute prohibited physician partnerships from directly owning pharmacies, but did not apply to an individual physician or a partnership of physicians who own stock in a corporation which owns and operates a pharamacy. *Magan Medical Clinic v. California State Bd. of Medical Examiners, 249 Cal. App. 2d 124, 57 Cal. Rptr. 256, 262.*

Mich. Att'y Gen. 1977 State attorney general determined that, within limits, it was not illegal for physicians to refer patient specimens to clinical laboratories which they own or in which they have a financial interest. Opinion observes however that, under the Opinions and Reports of the Judicial Council Sec. 7, Paras. 21 and 22 (1972) [now Opinions 8.03 and 8.032] such referrals may be unethical. *Mich. Att'y Gen. Opinion No. 5229, 1977-78 Att'y. Gen. Op. 234.*

Journal 1997 Discusses the quality of neurological care and the ethical conflicts that are created by the drive to contain costs. Focuses on quality management and cost-containment programs and the conflicts created when neurologists attempt to reconcile the interests of patients and society. References Opinions 8.032 and 8.13. Bernat, *Quality of Neurological Care: Balancing Cost Control and Ethics*, 54 Arch. Neurol. 1341, 1343, 1345 (1997).

Journal 1995 Examines the metaphor of physicians as fiduciaries. Considers how the law holds physicians accountable in this regard. Discusses limits to this way of perceiving the physician-patient relationship in a changing health care environment. Quotes Preamble. Cites Opinion 8.03 (1986) [now Opinion 8.032]. Rodwin, *Strains in the Fiduciary Metaphor: Divided Physician Loyalties and Obligations in a Changing Health Care System*, XXI Am. J. Law & Med. 241, 246, 250 (1995).

Journal 1993 Discusses potential antitrust entanglements resulting from physician investment and self-referral. Argues that legislative efforts to curb or prohibit these activities are misdirected. Proposes a more effective solution to this problem—enforcement of existing laws. Quotes Opinion 8.032. Morreim, *Blessed Be the Tie That Binds? Antitrust Perils of Physician Investment and Self-Referral*, 14 J. Legal Med. 359, 367, 374, 377, 394, 409 (1993).

Journal 1993 Examines financial conflicts of interest involving physicians. Describes conflicts of interest and reasons for regulating them. Discusses ways to identify conflicts and possible remedies. References Opinion 8.032. Thompson, *Understanding Financial Conflicts of Interest*, 329 New Eng. J. Med. 573 (1993).

Journal 1992 Discusses the safe harbor regulations under the Medicare and Medicaid Antikickback Statute; examines the *Hanlester Network* case; and describes the problem of physician self-referral.

Concludes that a societal consensus is evolving against self-referral. References Opinion 8.032. Crane, *The Problem of Physician Self-Referral Under the Medicare and Medicaid Antikickback Statute: The Hanlester Network Case and the Safe Harbor Regulation*, 268 J.A.M.A. 85, 89, 90 (1992).

Journal 1992 Analyzes the Medicare Antifraud Statute and the safe harbor regulations in light of recent criticisms. Finds that critics have raised both valid and invalid concerns. Concludes that the antifraud statute is an appropriate way to deal with fraud, but that other steps also should be taken. Proposes certain modifications to the regulations. References Opinion 8.032. Farley, *The Medicare Antifraud Statute and Safe Harbor Regulations: Suggestions for Change*, 81 Georgetown L.J. 167, 184 (1992).

Journal 1992 Considers the responsibility of HIV-infected health care workers to protect patients from infection. Examines several issues related to this subject including mandatory testing, disclosure to co-workers and supervisors, and the degree to which the practice of an HIV-infected health care worker should be modified. Focuses on whether there is a duty to disclose HIV-positive status to patients. Concludes that courts likely will impose such a requirement when there is a substantial risk of HIV transmission. Quotes Opinions 8.03 (1989) [now Opinion 8.032], and 8.07 (1989) [now Opinion 8.03]. References Opinion 9.131. Lieberman & Derse, *HIV-Positive Health Care Workers and the Obligation to Disclose: Do Patients Have a Right to Know?*, 13 J. Legal Med. 333, 353, 354 (1992).

Journal 1992 Examines a memorandum issued by the Chief Counsel of the Internal Revenue Service which clearly identified certain transactions that could jeopardize the tax exempt status of hospitals. Points out various criticisms of this memorandum. Concludes that the memorandum provides valuable guidance for hospitals in spite of its shortcomings. References Opinion 8.032. Mancino, *New GCM Suggests Rules for Ventures Between Nonprofit Hospitals and Doctors*, 76 J. Taxation 164, 167 (1992).

Journal 1992 Analyzes the controversy over physician ownership of health care facilities. Examines applicable federal law and regulations. Considers a study of physician joint ventures in Florida and finds that current legislation prohibiting or restricting such arrangements is inadequate. Concludes that future legislation should address this problem. Quotes Opinion 8.032. Mitchell & Scott, *Evidence on Complex Structures of Physician Joint Ventures*, 9 Yale J. Regulation 489, 503 (1992).

Journal 1992 Discusses the problem of physician joint ventures and examines their prevalence in Florida. Presents the results of a study looking at this issue. Finds that physician joint ventures are a common phenomenon in Florida. Concludes that these arrangements may cause physicians to prioritize economic incentives over patients' medical needs. References Opinion 8.032. Mitchell & Scott, *New Evidence of the Prevalence and Scope of Physician Joint Ventures*, 268 J.A.M.A. 80, 84 (1992).

Journal 1992 Examines the issue of physician joint ventures in the context of physical therapy and rehabilitation services. Presents the results of a study comparing service and treatment decisions in joint venture and non-joint venture facilities. Finds that facility utilization, patient cost, and physician profits were higher at the joint venture facilities. Concludes that the medical community, insurance companies, and policy makers should take note of these results. References Opinion 8.032. Mitchell & Scott, *Physician Ownership of Physical Therapy Services: Effects on Charges, Utilization, Profits, and Service Characteristics*, 268 J.A.M.A. 2055, 2058 (1992).

Journal 1992 Examines the problem of physician joint ventures in the context of radiation therapy services. Presents results of a study indicating that such arrangements increase the use and cost of these services and reduce access to care in inner city and rural areas. Concludes that physician joint ventures have negative consequences and proposes that carefully crafted legislation be enacted to ban such arrangements. Quotes Opinion 8.032. Mitchell & Sunshine, *Consequences of Physicians' Ownership of Health Care Facilities—Joint Ventures in Radiation Therapy*, 327 New Eng. J. Med. 1497, 1500 (1992).

Journal 1992 Examines the debate regarding physician self-referral. Focuses on the position of the American Medical Association. Argues in favor of the AMA's statement in general, but urges an even stronger and more comprehensive position in this context. References Opinion 8.032. Relman, *Self-Referral—What's at Stake?*, 327 New Eng. J. Med. 1522, 1524 (1992).

Journal 1992 Explores the problem of physician self-referral and overuse of physician-owned facilities. Presents the results of a study that examined the use of physician-owned testing and treatment facilities in workers' compensation cases. Concludes that in the cases studied, physician ownership of a facility increased the use and cost of services. Quotes Opinion 8.032. Swedlow, Johnson, Smithline, & Milstein, *Increased Costs and Rates of Use in the California Workers' Compensation System as a Result of Self-Referral By Physicians*, 327 New Eng. J. Med. 1502 (1992).

Journal 1991 Discusses conflict of interest problems that sometimes arise in the doctor-patient relationship. Explores the impact of *Moore v. Regents of the University of California*. Looks at the physician as a fiduciary and the law governing fiduciary relationships. Concludes that fiduciary concepts are a valuable basis for establishing ethical and legal guidelines for physician behavior. Quotes Opinions 2.19, 8.03 (1989) [now Opinion 8.032], and 8.06. Healey & Dowling, *Controlling Conflicts of Interest in the Doctor-Patient Relationship: Lessons From Moore v. Regents of the University of California*, 42 Mercer L. Rev. 989, 997, 998 (1991).

Journal 1991 Discusses the issue of HIV-infected surgeons in light of the New Jersey case decision in *Behringer v. Medical Center*. Summarizes the case and presents its implications. Considers future developments. References Opinions 8.032 and 9.131. Orentlicher, *HIV-Infected Surgeons: Behringer v. Medical Center*, 266 J.A.M.A. 1134, 1136 (1991).

Journal 1990 Discusses efforts of third party payors to control health care expenditures for beneficiaries. Focuses on use of financial incentives to encourage providers to minimize the amount of care provided. Also discusses monitoring of requests for payment to determine necessity of care provided. Raises questions regarding impact of cost control mechanisms on quality of care, observing that available evidence is equivocal. Evaluates importance of disclosure to beneficiaries of use of financial incentives to limit care as well as other cost control mechanisms. Concludes that financial incentives and other cost control techniques should be disclosed and that the rationale for such disclosure is compelling. Quotes Opinions 2.03, 2.09, and 8.03 [now Opinions 8.03 and 8.032]. Cites Opinions 2.19, 4.04, and 4.06. Hirshfeld, *Should Third Party Payors of Health Care Services Disclose Cost Control Mechanisms to Potential Beneficiaries?*, 14 Seton Hall Legis. J. 115, 130, 131, 144, 145, 146 (1990).

Journal 1990 Examines various cost control mechanisms utilized by prepaid health plans and other managed care programs and considers the impact of such mechanisms on clinical decision-making. Various reports, commentaries, and studies are evaluated with respect to the impact, if any, of financial incentives on the quality of patient care. Emphasis is placed on the possible existence of conflicts of interest on the part of health care providers in this context and discussion of legal and ethical duties and responsibilities is offered. Quotes Opinions 8.03 [now Opinions 8.03 and 8.032] and 8.13. Hirshfeld, *Defining Full and Fair Disclosure in Managed Care Contracts*, 60 The Citation 67, 70 (1990).

Journal 1990 Considers the arguments for and against banning physician self-referrals. Balances the "laissez-faire" concerns of individual freedom and personal choice with the "Prohibitionists" desire to protect patients from poor quality care and unnecessary referrals. Concludes that civil remedies should be emphasized by extending the doctrines of "bad faith" and "breach of contract" into this arena. References Opinion 8.032. Morreim, *Physician Investment and Self-Referral: Philosophical Analysis of a Contentious Debate*, 15 J. Med. & Phil. 425, 428, 429, 430, 431 (1990).

Journal 1985 Focuses on the importance of patient autonomy in medical decisionmaking. Initially describes how existing doctrines protect the value of autonomy in the context of the physician-patient relationship, then examines various problems in the current protective scheme. Case law is evaluated wherein enhanced protection is afforded to patient autonomy. Concludes by recommending the creation of an independent articulable protected interest in patient autonomy. Quotes Principles II and IV. Cites Opinions 4.04 (1984) [now Opinions 8.03 and 8.032] and 6.03 (1984) [now Opinion 6.02]. Shultz, *From Informed Consent to Patient Choice: A New Protected Interest*, 95 Yale L. J. 219, 275 (1985).

8.035 Conflicts of Interest in Home Health Care

Physicians who refer patients to home care providers or any other outside facility should avoid possible conflicts of interest by not accepting payment from those providers or facilities for referrals or as compensation for their cognitive services in prescribing, monitoring, or revising a patient's course of treatment. Payment for these cognitive services is acceptable when it comes from patients, who are the beneficiaries of the physician's services, or from the patients' designated third-party payers.

In accordance with Opinion 8.032, physicians may refer patients to home care facilities in which they have an ownership interest if they actively participate on-site in the care provided to patients. Since the appropriate frequency and duration of home visits is a medical decision that should be made on a case-by-case basis, there is no specific minimum number of home visits that may be identified as a conclusive test of the physician's involvement in the patient's home care regimen. Although different patients will have different needs, physicians who directly provide care in the patient's home on at least every fourth visit may presumptively be considered to have made home care a true extension of practice. (II, III, IV)

Issued June 1994 based on the report, "Conflicts of Interest: Update on Home Care," adopted December 1993.

8.04   Consultation

Physicians should obtain consultation whenever they believe that it would be medically indicated in the care of the patient or when requested by the patient or the patient's representative. When a patient is referred to a consultant, the referring physician should provide a history of the case and such other information as the consultant may need, calling to the attention of the consultant any specific questions about which guidance is sought, and the consultant should advise the referring physician of the results of the consultant's examination and recommendations. (V)

Issued prior to April 1977.

Updated June 1992 and June 1996.

D.S.C. 1968 Military dependent sued government physicians under Federal Tort Claims Act where child with acute abdominal pain was twice referred to naval hospital with diagnosis of possible appendicitis and twice sent home without treatment, eventually suffering ruptured appendix and serious complications. In finding for the plaintiff, the court quoted Principle 8 (1957) [now Principle V and Opinion 8.04] in considering whether the physicians had a duty to seek consultation in such a situation. *Steeves v. United States, 294 F. Supp. 446, 454.*

Wash. 1951 Plaintiff, a charitable, not for profit medical corporation, offered prepaid health care services to members and their families. Suit was filed against county medical society and others for damages and injunction for defendants' alleged efforts to monopolize prepaid medical care in area and unlawfully restrain competition by plaintiff and its physicians. Defendants alleged as affirmative defense that their efforts were designed to curb "unethical" prepaid contract practice by plaintiff. Court examined at length American Medical Association's position regarding "contract practice" including Principles Ch. III, Art. VI, Secs. 3 and 4 (1947) [now Principle VI and Opinions 8.05 and 9.06] concluding nothing in plaintiff's practice violated the Association's ethical guidelines. Further, quoting Principles Ch. III, Art. III, Sec.1 (1947) [now Opinion 8.04] dealing with consultations, court noted that defendants' efforts impeded plaintiff's physicians from obtaining consultations. Court concluded defendants' actions constituted unlawful, monopolistic behavior and issued an injunction, although it declined to award damages. *Group Health Coop. v. King County Medical Soc'y, 39 Wash. 2d 586, 237 P.2d 737, 744, 750-51, 759-60.*

Journal 1994 Focuses on physicians' legal and ethical duties to pregnant women to provide medical information relevant to patient choice regarding abortion and to make referrals for services that physicians are unable or unwilling to perform. Argues that physicians' own moral views on abortion do not excuse obligations to facilitate choice for patients. Concludes that medical educators, professional associations, women's groups, and state legislatures should address these issues. Cites Opinions 3.04 and 8.04. Law, *Silent No More: Physicians' Legal and Ethical Obligations to Patients Seeking Abortions*, 21 N.Y.U. Rev. L. & Soc. Change 279, 289, 290, 300 (1994).

8.041 Second Opinions

Physicians should recommend that a patient obtain a second opinion whenever they believe it would be helpful in the care of the patient. When recommending a second opinion, physicians should explain the reasons for the recommendation and inform their patients that patients are free to choose a second-opinion physician on their own or with the assistance of the first physician. Patients are also free to obtain second opinions on their own initiative, with or without their physician's knowledge.

With the patient's consent, the first physician should provide a history of the case and such other information as the second-opinion physician may need, including the recommendations about management. The second-opinion physician should maintain the confidentiality of the evaluation and should report to the first physician if the consent of the patient has been obtained.

After evaluating the patient, a second-opinion physician should provide the patient with a clear understanding of the opinion, whether or not it agrees with the recommendations of the first physician.

When a patient initiates a second opinion, it is inappropriate for the primary physician to terminate the patient-physician relationship solely because of the patient's decision to obtain a second opinion.

In some cases, patients may ask the second-opinion physician to provide the needed medical care. In general, second-opinion physicians are free to assume responsibility for the care of the patient. It is not unethical to enter into a patient-physician relationship with a patient who has been receiving care from another physician. By accepting second-opinion patients for treatment, physicians affirm the right of patients to have free choice in the selection of their physicians.

There are situations in which physicians may choose not to treat patients for whom they provide second opinions. Physicians may decide not to treat the patient in order to avoid any perceived conflict of interest or loss of objectivity in rendering the requested second opinion. However, the concern about conflicts of interest does not require physicians to decline to treat second-opinion patients. This inherent conflict in the practice of medicine is resolved by the responsible exercise of professional judgment.

Physicians may agree not to treat second-opinion patients as part of their arrangements with insurers or other third party payers. Physicians who enter into such contractual agreements must honor their commitments.

Physicians must decide independently of their colleagues whether to treat second-opinion patients. Physicians may not establish an agreement or understanding among themselves that they will refuse to treat each others' patients when asked to provide a second opinion. Such agreements compromise the ability of patients to receive care from the physicians of their choice and are therefore not only unethical but also unlawful. (IV, V)

Issued June 1992.

Updated June 1996.

8.05 Contractual Relationships

The contractual relationships that physicians assume when they join or affiliate with group practices or agree to provide services to the patients of an insurance plan are varied.

Income arrangements may include hourly wages for physicians working part time, annual salaries for those working full time, and share of group income for physicians who are partners in groups that are somewhat autonomous and contract with plans to provide the required medical care. Arrangements also usually include a range of fringe benefits, such as paid vacations, insurance, and pension plans.

Physicians may work directly for plans or may be employed by the medical group or the hospital that has contracted with the plan to provide services. In the operation of such plans, physicians should not be subjected to lay interference in professional medical matters and their primary responsibility should be to the patients they serve. (VI)

Issued prior to April 1977.

Updated June 1994 and June 1996.

1st Cir. 1984 Plaintiff-physicians sued defendant-insurer, alleging defendant's ban on "balance billing" practice violated antitrust law. That practice required defendant to pay the physicians treating defendant's insureds only if the physicians agreed not to make any additional charges to the insureds. In holding that defendant's billing practice did not violate antitrust law, the court noted in passing a 1954 law journal article that cited, with an incorrect reference, Principles Ch. III, Art. VI, Sec. 3 (1947) in arguing that "selling services to third parties...might interfere with the absolute ethical obligation that a doctor owes to the patient." The specific concept treated by this Principle is no longer directly treated although Opinion 8.05 reflects similar concerns. *Kartell v. Blue Shield of Mass., Inc., 749 F.2d 922, 926, cert. denied, 471 U.S. 1029 (1985).*

2d Cir. 1980 Federal Trade Commission ordered American Medical Association and others to cease, with some exceptions, imposing restraints on advertising and "contract practice" by physicians, as well as on business relations between physicians and laypersons. Commission found restraints violated 15 U.S.C. Sec. 45(a)(1). See 94 F.T.C. 701 (1979). Association petitioned for judicial review of Commission's order. Court reviewed order, noting specific ethical pronouncements of Association which Commission found improper, including the following: restrictions upon advertising and solicitation, Principle 5 (1957) and Opinions and Reports of the Judicial Council Sec. 5, Para. 11 (1971) [now Opinion 5.02]; restrictions on "contract practice," Principle 6 (1957) and Opinions and Reports of the Judicial Council Sec. 6, Paras. 3, 4, and 5 (1971) [now Opinion 8.05]; and restrictions on business organizations and relations with laypersons, Opinions and Reports of the Judicial Council Sec. 6, Paras. 14 and 15 (1971). Court rejected Association's argument that its ethical rules did not provide impetus for local and state medical societies to act against physicians violating its rules. Further, court rejected Association's position that liability should be precluded because of revisions in the Opinions in 1977 and the Principles in 1980. Specifically, the court found that removal of the ban on patient solicitation and changes reflected in Principles II and IV (1980) did not render Commission's order moot. The order was therefore enforced with modifications. Dissenting judge, referring to 1980 revisions in Principles and to Opinions and Reports of the Judicial Council 4.05 and 6.00 (1977) [now Opinions 5.02 and 8.05], concluded order should not be enforced on grounds of mootness. *American Medical Ass'n v. FTC, 638 F.2d 443, 446, 446 n.1, 448, 449, 449 n.5, 450, 451, 455-57, aff'd, 455 U.S. 676 (1982).*

7th Cir. 1984 Plaintiff brought medical malpractice suit against several physicians appointed to the Veterans Administration Department of Medicine and Surgery. The court held that "strict control" test for determining whether defendants ought to be considered employees or independent contractors under the Federal Tort Claims Act was not appropriate because the ethical obligation of a physician to a patient, evidenced by Principle 6 (1957) [now Opinions 8.03 and 8.05], required that independent judgment be exercised, preventing a physician from being "strictly controlled" by the Veterans Administration. *Quilico v. Kaplan, 749 F.2d 480, 483-84.*

10th Cir. 1983 Pursuant to the Federal Tort Claims Act, plaintiff sued the federal government for the negligence of a neurosurgeon, allegedly an employee of a Veteran's Administration hospital. Plaintiff argued that applying the traditional control test to determine a physician's employment status was inappropriate because physicians are bound by Principle 6 (1957) [now Opinions 8.03 and 8.05] requiring them to have "free and complete exercise of [their] medical judgment and skill...." However, the court did not reach the merits of that argument because the contractual agreement between the neurosurgeon and the VA hospital was "outside the parameters of an employer-employee relationship with the government," thus precluding plaintiff's claim. *Lurch v. United States, 719 F.2d 333, 337, cert. denied, 466 U.S. 927. (1984).*

D.C. Cir. 1942 Medical associations appealed conviction on charges of conspiracy to restrain trade or commerce where associations attempted to prevent competition by elimination of prepaid, low cost medical and hospital care. Principles Ch. III, Art. VI, Secs. 2 and 3 [now Opinion 8.05] limiting "contract practice" had been used as a basis to discipline members of medical association employed by prepaid medical organization. The court held that the associations were subject to the Sherman Antitrust Act and that the evidence sustained the conviction. *American Medical Ass'n v. United States, 130 F.2d 233, 238-239 n.23, aff'd, 317 U.S. 519 (1943).*

Wash. 1951 Plaintiff, a charitable, not for profit medical corporation, offered prepaid health care services to members and their families. Suit was filed against county medical society and others for damages and injunction for defendants' alleged efforts to monopolize prepaid medical care in area and unlawfully restrain competition by plaintiff and its physicians. Defendants alleged as affirmative defense that their efforts were designed to curb "unethical" prepaid contract practice by plaintiff. Court examined at length American Medical Association's position regarding "contract practice" including Principles Ch. III, Art. VI, Secs. 3 and 4 (1947) [now Principle VI and Opinions 8.05 and 9.06] concluding nothing in plaintiff's practice violated the Association's ethical guidelines. Further, quoting Principles Ch. III, Art. III, Sec. 1 (1947) [now Opinion 8.04] dealing with consultations, court noted that defendants' efforts impeded plaintiff's physicians from obtaining consultations. Court concluded defendants' actions constituted unlawful, monopolistic behavior and issued an injunction, although it declined to award damages. *Group Health Coop. v. King County Medical Soc'y, 39 Wash. 2d 586, 237 P.2d 737, 744, 750-51, 759-60.*

8.051 Conflict of Interest Under Capitation

The application of capitation to physicians' practices can result in the provision of cost-effective, quality medical care. It is important to note, however, that the potential for conflict exists under such systems. Managed care organizations and the physicians who contract with them should attempt to minimize these conflicts and to ensure that capitation is applied in a manner consistent with the interests of patients.

(1) Physicians have an obligation to evaluate a health plan's capitation payments prior to contracting with that plan to ensure that the quality of patient care is not threatened by inadequate rates of capitation. Capitation payments should be calculated primarily on relevant medical factors, available outcomes data, the costs associated with involved providers, and consensus-oriented standards of necessary care. Furthermore, the predictable costs resulting from existing conditions of enrolled patients should be considered when determining the rate of capitation. Different populations of patients have different medical needs and the costs associated with those needs should be reflected in the per member per month payment. Physicians should seek agreements with plans that provide sufficient financial resources for all necessary care and should refuse to sign agreements that fail in this regard.

(2) Physicians must not assume inordinate levels of financial risk and should therefore consider a number of factors when deciding whether or not to sign a provider agreement. The size of the plan and the time period over

which the rate is figured should be considered by physicians evaluating a plan as well as in determinations of the per member per month payment. The capitation rate for large plans can be calculated more accurately than for smaller plans because of the mitigating influence of probability and the behavior of large systems. Similarly, length of time will influence the predictability of patient expenditures and should be considered accordingly. Capitation rates calculated for large plans over an extended period of time are able to be more accurate and are therefore preferable to those calculated for small groups over a short time period.

(3) Stop-loss plans should be in effect to prevent the potential of catastrophic expenses from influencing physician behavior. Physicians should attempt to ensure that such arrangements are finalized prior to signing an agreement to provide services in a health plan.

(4) Physicians must be prepared to discuss with patients any financial arrangements which could impact patient care. Physicians should avoid reimbursement systems that cannot be disclosed to patients without negatively affecting the patient-physician relationship. (I, II)

Issued June 1998 based on the report, "The Ethical Implications of Capitation," adopted June 1997.

8.052 Negotiating Discounts for Specialty Care

Patients are entitled to all the benefits outlined in their insurance plan. Therefore, it is unethical for a referring physician to restrict the referral options of patients who have chosen a plan that provides for access to an unlimited or broad selection of specialist physicians. It is also unethical to base the referral of these patients on a discount for the capitated patients in a primary care physician's practice. (I, II)

Issued June 1998 based on the report, "Ethical Issues in Negotiating Discounts for Specialty Care," adopted June 1996.

8.06 Drugs and Devices: Prescribing

(1) A physician should not be influenced in the prescribing of drugs, devices, or appliances by a direct or indirect financial interest in a pharmaceutical firm or other supplier. Whether the firm is a manufacturer, distributor, wholesaler, or repackager of the products involved is immaterial.

(2) A physician may own or operate a pharmacy but generally may not refer his or her patients to the pharmacy. However, a physician may refer patients to his or her pharmacy if there is a demonstrated need for the pharmacy in the community and alternative financing is unavailable (as defined in Opinion 8.032). Physicians may dispense drugs within their office practices provided there is no resulting exploitation of patients.

(3) A physician should not give patients prescriptions in code or enter into agreements with pharmacies or other suppliers regarding the filling of prescriptions by code.

(4) Patients are entitled to the same freedom of choice in selecting who will fill their prescription needs as they are in the choice of a physician. (See Opinions 9.06 and 8.03.) The prescription is a written direction for a therapeutic or corrective agent. A patient is entitled to a copy of the physician's prescription for drugs, eyeglasses, contact lenses, or other devices as required by the Principles of Medical Ethics and as required by law. The patient has the right to have the prescription filled wherever the patient wishes.

(5) Patients have an ethically and legally recognized right to prompt access to the information contained in their individual medical records. The prescription is an essential part of the patient's medical record. Physicians should not discourage patients from requesting a written prescription or urge them to fill prescriptions from an establishment which has a direct telephone line or which has entered into a business or other preferential arrangement with the physician with respect to the filling of the physician's prescriptions. (I, II, III, IV, V)

Issued prior to April 1977.

Updated June 1994 based on the report, "Conflicts of Interest: Physician Ownership of Medical Facilities," adopted December 1991 (JAMA. 1992; 267: 2366-2369).

E.D. N.Y. 1975 Medical laboratories sought injunction against city's award of exclusive contracts for Medicaid services. The court granted a preliminary injunction and held that the laboratories had a substantial probability of success on the merits of the claim that Medicaid recipients would be deprived of statutory right of free choice of providers. In balancing the equities, the court also noted that the contracts would create an ethical dilemma for physicians who are required to provide patients with free choice of ancillary services under Opinions and Reports of the Judicial Council Sec. 1, Paras. 6 and 14 (1971) [now Opinions 8.03, 8.06, and 9.06]. *Bay Ridge Diagnostic Laboratory, Inc. v. Dumpson, 400 F. Supp. 1104, 1109-10.*

Cal. App. 1967 Physician-stockholders of publicly-owned pharmaceutical corporations and physicians whose medical partnerships owned and operated pharmacies challenged statutory prohibition of physician membership, proprietory interest, and co-ownership of pharmacies. The court quoted Principles Ch. I, Sec. 6 (1947) and a 1960 Judicial Council rule, later included in Opinions and Reports of the Judicial Council Sec. 7, Para. 38 (1965) [now Opinions 8.03, 8.032, and 8.06] in its discussion of the potential conflict of interest created by such ownership. The court held that the statute prohibited physician partnerships from directly owning pharmacies but did not apply to an individual physician or a partnership of physicians who own stock in a corporation which owns and operates a pharamacy. *Magan Medical Clinic v. California State Bd. of Medical Examiners, 249 Cal. App. 2d 124, 57 Cal. Rptr. 256, 262.*

Minn. App. 1997 Patients brought suit against physician for prescribing a growth hormone drug while receiving kickbacks, in violation of the physician-patient fiduciary duty and the Minnesota Consumer Fraud Act. The distributor of the drug induced physicians to refer patients for the drug. The court cited Opinion 8.06 for the proposition that patients are entitled to receive medical opinions and referrals which are not motivated by physician gain. The court found, however, that the complaint sounded in medical malpractice and declined to allow a new cause of action based on breach of a fiduciary duty. Because the malpractice limitations had expired and the patients had failed to allege sufficient injury under the Consumer Fraud Act, the court affirmed dismissal with prejudice. *D.A.B v. Brown, 570 N.W. 2d 168, 170.*

Mo. Att'y Gen. 1982 State attorney general, citing Opinion 8.06 (1982), concluded that a physician who requires a patient to accept drugs dispensed by the physician and refuses to provide the patient with a prescription for the patient's use elsewhere violates state antitrust law and has engaged in professional "misconduct." A similar conclusion, again based in part on Opinion 8.06, was rendered regarding a physician who requires a patient to fill a prescription at a pharmacy in which the physician has a personal interest. *Missouri Att'y Gen. Op. No. 6 (July 8, 1982) (LEXIS, States library, Mo. file).*

Journal 1991 Discusses conflict of interest problems that sometimes arise in the doctor-patient relationship. Explores the impact of *Moore v. Regents of the University of California*. Looks at the physician as a fiduciary and the law governing fiduciary relationships. Concludes that fiduciary concepts are a valuable basis for establishing ethical and legal guidelines for physician behavior. Quotes Opinions 2.19, 8.03 (1989) [now Opinion 8.032], and 8.06. Healey & Dowling, *Controlling Conflicts of Interest in the Doctor-Patient Relationship: Lessons From Moore v. Regents of the University of California*, 42 Mercer L. Rev. 989, 997, 998 (1991).

8.061 Gifts to Physicians From Industry

Many gifts given to physicians by companies in the pharmaceutical, device, and medical equipment industries serve an important and socially beneficial function. For example, companies have long provided funds for educational seminars and conferences. However, there has been growing concern about certain gifts from industry to physicians. Some gifts that reflect customary practices of industry may not be consistent with the Principles of Medical Ethics. To avoid the acceptance of inappropriate gifts, physicians should observe the following guidelines:

(1) Any gifts accepted by physicians individually should primarily entail a benefit to patients and should not be of substantial value. Accordingly, textbooks, modest meals, and other gifts are appropriate if they serve a genuine educational function. Cash payments should not be accepted. The use of drug samples for personal or family use is permissible as long as these practices do not interfere with patient access to drug samples. It would not be acceptable for non-retired physicians to request free pharmaceuticals for personal use or use by family members.

(2) Individual gifts of minimal value are permissible as long as the gifts are related to the physician's work (e.g., pens and notepads).

(3) The Council on Ethical and Judicial Affairs defines a legitimate "conference" or "meeting" as any activity, held at an appropriate location where, (a) the gathering is primarily dedicated, in both time and effort, to promoting objective scientific and educational activities and discourse (one or more educational presentation(s) should be the highlight of the gathering), and (b) the main incentive for bringing attendees together is to further their knowledge on the topic(s) being presented. An appropriate disclosure of financial support or conflict of interest should be made.

(4) Subsidies to underwrite the costs of continuing medical education conferences or professional meetings can contribute to the improvement of patient care and therefore are permissible. Since the giving of a subsidy directly to a physician by a company's representative may create a relationship that could influence the use of the company's products, any subsidy should be accepted by the conference's sponsor who in turn can use the money to reduce the conference's registration fee. Payments to defray the costs of a conference should not be accepted directly from the company by the physicians attending the conference.

(5) Subsidies from industry should not be accepted directly or indirectly to pay for the costs of travel, lodging, or other personal expenses of physicians attending conferences or meetings, nor should subsidies be accepted to

compensate for the physicians' time. Subsidies for hospitality should not be accepted outside of modest meals or social events held as a part of a conference or meeting. It is appropriate for faculty at conferences or meetings to accept reasonable honoraria and to accept reimbursement for reasonable travel, lodging, and meal expenses. It is also appropriate for consultants who provide genuine services to receive reasonable compensation and to accept reimbursement for reasonable travel, lodging, and meal expenses. Token consulting or advisory arrangements cannot be used to justify the compensation of physicians for their time or their travel, lodging, and other out-of-pocket expenses.

(6) Scholarship or other special funds to permit medical students, residents, and fellows to attend carefully selected educational conferences may be permissible as long as the selection of students, residents, or fellows who will receive the funds is made by the academic or training institution. Carefully selected educational conferences are generally defined as the major educational, scientific or policymaking meetings of national, regional or specialty medical associations.

(7) No gifts should be accepted if there are strings attached. For example, physicians should not accept gifts if they are given in relation to the physician's prescribing practices. In addition, when companies underwrite medical conferences or lectures other than their own, responsibility for and control over the selection of content, faculty, educational methods, and materials should belong to the organizers of the conferences or lectures. (II)

Issued June 1992 based on the report, "Gifts to Physicians from Industry," adopted December 1990 (JAMA. 1991; 265: 501 and *Food and Drug Law Journal*. 1992; 47: 445-458).

Updated June 1996 and June 1998.

Journal 1997 Discusses the process for marketing new drugs, medical devices, or biologics. Considers issues such as whether insurers or payers will cover these products, how much each will cost, and whether marketing programs comply with government regulations. References Opinion 8.061. Reiss, *Commentary on Payment and Reimbursement Issues Affecting the Marketing of Drugs, Medical Devices, and Biologics, with Emphasis on the Anti-Kickback Statute and Stark II*, 52 Food & Drug L. J. 99,107 (1997).

Journal 1997 Explores the extent to which pharmaceutical drug samples are taken by physicians or other medical staff for personal use. Concludes that this practice is common and raises pertinent ethical issues. Quotes Opinion 8.061. Westfall, McCabe, & Nicholas, *Personal Use of Drug Samples by Physicians and Office Staff*, 278 J.A.M.A. 141, 142 (1997).

Journal 1994 Discusses the role of professional societies in establishing ethical guidelines for physicians in the context of using medical innovations and new technologies. Observes that these standards must be supplemented by additional external measures or incentives in order to be most effective. Concludes that professional societies are more successful at setting standards than ensuring acceptance and implementation of those standards by member professionals. Cites Opinions 1.01, 1.02, 8.061, 9.04, and 9.131. Orentlicher, *The Influence of a Professional Organization on Physician Behavior*, 57 Alb. L. Rev. 583, 592, 593, 594, 595, 596 (1994).

Journal 1993 Examines how the Food and Drug Administration (FDA) regulates marketing of new medical devices and its authority to do so. Describes how these regulations differ from those governing drugs. Proposes a course of action for the FDA and the medical device industry concerning this issue. References Opinion 8.061. Dennis, *Promotion of Devices: An Extension of FDA Drug Regulation or a New Frontier?*, 48 Food & Drug L. J. 87 (1993).

Journal 1992 Surveys federal and state antikickback and antireferral statutes pertaining to drug and device marketing activities. Considers the effectiveness of regulatory safe harbors. Reviews the AMA's ethical guidelines concerning gifts to physicians from industry. Quotes Opinion 6.04. References Opinion 8.061. Kirschenbaum & Kuhlik, *Federal and State Laws Affecting Discounts, Rebates, and Other Marketing Practices for Drugs and Devices*, 47 Food & Drug L. J. 533, 560 (1992).

Journal 1992 Discusses the extent of the Food and Drug Administration's (FDA) authority to regulate oral sales promotion of pharmaceuticals. Explores the debate over the extent of the FDA's power to regulate. References Opinion 8.061. Noah, *Death of a Salesman: To What Extent Can the FDA Regulate the Promotional Statements of Pharmaceutical Sales Representatives?*, 47 Food & Drug L. J. 309, 316 (1992).

Journal 1992 Reviews concerns about commercial involvement in and funding of continuing medical education. Discusses CME requirements, accumulation of CME credits, and changes in standards governing commercial sponsorship. References Opinions 8.061 and 9.011. Wentz, Osteen, & Gannon, *Continuing Medical Education: Unabated Debate*, 268 J.A.M.A. 1118 (1992).

Journal 1991 Examines legal, ethical, and economic concerns surrounding pharmaceutical company promotions. Focuses on the "gift-giving relationship between physicians and pharmaceutical companies." Offers guidance to governmental units in regulating these activities. Concludes that pharmaceutical freebies can serve a positive role in health care if adequately regulated. Quotes Opinions 8.061 and 8.08. Note, *The Economic Wisdom of Regulating Pharmaceutical "Freebies,"* 1991 Duke L.J. 206, 216, 233, 234 (1991).

Journal 1991 Discusses commercial support of continuing medical education. Explains ethical guidelines for accepting such assistance and how those guidelines have changed. References Opinions 8.061 and 9.011. Wentz, Osteen, & Gannon, *Refocusing Support and Direction*, 266 J.A.M.A. 953 (1991).

8.07   Gifts to Physicians: Offers of Indemnity

Physicians should prescribe drugs, devices, and other treatments based solely upon medical considerations and patient needs. A third party's offer to indemnify a physician for lawsuits arising from the physician's prescription or use of the third party's drug, device, or other product, introduces inappropriate factors into medical decision making. Such offers, regardless of their limitations, therefore constitute unacceptable gifts.

This opinion does not address contractual assignments of liability between employers or in research arrangements, nor does it address government indemnification plans. (II)

Issued June 1992.

Updated June 1994.

8.08   Informed Consent

The patient's right of self-decision can be effectively exercised only if the patient possesses enough information to enable an intelligent choice. The patient should make his or her own determination on treatment. The physician's obligation is to present the medical facts accurately to the patient or to the individual responsible for the patient's care and to make recommendations for management in accordance with good medical practice. The physician has an ethical obligation to help the patient make choices from among the therapeutic alternatives consistent with good medical practice. Informed consent is a basic social policy for which exceptions are permitted: (1) where the patient is unconscious or otherwise incapable of consenting and harm from failure to treat is imminent or (2) when risk-disclosure poses such a serious psychological threat of detriment to the patient as to be medically contraindicated. Social policy does not accept the paternalistic view that the physician may remain silent because divulgence might prompt the patient to forego needed therapy. Rational, informed patients should not be expected to act uniformly, even under similar circumstances, in agreeing to or refusing treatment. (I, II, III, IV, V)

Issued March 1981.

W. Va. 1995 West Virginia Board of Medicine received a complaint from patient that physician was using depossession treatment. The hearing examiner in part found that there had been a lack of informed consent for such treatment. The Board changed the examiner's report and added sanctions. In doing so, it quoted Opinion 8.08. On appeal, the circuit court reversed, finding the Board's order arbitrary and an abuse of discretion. The appellate court agreed that the Board abused its discretion, but remanded the case for consideration of the issue of informed consent for depossession treatment. *Modi v. West Virginia Board of Medicine*, 465 S.E.2d 230, 236.

Journal 1997 Examines the evolution of the Indiana health care system. Discusses developments in Indiana jurisprudence regarding the physician-patient relationship. Explores various challenges facing the relationship and recognizes the need for legal rules to help address these challenges. Quotes Opinion 8.08. Cites Opinions 2.20, 9.06, and 9.12. Kinney & Selby, *History and Jurisprudence of the Physician-Patient Relationship in Indiana*, 30 Ind. L. Rev. 263, 269, 272, 276 (1997).

Journal 1997 Explores the meaning of cardiopulmonary resuscitation and legal issues involving DNR orders. Considers problems created by DNR orders in operating rooms in light of patients' rights. Concludes that hospitals must adopt clear policies for their surgical teams to follow. Quotes Opinion 8.08. References Opinion 2.22. Lonchyna, *To Resuscitate or Not . . . In the Operating Room: The Need for Hospital Policies for Surgeons Regarding DNR Orders*, 6 Annals Health L. 209, 215, 217 (1997).

Journal 1996 Examines the constitutional implications of government-subsidized speech. Proposes two key characterization questions that should be answered when undertaking legal analysis. Observes, among other things, that potential ethical conflicts may exist when governmental subsidies are utilized to control the discourse between physicians and their patients. Quotes Opinion 8.08. Post, *Subsidized Speech*, 106 Yale L. J. 151, 173 (1996).

Journal 1996 Discusses new abortion legislation in Utah. Notes that patient consent must be obtained in accordance with AMA ethical standards, requiring physicians to provide all relevant data. Concludes that new laws require more detailed and comprehensive information be given to women. Quotes Opinion 8.08. Schnibbe, *Recent Legislative Developments in Utah Law: Family Law*, 1996 Utah L. Rev. 1335, 1394 (1996).

Journal 1996 Considers the ethical requirement for physicians to receive informed consent from patients before beginning treatment. Reviews the case of *Jacobson v. Massachusetts*, discussing its impact on informed consent and vaccination policy in the United States. Quotes Fundamental Elements (2). References Opinion 8.08. Severyn, *Jacobson v. Massachusetts: Impact on Informed Consent and Vaccine Policy*, 5 J. Pharmacy & L. 249, 253, 274 (1996).

Journal 1995 Observes that physicians are unable to obtain informed consent because they can not guess which treatment alternatives will best serve an individual patient's interests. Suggests that this situation would be improved if patients were paired with physicians who share their personal values. Quotes Opinion 8.08. Veatch, *Abandoning Informed Consent*, 25 Hastings Center Rep. 5, 6 (March/April 1995).

Journal 1994 Discusses how physicians historically have taken too much license with patients' bodies and placed greater value on longevity than on quality of life. Argues that patients should be the ultimate decisionmakers in matters that affect their lives. Suggests that greater emphasis should be given to physician disclosure obligations in order to improve the quality of patient consent. Quotes Opinion 8.07 (1981) [now Opinion 8.08]. Katz, *Informed Consent—Must It Remain a Fairy Tale?*, 10 J. Contemp. Health L. & Pol'y 69, 80 (1994).

Journal 1994 Reviews the evolution of the physician-patient relationship. Describes legal responses to increasing awareness of the importance of ensuring patient autonomy. Examines the changing health care delivery environment. Concludes with a discussion of the impact of these changes on patient participation in medical decision-making. Quotes Preamble, Principles I, II, III, IV, V, and VI, Fundamental Elements (1) and (2), and Opinions 1.02 and 8.07 (1981) [now Opinion 8.08]. Cites Opinion 1.01. Szczygiel, *Beyond Informed Consent, 21 Ohio N.U.L. Rev. 171, 217, 218, 220, 225, 226, 256 (1994).*

Journal 1993 Considers how patient self-determination may be affected by cardiopulmonary resuscitation and Do-Not-Resuscitate policies. Proposes a traditional informed consent model for medical decision making in this context. Opposes a "futility" exception to informed consent as being violative of a physician's fiduciary duties to patients. Cites Opinion 8.07 (1986) [now Opinion 8.08]. References Opinion 2.22. Boozang, *Death Wish: Resuscitating Self-Determination for the Critically Ill, 35 Ariz. L. Rev. 23, 24, 28, 52 (1993).*

Journal 1993 Discusses physicians' duty to disclose medical treatment alternatives to patients that are not readily available. Proposes that based on the historical development and legal requirements of the informed consent doctrine, physicians should be required to inform patients of nonreadily available alternatives or face liability for breach of such obligation. Quotes Principles I, II, III, IV, and V and Opinion 8.08. Note, *Informed Choice: Physicians' Duty to Disclose Nonreadily Available Alternatives, 43 Case W. Res. L. Rev. 491, 491, 498-499, 508, 509 (1993).*

Journal 1993 Examines the case of *Rust v. Sullivan*, in which the Supreme Court sustained regulations barring abortion counseling and referral at federally-funded clinics. Criticizes the Court's deference to the executive branch and its failure to classify the regulations as violative of constitutional rights to free speech. Quotes Opinion 8.08. Note, *Rust on the Constitution: Politics and Gag Rules, 37 How. L.J. 83, 96 (1993).*

Journal 1993 Critiques the Supreme Court's decision in *Rust v. Sullivan*, which upheld regulations prohibiting employees of Title X-funded clinics from discussing abortions with patients. Focuses on the Court's constitutional analysis and how the control of knowledge affects the oppression and liberation of subordinated groups. Advocates an affirmative government obligation to provide abortion counseling to Title X patients. Cites Opinion 8.08. Roberts, *Rust v. Sullivan and the Control of Knowledge, 61 Geo. Wash. L. Rev. 587, 641 (1993).*

Journal 1993 Discusses legal attempts to control reproduction by HIV-positive women. Considers how control over childbearing and HIV testing infringes on basic individual rights. Suggests that controls will not achieve the goal of lessening children's suffering, but will discourage HIV-positive women from seeking health care services. Quotes Opinion 8.08. Sangree, *Control of Childbearing by HIV-Positive Women: Some Responses to Emerging Legal Policies, 41 Buff. L. Rev. 309, 362 (1993).*

Journal 1992 Examines the constitutionality of certain restrictions on speech in federally funded programs. Argues that government's selective funding of institutions, programs, and the like may restrict the free flow of ideas. Advocates greater first amendment protections in these situations. Quotes Opinion 8.08. Cole, *Beyond Unconstitutional Conditions: Charting Spheres of Neutrality in Government-Funded Speech, 67 N.Y.U. L. Rev. 675, 744 (1992).*

Journal 1992 Discusses the problem of protecting the privacy and confidentiality of public figures in light of contemporary tabloid journalism. Argues that current tort law does not adequately address this problem and advocates a new cause of action based on breach of confidentiality. Quotes Opinion 8.08. Harvey, *Confidentiality: A Measured Response to the Failure of Privacy, 140 Univ. Pa. L. Rev. 2385, 2454 (1992).*

Journal 1992 Analyzes the case of *Rust v. Sullivan* in which the U.S. Supreme Court let stand regulations restricting abortion counseling in federally funded clinics. Considers the extent to which governmental entities may limit the right to an abortion. Examines the history of the right to choose and how that right has been interpreted in recent years. Concludes that *Rust* limits this right by expanding government powers. Cites Opinion 8.08. Note, *Constitutional Law—Judicial Deference—Supreme Court Will Defer to "Reasonable" Abortion Restrictions, 14 Univ. Ark. Little Rock 557, 573 (1992).*

Journal 1992 Discusses limitations on abortion counseling in federally funded clinics in light of the U.S. Supreme Court decision in *Rust v. Sullivan*. Summarizes the regulations limiting this type of counseling and the relevant history. Considers the effect of *Rust* on physicians, clinic patients, and legislators. Concludes that the *Rust* decision improperly limits freedom of speech. Cites Opinion 8.08. Note, *The Policy Against Federal Funding for Abortions Extends Into the Realm of Free Speech After Rust v. Sullivan, 19 Pepperdine L. Rev. 637, 681 (1992)*.

Journal 1991 Discusses the manner in which a changing economy and an evolving health care system require society to expand its understanding of the physician-patient relationship. Argues that physicians must offer patients sufficient information about available medical services, including cost. Concludes that such open discussion may become part of the standard of care. References Opinions 8.08 and 8.12. Morreim, *Economic Disclosure and Economic Advocacy: New Duties in the Medical Standard of Care, 12 J. Legal Med. 275, 306 (1991)*.

Journal 1991 Considers how administrative restrictions on abortion counseling in Title X-funded clinics were affected by the Supreme Court's decision in *Rust v. Sullivan*. Concludes that *Rust* expands the powers of administrative agencies and narrows first amendment free speech rights and fifth amendment due process rights. Cites Opinion 8.08. Note, *Administrative Agencies Get Their Way Over Constitutional Rights in Rust v. Sullivan, 28 Willamette L. Rev. 173, 193 (1991)*.

Journal 1991 Examines legal, ethical, and economic concerns surrounding pharmaceutical company promotions. Focuses on the "gift-giving relationship between physicians and pharmaceutical companies." Offers guidance to governmental units in regulating these activities. Concludes that pharmaceutical freebies can serve a positive role in health care if adequately regulated. Quotes Opinions 8.061 and 8.08. Note, *The Economic Wisdom of Regulating Pharmaceutical "Freebies," 1991 Duke L.J. 206, 216, 233, 234 (1991)*.

Journal 1990 Examines Minnesota's "Crack Baby" law as a response to the increasing problem of drug abuse. Focuses on how the law affects the rights of women. Discusses informed consent, personal autonomy, and the right to privacy in this context. Also considers the rights of the unborn. Concludes that Minnesota's "Crack Baby" law endangers basic constitutional rights of women. Quotes Opinion 8.07 (1986) [now Opinion 8.08]. Johnson, *Minnesota's "Crack Baby" Law: Weapon of War or Link in a Chain?, 8 Law & Ineq. 485, 494, 495, 496 (1990)*.

Journal 1985 Focuses on the importance of patient autonomy in medical decisionmaking. Initially describes how existing doctrines protect the value of autonomy in the context of the physician-patient relationship, then examines various problems in the current protective scheme. Case law is evaluated wherein enhanced protection is afforded to patient autonomy. Concludes by recommending the creation of an independent articulable protected interest in patient autonomy. Quotes Principles II and IV. Cites Opinions 4.04 (1984) [now Opinion 8.08] and 6.03 (1984) [now Opinion 6.02]. Shultz, *From Informed Consent to Patient Choice: A New Protected Interest, 95 Yale L. J. 219, 275 (1985)*.

Journal 1983 Discusses both moral and legal dilemmas in the use of placebos in treating patients. Relevant moral problems include inherent deception, violation of patient autonomy, and possible harm resulting from placebo therapy. Also addressed are various medical legal risks, including liability for fraud, malpractice, breach of contract, and violation of informed consent requirements. Concludes that, while arguments against placebo therapy are noble, a complete ban of placebo therapy is impractical and undesirable. Recommends careful control of placebo therapy through the exercise of a high degree of respect for the rights and sensibilities of the patient. Quotes Opinions 8.07 (1982) [now Opinion 8.08] and 8.11 (1982) [now Opinion 8.12]. Kapp, *Placebo Therapy and the Law: Prescribe With Care, 8 Am. J. Law & Med. 371, 391 (1983)*.

8.085 Waiver of Informed Consent for Research in Emergency Situations

The current state of emergency medicine and research has resulted in the application of standard treatments that often have not been scientifically evaluated for safety and effectiveness and may render unsatisfactory outcomes. Given the insufficiency of standard treatment alternatives it is appropriate, in certain situations and with special safeguards, to provide experimental treatments without obtaining the informed consent of the subject. However, in order to protect the rights and welfare of the subjects several conditions must be met:

(1) This type of research is limited to emergency, life-threatening situations, and may involve only experimental treatments that are ready for trials involving human subjects.

(2) The subject must lack the capacity to give informed consent for participation in the research.

(3) The window of opportunity for intervention must be so narrow as to make obtaining surrogate consent unfeasible.

(4) Obtaining prospective informed consent for the protocol must not be feasible (*i.e.*, the life threatening emergency situation could not have been anticipated).

(5) The experimental treatment must have a realistic probability of benefit equal to or greater than standard care.

(6) The risks associated with the research should be reasonable in light of the critical nature of the conditions and the risks associated with standard treatment.

(7) Where informed consent is waived, subjects or their representatives must be informed as soon as possible about inclusion in the study and asked to consent to further participation. Subjects or their representatives may choose to discontinue participation at any time after being fully informed about the possible consequences. Additionally, if the patient dies while participating in the research protocol, the patient's family or representative must be informed that the patient was involved in an experimental protocol.

(8) Community input should be sought prior to approval of the protocol, and public disclosure should be made of study results. Fair randomization of research subjects should be given thorough consideration. Moreover, an independent data monitoring board should be established to oversee the ongoing trial. (I, V)

Issued June 1998 based on the report, "Waiver of Informed Consent for Research in Emergency Situations," adopted June 1997.

8.09   Laboratory Services.

(1) A physician should not misrepresent or aid in the misrepresentation of laboratory services performed and supervised by a non-physician as the physician's professional services. Such situations could involve a laboratory owned by a physician who directs and manages its financial and business affairs with no professional medical services being provided; laboratory work being performed by technicians and directly supervised by a medical technologist with no participation by the physician; or the physician's name being used in connection with the laboratory so as to create the appearance that it is owned, operated, and supervised by a physician when this is not so.

(2) If a laboratory is owned, operated, and supervised by a non-physician in accordance with state law and performs tests exclusively for physicians who receive the results and make their own medical interpretations, the following considerations would apply:

The physician's ethical responsibility is to provide patients with high quality services. This includes services that the physician performs personally and those that are delegated to others. A physician should not utilize the services of any laboratory, irrespective of whether it is operated by a physician or non-physician, unless she or he has the utmost confidence in the quality of its services. A physician must always assume personal responsibility for the best interests of his or her patients. Medical judgment based upon inferior laboratory work is likewise inferior. Medical considerations, not cost, must be paramount when the physician chooses a laboratory. The physician who disregards quality as the primary criterion or who chooses a laboratory solely because it provides low cost laboratory services on which the patient is charged a profit, is not acting in the best interests of the patient. However, if reliable, quality laboratory services are available at lower cost, the patient should have the benefit of the savings. As a professional, the physician is entitled to fair compensation for his or her services. A physician should not charge a markup, commission, or profit on the services rendered by others. A markup is an excessive charge that exploits patients if it is nothing more than a tacked on amount for a service already provided and accounted for by the laboratory. A physician may make an acquisition charge or processing charge. The patient should be notified of any such charge in advance. (I, II, III, IV, V)

Issued prior to April 1977.

Updated June 1994.

8.10   Lien Laws

In states where there are lien laws, a physician may file a lien as a means of assuring payment of his or her fee provided the fee is fixed in amount and not contingent on the amount of settlement of the patient's claim against a third party. (I, VI)

Issued prior to April 1977.

8.11   Neglect of Patient

Physicians are free to choose whom they will serve. The physician should, however, respond to the best of his or her ability in cases of emergency where first aid treatment is essential. Once having undertaken a case, the physician should not neglect the patient. (I, VI)

Issued prior to April 1977.

Updated June 1996.

Ariz. 1965 Physician appealed denial of medical license which was based on alleged violations of local medical society rules and Principles 3, 5, and 10 (1957) [now Principles III and VII, and

Opinions 3.01, 8.11, and 9.06]. Alleged violations included treating a patient without first obtaining a prior treating physician's permission, inadequate patient care, performing operations without hospital privileges, and signing the medical record of a deceased patient who had been treated by interns. The court held that the evidence failed to show any clear violation of the Principles and that a local medical society had no right to prescribe a code of ethics for state licensing purposes. *Arizona State Bd. of Medical Examiners v. Clark*, 97 Ariz. 205, 398 P.2d 908, 914-915, 915 n.3.

Ariz. App. 1980 Malpractice suit against a paid "on call" physician for refusal to treat decedent resulting in delay in treatment. The court quoted Principle 5 (1957) [now Principle VI and Opinion 8.11] as establishing an ethical duty to provide emergency care. However, court distinguished any such ethical obligation from its holding that physician had a contractual duty to treat emergency patients to the best of his ability. *Hiser v. Randolph*, 126 Ariz. 608, 617 P.2d 774, 776 n.1, 777, 778.

Cal. App. 1978 Surviving spouse sued physicians who were on emergency surgical call panel for malpractice where patient died during surgery. Although defendants claimed immunity under state Good Samaritan statute, the court held the statute inapplicable since the legislative purpose was to encourage physicians to render care on an irregular basis to unattended persons discovered by chance at the scene of an emergency. In so holding, the court noted that Principle 5 (1957) [now Principle VI and Opinions 8.11 and 9.06] imposed an ethical duty to render emergency medical care. *Colby v. Schwartz*, 78 Cal. App. 3d 885, 144 Cal. Rptr. 624, 627 n.2.

Ill. App. 1997 Physician was found to be in civil contempt for violating a covenant not to compete by performing administrative functions from his home office. The trial court ordered the physician to desist from practicing medicine within the restricted area. The appellate court, in reversing, found that although the language of the agreement was ambiguous, it could be construed to prohibit the physician from practicing medicine. However, the court found that the practice of medicine does not include activities which are administrative or managerial in nature. Further, the court, quoting from Opinion 8.11, found that physicians have a legal and ethical duty to care for their patients, and may not neglect patients once they begin treatment. The court held that a finding of contempt for violating an agreement not to compete cannot be supported where physicians do not examine patients, but merely address medically related questions by phone. *Bloomington Urological Associates v. Scaglia*, Ill. App. 3d, 686 N.E. 2d 389, 394.

Ky. App. 1989 Malpractice suit was initiated against physician for failure to treat plaintiff's brother where defendant had repeatedly rebuffed plaintiff's request for emergency assistance and told him to "get in line" or "sign in." Plaintiff removed his brother to another hospital where he subsequently died of heart attack. Plaintiff argued that defendant was under a duty to treat based upon, inter alia, the AMA "Code of Ethics" [apparently Principle VI and Opinion 8.11]. The court rejected the argument, finding that a breach of ethical standards may establish grounds for professional discipline, but not a civil cause of action, and held that defendant was under no legal duty to treat. *Noble v. Sartori*, 1989 Ky. App. LEXIS 67.

Journal 1995 Argues that nonabandonment should be a core physician obligation. Suggests that if nonabandonment is better incorporated into medical ethics, medicine will become more humanized and responsive to everyday physician-patient problems. Quotes Opinion 8.10 (1986) [now Opinion 8.11]. Quill & Cassel, *Nonabandonment: A Central Obligation for Physicians*, 10 *Trends in Health Care, Law & Ethics* 25, 27 (Winter/Spring 1995).

Journal 1995 Provides legal and medical definitions of physician-assisted suicide and euthanasia. Offers relevant historical perspectives and provides comprehensive ethical and legal discussion of these compelling social issues. Highlights important legislative developments, including the Oregon Death with Dignity Act, and analyzes significant judicial opinions. Advocates legal tolerance of physician-assisted suicide and euthanasia. Quotes Principles III, IV, and VI and Opinions 2.21 and 9.12. Cites Opinions 2.20 and 8.11. Stone & Winslade, *Physician-Assisted Suicide and Euthanasia in the United States: Legal and Ethical Observations*, 16 J. Legal Med. 481, 483, 490, 497, 498, 499 (1995).

Journal 1993 Explores the idea of reverse informed consent, which would impose a duty on patients to inform health care professionals of their infectious status. Concludes that such a duty is justified. Quotes Principles IV and VI and Opinions 8.11 and 9.131. Oddi, *Reverse Informed Consent: The Unreasonably Dangerous Patient*, 46 Vand. L. Rev. 1417, 1449, 1463, 1465, 1479 (1993).

Journal 1988 Discusses the question of whether health professionals are obligated to subject themselves to the risks that attend treating patients with communicable diseases, particularly

AIDS. Examines the ethical pronouncements and codes of the nursing and medical professions in this respect, noting that the most recent statements of professional values imply the existence of an obligation to treat HIV-infectious patients. Offers a discussion of the evolution of this viewpoint. Quotes Opinion 8.10 (1986) [now Opinion 8.11] and Principle VI. Cites Opinion 9.11 (1986) [now Opinion 9.12]. Freedman, *Health Professions, Codes, and the Right to Refuse to Treat HIV-Infectious Patients*, 18 Hastings Center Rep. 20 (Supp.), 23, 24 (April/May 1988).

Journal 1987 Considers arguments for and against active voluntary euthanasia, including arguments based on self-determination and various slippery-slope scenarios. Concludes that a policy or practice of active voluntary euthanasia is not desirable, linking a moral prohibition against active voluntary euthanasia to the moral prohibition against physicians actively participating in capital punishment. In place of any practice of active voluntary euthanasia, recommends increased use of hospices, greater emphasis on training physicians to care for the dying patient, and further research aimed at producing symptomatic relief in dying patients. Cites Opinions 2.06, 8.10 (1986) [now Opinion 8.11], and 9.06. Shewmon, *Active Voluntary Euthanasia: A Needless Pandora's Box*, 3 Issues in Law and Med. 219, 220, 222, 243 (1987).

Journal 1986 Addresses the problem of "patient dumping" and explores the various reasons underlying this practice. Examines applicable common law and statutory law, emphasizing the antidumping provisions of COBRA. Weaknesses in this federal legislative scheme are highlighted and recommendations for strengthening the statute and maximizing access to emergency medical care are offered. Quotes Principle VI and Opinion 8.10 (1986) [now Opinion 8.11]. Note, *Preventing Patient Dumping: Sharpening the COBRA's Fangs*, 61 N. Y. U. L. Rev. 1186, 1189-90 (1986).

8.115 Termination of the Physician-Patient Relationship.

Physicians have an obligation to support continuity of care for their patients. While physicians have the option of withdrawing from a case, they cannot do so without giving notice to the patient, the relatives, or responsible friends sufficiently long in advance of withdrawal to permit another medical attendant to be secured. (I, VI)

Issued June 1996 (formerly included in Opinion 8.11).

Mass. Super. 1993 Plaintiff sought to enjoin defendant-physician from contacting patients that defendant treated while employed with plaintiff. The court denied the injunction, noting that under Opinion 8.11 [now Opinion 8.115] defendant has a duty to notify his patients before withdrawing from a case and an injunction would force defendant to choose between violating professional ethics or violating a court order. *Plastic Surgical Servs. of New England, P.C. v. Hall*, 1993 WL 818637.

Journal 1997 Compares past ethical opinions to current opinions and notes the differences. Comments on the forces that have changed medical ethics through the years. Notes differing theories on the future course of medical ethics. Quotes Fundamental Elements (Preamble) and Opinions 5.05, 5.057, 7.01, 8.12, 9.12, and 9.131. Cites Fundamental Elements (5) and Opinions 8.115 and 8.13. Buchanan, *Medical Ethics at the Millennium: A Brief Retrospective*, 26 Colo. Law. 141, 142, 143, 144, 145 (1997).

8.12 Patient Information

It is a fundamental ethical requirement that a physician should at all times deal honestly and openly with patients. Patients have a right to know their past and present medical status and to be free of any mistaken beliefs concerning their conditions. Situations occasionally occur in which a patient suffers significant medical complications that may have resulted from the physician's mistake or judgment. In these situations, the physician is ethically required to inform the patient of all the facts necessary to ensure understanding of what has occurred. Only through full disclosure is a patient able to make informed decisions regarding future medical care.

Ethical responsibility includes informing patients of changes in their diagnoses resulting from retrospective review of test results or any other information. This obligation holds even though the patient's medical treatment or therapeutic options may not be altered by the new information.

Concern regarding legal liability which might result following truthful disclosure should not affect the physician's honesty with a patient. (I, II, III, IV)

Issued March 1981.

Updated June 1994.

Minn. 1970 Defendant-physician appealed order to answer interrogatories, claiming that a medical malpractice plaintiff is prohibited from compelling expert testimony from a defendant to prove a charge of malpractice without calling other medical witnesses. In holding that a defendant could be compelled to provide expert medical opinion in response to interrogatories, the court quoted Principle 1 (1957) [now Principle II and Opinion 8.12] for the proposition that physicians owe a duty of disclosure to their patients. *Anderson v. Florence*, 288 Minn. 351, 181 N.W.2d 873, 880, 880 n.7.

Journal 1997 Compares past ethical opinions to current opinions and notes the differences. Comments on the forces that have changed medical ethics through the years. Notes differing theories on the future course of medical ethics. Quotes Fundamental Elements (Preamble) and Opinions 5.05, 5.057, 7.01, 8.12, 9.12, and 9.131. Cites Fundamental Elements (5) and Opinions 8.115 and 8.13. Buchanan, *Medical Ethics at the Millennium: A Brief Retrospective*, 26 Colo. Law. 141, 142, 143, 144, 145 (1997).

Journal 1996 Presents clinical problem-solving scenarios. Notes the AMA's instruction that physicians deal openly and honestly with patients. Considers the physician's role as educator and counselor. Opines that physicians must ensure that patients have the ability to make informed decisions. Quotes Opinion 8.12. Sirmon & Kreisberg, *The Invisible Patient*, 334 New Eng. J. Med. 908, 910, 911 (1996).

Journal 1991 Discusses the manner in which a changing economy and an evolving health care system require society to expand its understanding of the physician-patient relationship. Argues that physicians must offer patients sufficient information about available medical services, including cost. Concludes that such open discussion may become part of the standard of care. References Opinions 8.08 and 8.12. Morreim, *Economic Disclosure and Economic Advocacy: New Duties in the Medical Standard of Care*, 12 J. Legal Med. 275, 306 (1991).

Journal 1983 Discusses both moral and legal dilemmas in the use of placebos in treating patients. Relevant moral problems include inherent deception, violation of patient autonomy, and possible harm resulting from placebo therapy. Also addressed are various medical legal risks, including liability for fraud, malpractice, breach of contract, and violation of informed consent requirements. Concludes that, while arguments against placebo therapy are noble, a complete ban of placebo therapy is impractical and undesirable. Recommends careful control of placebo therapy through the exercise of a high degree of respect for the rights and sensibilities of the patient. Quotes Opinions 8.07 (1982) [now Opinion 8.08] and 8.11 (1982) [now Opinion 8.12]. Kapp, *Placebo Therapy and the Law: Prescribe With Care*, 8 Am. J. Law & Med. 371, 391 (1983).

8.13   **The previous Opinion 8.13, Referral of Patients-Disclosure of Limitations,** was changed to Opinion 8.132 in June 1996.

8.13 Managed Care

The expansion of managed care has brought a variety of changes to medicine including new and different reimbursement systems for physicians with complex referral restrictions and benefits packages for patients. Some of these changes have raised concerns that a physician's ability to practice ethical medicine will be adversely affected by the modifications in the system. In response to these concerns, the following points were developed to provide physicians with general guidelines that will assist them in fulfilling their ethical responsibilities to patients given the changes heralded by managed care.

(1) The duty of patient advocacy is a fundamental element of the physician-patient relationship that should not be altered by the system of health care delivery in which physicians practice. Physicians must continue to place the interests of their patients first.

(2) When managed care plans place restrictions on the care that physicians in the plan may provide to their patients, the following principles should be followed:

(a) Any broad allocation guidelines that restrict care and choices - which go beyond the cost/benefit judgments made by physicians as a part of their normal professional responsibilities - should be established at a policy making level so that individual physicians are not asked to engage in bedside rationing.

(b) Regardless of any allocation guidelines or gatekeeper directives, physicians must advocate for any care they believe will materially benefit their patients.

(c) Physicians should be given an active role in contributing their expertise to any allocation process and should advocate for guidelines that are sensitive to differences among patients. Managed care plans should create structures similar to hospital medical staffs that allow physicians to have meaningful input into the plan's development of allocation guidelines. Guidelines for allocating health care should be reviewed on a regular basis and updated to reflect advances in medical knowledge and changes in relative costs.

(d) Adequate appellate mechanisms for both patients and physicians should be in place to address disputes regarding medically necessary care. In some circumstances, physicians have an obligation to initiate appeals on behalf of their patients. Cases may arise in which a health plan has an allocation guideline that is generally fair but in particular circumstances results in unfair denials of care, i.e., denial of care that, in the physician's judgment, would materially benefit the patient. In such cases, the physician's duty as patient advocate requires that the physician challenge the denial and argue for the provision of treatment in the specific case. Cases may also arise when a health plan has an allocation guideline that is generally unfair in its operations. In such cases, the physician's duty as patient advocate requires not only a challenge to any denials of treatment from the guideline but also advocacy at the health plan's policy-making level to seek an elimination or modification of the guideline.

Issued December 1989.

Updated March 1992 based on the report, "Sexual Misconduct in the Practice of Medicine," adopted December 1990 (JAMA. 1991; 266: 2741-2745).

Cal. 1995 Patient sued ultrasound technician, who sexually assaulted her, and hospital for professional negligence, battery, and intentional and negligent infliction of emotional distress. In differentiating between the physician-patient relationship and the technician-patient relationship, the court cited AMA Council on Ethical and Judicial Affairs, Sexual Misconduct in the Practice of Medicine, 266 JAMA 2741 (1991) [now Opinion 8.14]. Finding that the technician's acts did not arise from any events or conditions of his employment, the court held that the hospital was not liable under respondeat superior. *Lisa M. v. Henry Mayo Newhall Memorial Hosp.*, 12 Cal. 4th 291, 907 P.2d 358, 48 Cal. Rptr. 2d 510, 517.

Cal. App. 1992 Physician who had sexual relationship with patient brought a mandamus action challenging discipline imposed by Medical Board. The court concluded that a sexual relationship between physician and patient was alone an insufficient basis for discipline. An expert witness, referring to Opinion 8.14, testified that it is unethical for a physician to have a sexual relationship with a patient. However, focusing on the applicable state statute, the court found the relationship must affect the functions and duties of a physician to be a basis for discipline. *Gromis v. Medical Board*, 8 Cal. App. 4th 589, 10 Cal. Rptr. 2d 452, 455 n.3, reh'g denied, 1992 Cal. App. LEXIS 1047, and review denied, 1992 Cal. LEXIS 5101.

Md. App. 1992 Patient's husband sought damages from defendant psychiatrist because of the sexual relationship initiated during treatment of the patient by the defendant. Although the court held that the plaintiff in this case could not recover damages in tort for disruption of a marriage, it cited favorably Opinion 8.14 (1989) for its declaration that "sexual misconduct in the practice of medicine" is unethical. *Homer v. Long*, 90 Md. App. 1, 3 n.1 , 599 A.2d 1193, 1193 n.1.

Ohio 1991 State medical board revoked license of physician who had consensual sexual relations with his patient. The court upheld the board's ruling that this violated Principles I, II and IV. Dissenting judge, citing AMA Council on Ethical and Judicial Affairs, Sexual Misconduct in the Practice of Medicine, 266 JAMA 2741 [now Opinion 8.14], argued that until 1991, the AMA did not clearly deem sexual contact with a patient unethical. *Pons v. Ohio State Medical Bd.*, 66 Ohio St. 3d 619, 623, 625, 614 N.E.2d 748, 752, 753.

Journal 1997 Examines the balance needed between clinical objectivity and physician-patient bonding. Discusses personal boundaries and methods of coping with transgressions by both physicians and patients. Advocates a focus on communication with patients to allow physicians to maintain both an empathetic and objective relationship. References Opinion 8.14. Farber, Novack, & O'Brien, *Love, Boundaries, and the Physician-Patient Relationship*, 157 Arch. Intern. Med. 2291, 2292, 2293, 2294 (1997).

Journal 1996 Discusses the ethical implications of sexual misconduct in the medical field. Examines the current civil and criminal tools used to curb physician-patient misconduct. Notes the inadequacy of physician reporting. Proposes a statutory approach to discipline physicians who abuse their fiduciary duties. Quotes Principle II. References Opinion 8.14. Note, *Sexual Conduct Within the Physician-Patient Relationship: A Statutory Framework for Disciplining this Breach of Fiduciary Duty*, 1 Widener L. Symp. J. 501, 507 (1996).

Journal 1994 Explores the negative consequences of physician-patient sexual relationships. Proposes a model for balancing interests in protecting patients from harm with insulating consensual intimate relationships from unreasonable societal intrusion. Suggests that sexual contact be prohibited during the physician-patient relationship and for a period of time thereafter. Quotes Opinion 8.14. Appelbaum, Jorgenson, & Sutherland, *Sexual Relationships Between Physicians and Patients*, 154 Arch. Intern. Med. 2561, 2561 (1994).

Journal 1993 Examines the potential problems created by attorney-client sexual relations and the need for ethical guidelines. Considers ethical guidelines of other professions. Discusses malpractice case law, ethics opinions, and discipline cases. Examines ethical rules being debated in various states and proposes a model rule. References Opinion 8.14. Davis & Grimaldi, *Sexual Confusion: Attorney-Client Sex and the Need for a Clear Ethical Rule*, 7 Notre Dame J. Law, Ethics, & Pub. Pol. 57, 61 (1993).

Journal 1993 Discusses family privacy rights and a physician's ethical responsibility to report violence. Considers the meaning of justice, self respect, and the fundamental principles of physician ethics. Concludes that physicians have an ethical duty to intervene in domestic violence so long as such intervention does not breach confidentiality or violate patient autonomy. Quotes Principle IV and Opinion 5.05. References Opinions 8.14 and 9.131. Jecker, *Privacy Beliefs and the Violent Family: Extending the Ethical Argument for Physician Intervention*, 269 J.A.M.A. 776, 778, 779 (1993).

Journal 1993 Discusses the potential impact on health care practitioners of the AMA's prohibition against sexual relations between physicians and patients. Focuses on how the prohibition will influence disciplinary actions. Cites Opinion 8.14. Johnson, *Judicial Review of Disciplinary Action for Sexual Misconduct in the Practice of Medicine*, 270 J.A.M.A. 1596 (1993).

Journal 1993 Discusses potential problems caused by attorney-client sexual relations. Examines various means to check such conduct including civil suits and disciplinary actions. Reviews recently enacted legislation on this issue. Proposes a new rule that would prohibit attorney-client sexual relations. References Opinion 8.14. Livingston, *When Libido Subverts Credo: Regulation of Attorney-Client Sexual Relations*, 62 Fordham L. Rev. 5, 55 (1993).

Journal 1993 Evaluates self-policing mechanisms for addressing incompetent and unethical behavior in the medical profession. Discusses the problems physicians may encounter by exposing the errant colleague, such as harm to the reporting physician's reputation and the fear of litigation. States that problems involving physician competency and unethical behavior should be investigated, and that physicians should take personal responsibility for reporting problems they observe. References Principle II and Opinions 8.14 and 9.031. Morreim, *Am I My Brother's Warden? Responding to the Unethical or Incompetent Colleague*, 23 Hastings Center Rep. 19, 23 (May/June 1993).

Journal 1993 Discusses the medical profession's ethical prohibition on physician-patient sexual contact. Evaluates judicial application of the code of medical ethics in matters involving sexual contact. Concludes that legislatures and courts should give greater weight to the ethical code when defining standards of conduct for physician-patient sexual contact. Quotes Opinion 8.14. Note, *Physician-Patient Sexual Contact: The Battle Between the State and the Medical Profession*, 50 Wash. & Lee L. Rev. 1725, 1725-26, 1734, 1752 (1993).

Journal 1992 Discusses the problem of sex in the attorney-client relationship. Compares this relationship to that of physician and patient and argues that similar standards should apply. Proposes an explicit ban on sexual involvement between attorneys and their clients and advocates promulgation of a "bright line" rule. References Opinion 8.14. Goldberg, *Sex and the Attorney-Client Relationship: An Argument for a Prophylactic Rule*, 26 Akron L. Rev. 45 (1992).

Journal 1992 Discusses the problem of sexual relations between attorneys and their clients. Examines the similarities and differences between the physician-patient and the lawyer-client relationship. Concludes that concerns about sexual misconduct in each relationship are valid. Advocates a rebuttable presumption that sexual contact between attorneys and clients is wrongful. Cites Opinion 8.14. Gutheil, Jorgenson, & Sutherland, *Prohibiting Lawyer-Client Sex*, 20 Bull. Am. Acad. Psychiatry Law 365 (1992).

Journal 1992 Discusses patients' allegations of sexual abuse by physicians. Considers the ways in which state medical boards address this problem. Finds increasing reliance upon psychiatric testimony. Proposes that states adopt clear standards governing the admissibility of psychiatric testimony in administrative hearings. Quotes Opinion 8.14. Hyams, *Expert Psychiatric Evidence in Sexual Misconduct Cases Before State Medical Boards*, XVIII Am. J. Law & Med. 171, 173, 174 (1992).

8.15   Substance Abuse

It is unethical for a physician to practice medicine while under the influence of a controlled substance, alcohol, or other chemical agents which impair the ability to practice medicine. (I)

Issued December 1986.

Journal 1994 Discusses the issue of whom physicians must serve first: themselves, their patients, insurers, or society. Explores attempts by the legal system to resolve this issue within the framework of risks that may arise in the physician-patient relationship. Focuses on risks arising out of provider economic arrangements and risks arising out of other individual physician characteristics. Quotes Opinions 8.03 and 9.13. Cites Opinion 8.15. Bobinski, *Autonomy and Privacy: Protecting Patients from Their Physicians*, 55 U. Pitt. L. Rev. 291, 302, 313 (1994).

8.16   Substitution of Surgeon Without Patient's Knowledge or Consent

A surgeon who allows a substitute to operate on his or her patient without the patient's knowledge and consent is deceitful. The patient is entitled to choose his or her own physician and should be permitted to acquiesce to or refuse the substitution.

The surgeon's obligation to the patient requires the surgeon to perform the surgical operation: (1) within the scope of authority granted by the consent to the operation; (2) in accordance with the terms of the contractual relationship; (3) with complete disclosure of facts relevant to the need and the performance of the operation; and (4) utilizing best skill.

It should be noted that it is the operating surgeon to whom the patient grants consent to perform the operation. The patient is entitled to the services of the particular surgeon with whom he or she contracts. The operating surgeon, in accepting the patient, is obligated to utilize his or her personal talents in the performance of the operation to the extent required by the agreement creating the physician-patient relationship. The surgeon cannot properly delegate to another the duties which he or she is required to perform personally.

Under the normal and customary arrangement with patients, and with reference to the usual form of consent to operation, the operating surgeon is obligated to perform the operation but may be assisted by residents or other surgeons. With the consent of the patient, it is not unethical for the operating surgeon to delegate the performance of certain aspects of the operation to the assistant provided this is done under the surgeon's participatory supervision, i.e., the surgeon must scrub. If a resident or other physician is to perform the operation under non-participatory supervision, it is necessary to make a full disclosure of this fact to the patient, and this should be evidenced by an appropriate statement contained in the consent. Under these circumstances, it is the resident or other physician who becomes the operating surgeon. (I, II, IV, V)

Issued prior to April 1977.

Updated June 1994.

Ala. 1985 Patient sued physicians alleging fraud and conspiracy to commit fraud. The court clarified its previous holding in the case (461 So. 2d 775) that a new trial was ordered only on fraud and conspiracy to commit fraud theories. The court also noted that the trier of fact would need to decide whether the Current Opinions of the Judicial Council of the American Medical Association pamphlet was properly excluded under the "learned treatise" doctrine and whether, if properly authenticated, it might be admissible at a new trial as to the issue of whether "ghost surgery," condemned by Opinion 8.12 (1984) [now Opinion 8.16], constitutes fraud. *McMurray v. Johnson, 481 So. 2d 887, 889.*

N.J. 1983 Patient who consented to surgery by one surgeon, but was actually operated on by another, sued both surgeons. Pursuant to state law, patient submitted case to malpractice panel which found no basis to patient's claims and jury returned verdict for defendant surgeons. In holding that failure to permit plaintiff to show possible bias of panel doctor and to impeach the testimony constituted reversible error, the court quoted Opinion 8.12 (1982) [now Opinion 8.16] indicating that substitution of one surgeon for another without patient consent is a deceit and deviates from standard medical care, constituting the violation of a legal obligation as well as a tenet of the medical profession. *Perna v. Pirozzi, 92 N.J. 446, 457 A.2d 431, 434, 440, n.3.*

N.J. Super. 1991 Two physicians were sued by a patient claiming that one of the physician-surgeons had committed "ghost surgery" battery. The court acknowledged the rule in Perna v. Pirozzi, 92 N.J. 446, 457 A.2d 431 (1983). The court there, taking judicial notice of the standard of care set out by Opinion 8.12 (1982) [now Opinion 8.16], held that an intent to injure is not required to establish battery when a medical procedure is performed by a "substitute" physician. However, the court here held that the plaintiff had failed to establish by competent medical opinion that one of the physicians was an unauthorized operating surgeon. Furthermore, the court stated that to hold otherwise would create a punitive damage claim based on a patient's lay opinion concerning the proper role of an authorized surgeon in team surgery. *Monturi v. Englewood Hosp., 246 N.J. Super. 547, 552, 588 A.2d 408, 410, 411.*

N.J. Super. 1982 In a medical malpractice suit against a surgeon for negligence and for allowing a different surgeon to operate on plaintiff without plaintiff's express consent, the court noted Opinions and Reports of the Judicial Council Sec. 1, Para. 5 (1969) [now Opinion 8.16] as quoted in 209 J.A.M.A. 94748 (1969) that it is fraudulent and deceitful for a surgeon to allow another surgeon to operate on a patient without that patient's consent. The court ultimately concluded that "the doctrine of informed consent is a theory of professional liability independent from malpractice," and thus was not relevant to the case at bar. *Perna v. Pirozzi, 182 N.J. Super. 510, 442 A.2d 1016, 1019, rev'd, 92 N.J. 446, 457 A.2d 431 (1983).*

Okla. App. 1974 Owner of a bull sued veterinarian for malpractice and failure to disclose possible adverse reactions to penicillin. The appellate court held that the veterinarian was liable for damages to the plaintiff resulting from the death of the bull. In so holding, the court noted Opinions and Reports of the Judicial Council Sec. 1, Para. 5 (1969) [now Opinion 8.16] which, inter alia, requires a surgeon to make a complete disclosure of all facts relevant to the operation to be performed. *Hull v. Tate, No. 46443 (Okla. Ct. App. April 16, 1974) (LEXIS, States library, Okla. file), rev'd, No. 46443 (Okla. Sup. Ct. Oct. 29, 1974) (LEXIS, States library, Okla. file).*

Pa. Super. 1996 Physician told patient he would perform necessary surgery. As a result of the surgery, patient developed a drop foot which would drag whenever he walked. The patient later discovered that his treating physician did not appear for or participate in his surgery. When the hospital was unable to reach the physician, it contacted his office where another physician instructed the hospital to perform the surgery with a third physician. All of this was done without patient's consent and was not disclosed after recovery. Patient sued the physician for failure to perform the surgery and for directing or permitting a third party to perform the surgery. The court quoted from Opinion 8.12 (1982) [now Opinion 8.16] which provides that the patient is entitled to choose his or her physician and should be permitted to acquiesce in or refuse to accept any substitutions. *Grabowski v. Quigley, 454 Pa. Super. 27, 684 A.2d 610, 617.*

Journal 1996 Considers how practice guidelines may be used in malpractice litigation as inculpatory or exculpatory evidence. Concludes that use of guidelines as inculpatory evidence should not be eliminated until there is evidence of undesirable effects. Quotes Opinion 8.16. Hyams, Shapiro, & Brennan, *Medical Practice Guidelines in Malpractice Litigation: An Early Retrospective,* 21 J. Health Pol. Pol'y & L. 289, 298 (1996).

Journal 1996 Discusses tort liability in cases of substitution of surgeons without patient consent. Explores whether substitutions are a battery thereby allowing recovery, regardless of outcome. Concludes that "ghost surgery" should not automatically constitute a battery but that courts should allow recovery for infliction of emotional distress stemming from the substitution. Quotes Opinion 8.12 (1982) [now Opinion 8.16]. Lundmark, *Surgery by an Unauthorized Surgeon as a Battery,* 10 J. L. & Health 287, 293 (1996).

8.17   Use of Restraints

All individuals have a fundamental right to be free from unreasonable bodily restraint. Physical and chemical restraints should therefore be used only in the best interest of the patient and in accordance with the following guidelines:

(1) The use of restraints, except in emergencies, may be implemented only upon the explicit order of a physician, in conformance with reasonable professional judgment.

(2) Judgment should be exercised in issuing pro re nata (PRN) orders for the use of physical or chemical restraints, and the implementation of such orders should be frequently reviewed and documented by the physician.

(3) The use of restraints should not be punitive, nor should they be used for convenience or as an alternative to reasonable staffing.

(4) Restraints should be used only in accordance with appropriate clinical indications.

(5) As with all therapeutic interventions, informed consent by the patient or surrogate decisionmaker is a key element in the application of physical and chemical restraints, and should be incorporated into institutional policy.

(6) In certain limited situations, it may be appropriate to restrain a patient involuntarily. For example, restraints may be needed for the safety of the patient or others in the area. When restraints are used involuntarily, the restraints should be removed when they are no longer needed. (I, IV)

Issued March 1992 based on the report, "Guidelines for the Use of Restraints in Long Term Care Facilities," adopted June 1989.

8.18   Informing Families of a Patient's Death

Disclosing the death of a patient to the patient's family is a duty which goes to the very heart of the physician-patient relationship and should not be readily delegated to others by the attending physician. The emotional needs of the family and the integrity of the physician-patient relationship must at all times be given foremost consideration.

Physicians in residency training may be asked to participate in the communication of information about a patient's death, if that request is commensurate with the physician's prior training or experience and previous close personal relationship with the family.

It would not be appropriate for the attending physician or resident to request that a medical student notify family members of a patient's death. Medical students should be trained in issues of death and dying, and should be encouraged to accompany attending physicians when news of a patient's death is conveyed to the family members. (I, IV)

Issued March 1992 based on the report, "Informing Families of a Patient's Death: Guidelines for the Involvement of Medical Students," adopted December 1989.

Updated June 1994.

Journal 1995 Examines four essential principles of bioethics: patient autonomy; nonmaleficence; beneficence; and justice. Describes the application of these principles in clinical settings according to bioethical norms and AMA opinions. Concludes that such an approach promotes compassionate medical caregiving and that laws should reflect these values. Quotes Opinions 2.01 and 8.18. References Opinion 2.211. Cohen, *Toward a Bioethics of Compassion, 28 Ind. L. Rev. 667, 673, 681-82, 683 (1995)*.

8.19 Self-Treatment or Treatment of Immediate Family Members

Physicians generally should not treat themselves or members of their immediate families. Professional objectivity may be compromised when an immediate family member or the physician is the patient; the physician's personal feelings may unduly influence his or her professional medical judgment, thereby interfering with the care being delivered. Physicians may fail to probe sensitive areas when taking the medical history or may fail to perform intimate parts of the physical examination. Similarly, patients may feel uncomfortable disclosing sensitive information or undergoing an intimate examination when the physician is an immediate family member. This discomfort is particularly the case when the patient is a minor child, and sensitive or intimate care should especially be avoided for such patients. When treating themselves or immediate family members, physicians may be inclined to treat problems that are beyond their expertise or training. If tensions develop in a physician's professional relationship with a family member, perhaps as a result of a negative medical outcome, such difficulties may be carried over into the family member's personal relationship with the physician.

Concerns regarding patient autonomy and informed consent are also relevant when physicians attempt to treat members of their immediate family. Family members may be reluctant to state their preference for another physician or decline a recommendation for fear of offending the physician. In particular, minor children will generally not feel free to refuse care from their parents. Likewise, physicians may feel obligated to provide care to immediate family members even if they feel uncomfortable providing care.

It would not always be inappropriate to undertake self-treatment or treatment of immediate family members. In emergency settings or isolated settings where there is no other qualified physician available, physicians should not hesitate to treat themselves or family members until another physician becomes available. In addition, while physicians should not serve as a primary or regular care provider for immediate family members, there are situations in which routine care is acceptable for short-term, minor problems.

Except in emergencies, it is not appropriate for physicians to write prescriptions for controlled substances for themselves or immediate family members. (I, II, IV)

Issued June 1993.

Opinions on Professional Rights and Responsibilities

Accreditation

Physicians who engage in activities that involve the accreditation, approval, or certification of institutions, facilities, and programs that provide patient care or medical education or certify the attainment of specialized professional competence have the ethical responsibility to apply standards that are relevant, fair, reasonable, and nondiscriminatory. The accreditation of institutions and facilities that provide patient care should be based upon standards that focus upon the quality of patient care achieved. Standards used in the accreditation of patient care and medical education, or the certification of specialized professional attainment should not be adopted or used as a means of economic regulation. (II, IV, VII)

Issued December 1982.

Continuing Medical Education

Physicians should strive to further their medical education throughout their careers, for only by participating in continuing medical education (CME) can they continue to serve patients to the best of their abilities and live up to professional standards of excellence. Fulfillment of mandatory state CME requirements does not necessarily fulfill the physician's ethical obligation to maintain his or her medical expertise.

Attendees. Guidelines for physicians attending a CME conference or activity are as follows:

(1) The physician choosing among CME activities should assess their educational value and select only those activities which are of high quality and appropriate for the physician's educational needs. When selecting formal CME activities, the physician should, at a minimum, choose only those activities that (a) are offered by sponsors accredited by the Accreditation Council for Continuing Medical Education (ACCME), the American Academy of Family Physicians (AAFP), or a state medical society; (b) contain information on subjects relevant to the physician's needs; (c) are responsibly conducted by qualified faculty; and (d) conform to Opinion 8.061, "Gifts to Physicians from Industry."

(2) The educational value of the CME conference or activity must be the primary consideration in the physician's decision to attend or participate. Though amenities unrelated to the educational purpose of the activity may play a role in the physician's decision to participate, this role should be secondary to the educational content of the conference.

(3) Physicians should claim credit commensurate with only the actual time spent attending a CME activity or in studying a CME enduring material.

(4) Attending promotional activities put on by industry or their designees is not unethical as long as the conference conforms to Opinion 8.061, "Gifts to Physicians from Industry" and is clearly identified as promotional to all participants.

Faculty. Guidelines for physicians serving as presenters, moderators, or other faculty at a CME conference are as follows:

(1) Physicians serving as presenters, moderators, or other faculty at a CME conference should ensure that (a) research findings and therapeutic recommendations are based on scientifically accurate, up-to-date information and are presented in a balanced, objective manner and (b) the content of their presentation is not modified or influenced by representatives of industry or other financial contributors, and they do not employ materials whose content is shaped by industry. Faculty may, however, use scientific data generated from industry-sponsored research, and they may also accept technical assistance from industry in preparing slides or other presentation materials, as long as this assistance is of only nominal monetary value and the company has no input in the actual content of the material.

(2) When invited to present at non-CME activities that are primarily promotional, faculty should avoid participation unless the activity is clearly identified as promotional in its program announcements and other advertising.

(3) All conflicts of interest or biases, such as a financial connection to a particular commercial firm or product, should be disclosed by faculty members to the activity's sponsor and to the audience. Faculty may accept reasonable honoraria and reimbursement for expenses in accordance with Opinion 8.061, "Gifts to Physicians from Industry."

Sponsors. Guidelines for physicians involved in the sponsorship of CME activities are as follows:

(1) Physicians involved in the sponsorship of CME activities should ensure that (a) the program is balanced, with faculty members presenting a broad range of scientifically supportable viewpoints related to the topic at hand; (b) representatives of industry or other financial contributors do not exert control over the choice of moderators, presenters, or other faculty, or modify the content of faculty presentations. Funding from industry or others may be accepted in accordance with Opinion 8.061, "Gifts to Physicians from Industry."

(2) Sponsors should not promote CME activities in a way that encourages attendees to violate the guidelines of the Council on Ethical and Judicial Affairs, including Opinion 8.061, "Gifts to Physicians from Industry," or the principles established for the American Medical Association's

Physician Recognition Award. CME activities should be developed and promoted consistent with guideline (2) for Attendees.

(3) Any non-CME activity that is primarily promotional must be identified as such to faculty and participants, both in its advertising and at the conference itself.

(4) The entity presenting the program should not profit unfairly or charge a fee which is excessive for the content and length of the program.

(5) The program, content, duration, and ancillary activities should be consistent with the ideals of the AMA CME program. (I, V)

Issued December 1993.

Journal 1992 Reviews concerns about commercial involvement in and funding of continuing medical education. Discusses CME requirements, accumulation of CME credits, and changes in standards governing commercial sponsorship. References Opinions 8.061 and 9.011. Wentz, Osteen, & Cannon, *Continuing Medical Education: Unabated Debate,* 268 J.A.M.A. 1118 (1992).

Journal 1991 Discusses commercial support of continuing medical education. Explains ethical guidelines for accepting such assistance and how those guidelines have changed. References Opinions 8.061 and 9.011. Wentz, Osteen, & Gannon, *Refocusing Support and Direction,* 266 J.A.M.A. 953 (1991).

9.02   **Opinion 9.02, Agreements Restricting the Practice of Medicine,** was deleted in June 1998 and replaced with the opinion below.

9.02   **Restrictive Covenants and the Practice of Medicine**

Covenants-not-to-compete restrict competition, disrupt continuity of care, and potentially deprive the public of medical services. The Council on Ethical and Judicial Affairs discourages any agreement which restricts the right of a physician to practice medicine for a specified period of time or in a specified area upon termination of an employment, partnership or corporate agreement. Restrictive covenants are unethical if they are excessive in geographic scope or duration in the circumstances presented, or if they fail to make reasonable accommodation of patients' choice of physician. (VI, VII)

Issued prior to April 1977.

Updated June 1994 and June 1998.

N.D. Ill. 1996 A corporation which provided hair transplants brought suit against a physician group under contract to provide medical services to the corporation. The complaint alleged that the defendants had breached the contract in bad faith by attempting to start their own company, by hiring staff members away, and by threatening to enforce noncompetition covenants in their contracts should any physicians attempt to remain with the corporation. The court referred to Opinion 9.02 as explicitly discouraging the use of restrictive covenants in contracts with physicians. Additionally, with apparent reference to Opinion 7.03, the court noted that defendants had not sent notices advising patients of the departure of physicians from the corporation, or of the departing physicians' new practice locations. *Cleveland Hair Clinic, Inc. v. Puig,* 968 F. Supp. 1227, 1246.

Ariz. App. 1989 Plaintiff, an orthopaedic surgeon formerly employed by defendant, appealed a lower court's grant of a preliminary injunction which enforced the restrictive covenant in plaintiff's employment contract with defendant. Plaintiff asserted that Opinion 9.02 discouraged the use of such restrictive covenants and thus the covenant at issue should be declared per se unenforceable. The appellate court declined to make that declaration, noting that not all restrictive covenants are contrary to public policy and that the lower court had appropriately modified the terms of the covenant. *Phoenix Orthopaedic Surgeons, Ltd. v. Peairs, 164 Ariz. 54, 60, 790 P.2d 752, 758.*

Ga. 1988 Following termination of employment contract between the employer, a provider of psychiatric services, and a physician, the employer filed suit seeking an injunction to enforce a covenant not to compete. Supreme court, without opinion, upheld trial court's order granting an injunction. Dissenting judge, quoting Opinion 9.02 (1986) reasoned that restrictive covenants in such physician employment agreements are "illegal per se as against public policy irrespective of whether the covenant is reasonable." *Shankman v. Coastal Psychiatric Assocs., 258 Ga. 294, 295, 368 S.E.2d 753, 754 (dissent).*

Ind. App. 1987 Medical corporation sued physician who was former employee at will pursuant to covenant not to compete in employment contract seeking an injunction or liquidated damages. Court upheld covenant against physician's claim that enforcement was inappropriate where he had been terminated without good cause. Concurring judge, citing Opinion 9.02 (1986), expressed view that such covenants should be unenforceable as against public policy. *Gomez v. Chua Medical Corp., 510 N.E.2d 191, 197.*

Kan. App. 1985 Members of a medical partnership sought an injunction to enforce a covenant not to compete against defendant-physician, a former partner. Defendant asserted that the covenant was void as against public policy relying on Opinion 9.02 (1984). The court however ruled that the covenant was reasonable as defined by precedent and that it was bound to follow this precedent as opposed to the American Medical Association's position regarding such covenants. Defendant further argued enforcement of the covenant was precluded because the partnership had violated ethical norms, apparently referring to Opinions 6.03 and 6.04 (1984) [now Opinions 6.02 and 6.03] which were part of partnership contract. The court held defendant was estopped from complaining about the partnership's actions due to his own conduct. *Axtell Clinic v. Cranston, No. 56,745 (Kan. Ct. App. June 20, 1985) (LEXIS, States Library, Ka. file).*

Minn. 1983 Dispute arose between physician and clinic concerning covenant not to compete contained in employment contract entered into by physician after commencement of employment. Physician challenged enforceability of covenant due to lack of consideration to support it. The court agreed with physician and denied enforcement. In so ruling court did not reach issue of whether such covenants, in the context of medical practice, are against public policy. The court however noted that under Opinion 9.01 (1982) [now Opinion 9.02] the American Medical Association discourages such restrictive covenants. *Freeman v. Duluth Clinic, 334 N.W.2d 626, 631.*

N.J. 1978 Plaintiff and defendant, both physicians, had entered into an employment contract which included in its terms a restrictive covenant provision. When defendant failed to abide by the covenant upon termination of the employment contract, plaintiff sued to enforce the covenant. In affirming the lower court's decision to enforce the restrictive covenant, the appellate court quoted Current Opinion 4.63 (1977) [now Opinion 9.02] and stated that, although it hesitated to give weight to the rules of private organizations, even if it followed the Opinion the decision to uphold the covenant would be proper. *Karlin v. Weinberg, 77 N.J. 408, 390 A.2d 1161, 1168 n.6.*

N.J. Super. 1977 Plaintiff, a dermatologist who had previously employed defendant-dermatologist, sued to enforce a post-employment restrictive covenant signed by defendant. In holding the covenant enforceable, the court noted Opinion 4.63 (1977) [now Opinion 9.02] which at the time stated there was "no ethical proscription" against entering into a restrictive covenant if its terms are reasonable. Note that Opinion 9.02 now "discourages" such restrictive agreements. *Karlin v. Weinberg, 148 N.J. Super. 243, 372 A.2d 616, 618, aff'd, 77 N.J. 408, 390 A.2d 1161 (1978).*

Ohio App. 1991 Medical corporation sought an injunction to enforce a covenant not to compete against defendant-physician. The lower court granted summary judgment based on a referee's report which concluded that, under Principle VI and Opinions 6.11, 9.02, and 9.06 (1989) restrictive covenants were *per se* unenforceable as a matter of public policy. While recognizing a strong public interest in allowing open access to health care, the appellate court in reversing held that Opinion 9.02, which applied specifically to restrictive covenants, only "discouraged" such covenants. *Ohio Urology, Inc. v. Poll, 72 Ohio. App. 446, 450, 451, 594 N.E.2d 1027, 1030, 1031.*

Journal 1997 Examines noncompetition clauses in the medical field. Reviews policy concerns and historical and common-law analyses of agreements not to compete. Posits that, the more commercialized the medical profession becomes, the more noncompetition clauses infringe upon the physician-patient relationship and patients' rights. Quotes Opinions 9.02 and 9.06. Cites Preamble and Opinion 6.11. Comment, *Noncompetition Clauses in Physician Employment Contracts in Oregon*, 76 Or. L. Rev. 195, 204-06 (1997).

Journal 1997 Examines the judicial assessment of restrictive covenants within the legal and medical fields. Observes that courts tend to uphold physician, but not attorney, restrictive covenants. Concludes that covenants in medical practice should be treated in a manner similar to those in legal practice. Opinion 9.02. Levy, *Because Judges Went to Law School, Not Medical School: Restrictive Covenants in the Practices of Law and Medicine*, 30 J. Health & Hosp. L. 89, 92, 101 (1997).

Journal 1995 Analyzes South Carolina judicial treatment of covenants not to compete and liquidated damages provisions. Considers approaches in other jurisdictions and proposes guidelines for drafting contractual agreements. Quotes Opinion 9.06. Cites Opinion 9.01 (1982) [now Opinion 9.02]. Note, *Covenants Not to Compete and Liquidated Damages Clauses: Diagnosis and Treatment for Physicians*, 46 S.C. L. Rev. 505, 514 (1995).

Journal 1991 Considers the question of whether physicians should provide medical treatment to those who come to them for second opinions. Analyzes important ethical and legal guidelines. Concludes that each physician must individually decide whether to treat these patients. Quotes Opinions 6.11, 9.06, and 9.12. Cites Opinion 9.02. Ile, *Should Physicians Treat Patients Who Seek Second Opinions?*, 266 J.A.M.A. 273, 274 (1991).

Journal 1982 Discusses the legal status of restrictive covenants in employment contracts against the background of the American Medical Association's position discouraging such agreements as not serving the public interest. Observes that courts generally have upheld restrictive covenants if the limits are reasonable. Discusses several cases illustrating some of the elements that may impact the enforcement of restrictive covenants. Cites Opinion 9.01 (1982) [now Opinion 9.02]. Cooper, *Restrictive Covenants*, 248 J.A.M.A. 3091, 3091 (1982).

9.021 Covenants-Not-to-Compete for Physicians-in-Training

It is unethical for a teaching institution to seek a non-competition guarantee in return for fulfilling its educational obligations. Physicians-in-training (residents in programs approved by the Accreditation Council on Graduate Medical Education (ACGME), fellows in ACGME-approved fellowship programs, and fellows in programs approved by one of the American Board of Medical Specialty's specialty boards) should not be asked to sign covenants-not-to-compete as a condition of their entry into any residency or fellowship program. (VI, VII)

Issued June 1998 based on the report, "Covenants-Not-to-Compete for Physicians-in-training," adopted June 1997.

9.03 Civil Rights and Professional Responsibility

Opportunities in medical society activities or membership, medical education and training, employment and all other aspects of professional endeavors should not be denied to any duly licensed physician because of race, color, religion, creed, ethnic affiliation, national origin, sex, sexual orientation, age, or handicap. (IV)

Issued prior to April 1977.

Updated June 1994.

Journal 1996 Examines possible legal avenues for addressing claims of employment discrimination based upon sexual orientation. Concludes that lesbians and gay men need greater employment protection and an explicit statutory cause of action. Quotes Opinion 9.03. Gilmore, *Employment Protection for Lesbians and Gay Men,* 6 L. & Sex. 83, 95 (1996).

9.031   Reporting Impaired, Incompetent, or Unethical Colleagues

Physicians have an ethical obligation to report impaired, incompetent, and unethical colleagues in accordance with the legal requirements in each state and assisted by the following guidelines:

Impairment. Impairment should be reported to the hospital's in-house impairment program, if available. Otherwise, either the chief of an appropriate clinical service or the chief of the hospital staff should be alerted. Reports may also be made directly to an external impaired physician program. Practicing physicians who do not have hospital privileges should be reported directly to an impaired physician program, such as those run by medical societies, when appropriate. If none of these steps would facilitate the entrance of the impaired physician into an impairment program, then the impaired physician should be reported directly to the state licensing board.

Incompetence. Initial reports of incompetence should be made to the appropriate clinical authority who would be empowered to assess the potential impact on patient welfare and to facilitate remedial action. The hospital peer review body should be notified where appropriate. Incompetence which poses an immediate threat to the health of patients should be reported directly to the state licensing board. Incompetence by physicians without a hospital affiliation should be reported to the local or state medical society and/or the state licensing or disciplinary board.

Unethical conduct. With the exception of incompetence or impairment, unethical behavior should be reported in accordance with the following guidelines:

Unethical conduct that threatens patient care or welfare should be reported to the appropriate authority for a particular clinical service. Unethical behavior which violates state licensing provisions should be reported to the state licensing board or impaired physician programs, when appropriate. Unethical conduct which violates criminal statutes must be reported to the appropriate law enforcement authorities. All other unethical conduct should be reported to the local or state medical society.

Where the inappropriate behavior of a physician continues despite the initial report(s), the reporting physician should report to a higher or additional authority. The person or body receiving the initial report should notify the reporting physician when appropriate action has been taken. Physicians who receive reports of inappropriate behavior have an ethical duty to critically and objectively evaluate the reported information and to assure that identified deficiencies are either remedied or further reported to a higher or additional authority. Anonymous reports should receive appropriate review and confidential investigation. Physicians who are under scrutiny or charge should be protected by the rules of confidentiality until such charges are proven or until the physician is exonerated. (II)

Issued March 1992 based on the report, "Reporting Impaired, Incompetent, or Unethical Colleagues," adopted January 1992.

Updated June 1994 and June 1996.

Mich. App. 1968 Physician was properly dismissed from hospital staff for violating Principle 4 (1957) [now Principle II and Opinion 9.031] when on numerous occasions physician "vilified" other physicians, swore and screamed in the hospital, and quarreled with staff and hospital visitors. *Anderson v. Bd. of Trustees of Caro Community Hosp.*, 10 Mich. App. 348, 159 N.W.2d 347, 348-50.

Journal 1993 Evaluates self-policing mechanisms for addressing incompetent and unethical behavior in the medical profession. Discusses the problems physicians may encounter by exposing the errant colleague, such as harm to the reporting physician's reputation and the fear of litigation. States that problems involving physician competency and unethical behavior should be investigated, and that physicians should take personal responsibility for reporting problems they observe. References Principle II and Opinions 8.14 and 9.031. Morreim, *Am I My Brother's Warden? Responding to the Unethical or Incompetent Colleague*, 23 Hastings Center Rep. 19, 23 (May/June 1993).

9.032 Reporting Adverse Drug or Device Events

A physician who suspects the occurrence of an adverse reaction to a drug or medical device has an obligation to communicate that information to the broader medical community (e.g., through submitting a report or letter to a medical journal or informing the manufacturer of the suspect drug or device). In the case of a serious adverse event, the event should be reported to the Food and Drug Administration (FDA). Spontaneous reports of adverse events are irreplaceable as a source of valuable information about drugs and medical devices, particularly their rare or delayed effects, as well as their safety in vulnerable patient populations. Although premarketing and mandated postmarketing studies provide basic safeguards for the public health, they suffer from inherent deficiencies that limit their ability to detect rare or unexpected consequences of drug or medical device use. Physicians who prescribe and monitor the use of drugs and medical devices constitute the group best able to observe and communicate information about resulting adverse events.

Serious adverse events, such as those resulting in death, hospitalization, or medical or surgical intervention, are the most important to report and are the only adverse events for which the FDA desires a report. Certainty, or even reasonable likelihood, of a causal relationship between the drug or medical device and the serious adverse event will rarely exist and is not required before reporting the event to the FDA. Suspicion of such a relationship is sufficient to give rise to an obligation to participate in the reporting system. (I, V, VII)

Issued June 1994 based on the report, "Reporting Adverse Drug and Medical Device Events," adopted June 1993.

Updated June 1994.

Journal 1993 Explains MedWatch, an FDA program designed to facilitate the reporting of adverse events associated with the use of FDA-approved drugs and medical devices. Emphasizes that physicians are best able to provide such information. Quotes Opinion 9.032. Rheinstein, *MedWatch: The FDA Medical Products Reporting Program*, 48 Am. Fam. Physician 636, 636 (1993).

9.035   Gender Discrimination in the Medical Profession

Physician leaders in medical schools and other medical institutions should take immediate steps to increase the number of women in leadership positions as such positions become open. There is already a large enough pool of female physicians to provide strong candidates for such positions. Also, adjustments should be made to ensure that all physicians are equitably compensated for their work. Women and men in the same specialty with the same experience and doing the same work should be paid the same compensation.

Physicians in the workplace should actively develop the following: (a) retraining or other programs which facilitate the reentry of physicians who take time away from their careers to have a family; (b) on-site child care services for dependent children; (c) policies providing job security for physicians who are temporarily not in practice due to pregnancy or family obligations.

Physicians in the academic medical setting should strive to promote the following: (a) extension of tenure decisions through "stop the clock" programs, relaxation of the seven year rule, or part-time appointments that would give faculty members longer to achieve standards for promotion and tenure; (b) more reasonable guidelines regarding the appropriate quantity and timing of published material needed for promotion or tenure that would emphasize quality over quantity and that would encourage the pursuit of careers based on individual talent rather than tenure standards that undervalue teaching ability and overvalue research; (c) fair distribution of teaching, clinical, research, administrative responsibilities, and access to tenure tracks between men and women. Also, physicians in academic institutions should consider formally structuring the mentoring process, possibly matching students or faculty with advisors through a fair and visible system.

Where such policies do not exist or have not been followed, all medical workplaces and institutions should create strict policies to deal with sexual harassment. Grievance committees should have broad representation of both sexes and other groups. Such committees should have the power to enforce harassment policies and be accessible to those persons they are meant to serve.

Grantors of research funds and editors of scientific or medical journals should consider blind peer review of grant proposals and articles for publication to help prevent bias. However, grantors and editors will be able to consider the author's identity and give it appropriate weight. (II, VII)

Issued June 1994 based on the report, "Gender Discrimination in the Medical Profession," adopted June 1993.

Journal 1996 Considers the pharmaceutical industry's failure to test products on female subjects. Comments on the potential for harm. Notes legal difficulties women experience when attempting to prove a drug was not adequately tested. Posits that litigation can affect the behavior of pharmaceutical companies. References Opinion 9.035. Comment, *Tort Reform to Ensure the Inclusion of Fertile Women in Early Phases of Commercial Drug Research*, 3 U. Chi. L. Sch. Roundtable 355, 359 (1996).

Incompetence, corruption, or dishonest or unethical conduct on the part of members of the medical profession is reprehensible. In addition to posing a real or potential threat to patients, such conduct undermines the public's confidence in the profession. A physician should expose, without fear or loss of favor, incompetent or corrupt, dishonest or unethical conduct on the part of members of the profession. Questions of such conduct should be reported and reviewed in accordance with Opinion 9.031, "Reporting Impaired, Incompetent, or Unethical Colleagues."

Violation of governmental laws may subject the physician to civil or criminal liability. Expulsion from membership is the maximum penalty that may be imposed by a medical society upon a physician who violates the ethical standards involving a breach of moral duty or principle. However, medical societies have a civic and professional obligation to report to the appropriate governmental body or state board of medical examiners credible evidence that may come to their attention involving the alleged criminal conduct of any physician relating to the practice of medicine.

Although a physician charged with allegedly illegal conduct may be acquitted or exonerated in civil or criminal proceedings, this does not discharge a medical society from its obligation to initiate a disciplinary proceeding against a member with reference to the same conduct where there is credible evidence tending to establish unethical conduct.

The Council cannot pass judgment in advance on a situation that may later come before it on appeal. The Council cannot be an attorney for a society or a member thereof and later judge in the same factual situation. The local medical society has the initial obligation of determining all the facts and whether or not disciplinary action is indicated. Questions asking for a review of a proposed course of action or an evaluation of an existing factual situation should be presented to the appropriate official of the physician's local society. (II, III, VII)

Issued prior to April 1977.

Updated June 1994.

Cal. App. 1956 Physician-petitioner sought mandamus against local medical association whose bylaws provided for the expulsion of any member who violated the Principles. Petitioner had been expelled under the provision and the expulsion was affirmed by the American Medical Association's Judicial Council. The initial grounds for expulsion was alleged violation of Principles Ch. III, Art. IV, Sec.4 (1947) [now Opinions 9.04 and 9.07] for disparaging statements regarding another physician in a report used in judicial proceedings. In holding that application of the provision to petitioner was contrary to public policy, the court noted that the physician's statements had been made at the request of a civil litigant and enjoyed a statutory testimonial privilege. Further, the court found that the American Medical Association's right to formulate ethical principles did not extend to defining the duties of witnesses. Expulsion was also based on petitioner's critical comments about other physicians overheard by their patients in violation of Principles Ch. III, Art. IV, Sec.1 (1947) [now Principle II and Opinion 9.04]. The court found application of this Principle under the circumstances reasonable and not contrary to public policy. *Bernstein v. Alameda-Contra Costa Medical Ass'n, 139 Cal. App. 2d 241, 293 P.2d 862, 863, 863 nn.1, 2, 865 nn.4, 6, 866, 866 n.8, 867.*

Ohio 1980 A physician, charged with violating the state medical licensing statute by distributing controlled substances without a proper license and writing prescriptions for narcotics in the name of one person when they were intended for another, challenged the state medical board's decision to suspend his license and place him on two years probation. Under the statute, a physician could be disciplined for various activities including "violation of any provision of a code of ethics of a national professional organization" such as the American Medical Association. The board found in part that the physician's actions violated Principles 4 and 7 (1957) [now Principles II and III and Opinions 6.04 and 9.04]. The trial court reversed, holding that the board had insufficient evidence for its decision, and the court of appeals affirmed. On appeal, the supreme court held that expert testimony was not required at a hearing before a medical licensing board because they were experts and could determine for themselves whether the Principles had been violated. *Arlen v. State*, 61 Ohio St. 2d 168, 399 N.E.2d 1251, 1252, 1253-54.

Journal 1994 Discusses the role of professional societies in establishing ethical guidelines for physicians in the context of using medical innovations and new technologies. Observes that these standards must be supplemented by additional external measures or incentives in order to be most effective. Concludes that professional societies are more successful at setting standards than ensuring acceptance and implementation of those standards by member professionals. Cites Opinions 1.01, 1.02, 8.061, 9.04, and 9.131. Orentlicher, *The Influence of a Professional Organization on Physician Behavior*, 57 Alb. L. Rev. 583, 592, 593, 594, 595, 596 (1994).

9.05 Due Process

The basic principles of a fair and objective hearing should always be accorded to the physician or medical student whose professional conduct is being reviewed. The fundamental aspects of a fair hearing are a listing of specific charges, adequate notice of the right of a hearing, the opportunity to be present and to rebut the evidence, and the opportunity to present a defense. These principles apply when the hearing body is a medical society tribunal, medical staff committee, or other similar body composed of peers. The composition of committees sitting in judgment of medical students, residents, or fellows should include a significant number of persons at a similar level of training.

These principles of fair play apply in all disciplinary hearings and in any other type of hearing in which the reputation, professional status, or livelihood of the physician or medical student may be negatively impacted.

All physicians and medical students are urged to observe diligently these fundamental safeguards of due process whenever they are called upon to serve on a committee which will pass judgment on a peer. All medical societies and institutions are urged to review their constitutions and bylaws and/or policies to make sure that these instruments provide for such procedural safeguards. (II, III, VII)

Issued prior to April 1977.

Updated June 1994.

Ill. App. 1979 Physician sued professional association of orthopaedic surgeons after it denied his application for membership. Plaintiff claimed he was not fully informed of the basis of denial, received no notice or opportunity to attend the hearing in which his application was considered, and was neither allowed to hear adverse evidence nor present a defense. Since the association's by-laws required adherence to the Principles, including Opinion 6.18 (1977) [now Opinion 9.05], which demanded that due process be afforded a physician whose conduct is being reviewed, plaintiff alleged that the association had violated its own procedures in the application process. The court held that the applicant did not have a right to have his application considered according to the association's bylaws and could not obtain judicial review without a showing of economic necessity. *Treister v. American Academy of Orthopaedic Surgeons*, 78 Ill. App. 3d 746, 396 N.E.2d 1225, 1228, 1232, 1238.

Journal 1984 Discusses litigation by physicians in situations where medical staff privileges have been denied, curtailed, or revoked. Specific attention is devoted to litigation based on either Section 1 or Section 2 of the Sherman Act, which is the predominant federal antitrust legislative scheme. Section 1 prohibits restraint of trade practices while Section 2 prohibits monopolies. Offers an analysis of the relevant legal theories and practice considerations that form part of hospital privilege antitrust litigation but concludes that litigation based on the Sherman Act in this context generally has been unsuccessful due to stringent requirements of proof. Cites Opinion 9.04 (1982) [now Opinion 9.05]. Tabor, *The Battle for Hospital Privileges, 251 J.A.M.A. 1602, 1602 (1984)*.

Journal 1983 Describes special problems that may confront family physicians in the context of applying for hospital privileges. Offers a recommended approach to the application process which encourages physicians to document areas of residency training, become familiar with the hospital policies, guidelines, and procedures involved in applying for privileges, and solicit the support of staff physicians. Also summarizes individual rights within the context of the application process as well as protections afforded under concepts of due process of law. Quotes Opinion 9.04 (1981) [now Opinion 9.05]. Pugno, *Hospital Privileges for Family Physicians: Rights, Rationale, and Resources, 17 J. Fam. Practice 77, 79 (1983)*.

9.055   Disputes Between Medical Supervisors and Trainees

Clear policies for handling complaints from medical students, resident physicians, and other staff should be established. These policies should include adequate provisions for protecting the confidentiality of complainants whenever possible. Confidentiality of complainants should be protected when doing so does not hinder the subject's ability to respond to the complaint. Access to employment and evaluation files should be carefully monitored to remove the possibility of tampering. Resident physicians should be permitted access to their employment files and also the right to copy the contents thereof, within the provisions of applicable federal and state laws.

Medical students, resident physicians, and other staff should refuse to participate in patient care ordered by their supervisors in those rare cases in which they believe the orders reflect serious errors in clinical or ethical judgment, or physician impairment, that could result in a threat of imminent harm to the patient or to others. In these rare cases, the complainant may withdraw from the care ordered by the supervisor, provided withdrawal does not itself threaten the patient's immediate welfare. The complainant should communicate his or her concerns to the physician issuing the orders and, if necessary, to the appropriate persons for mediating such disputes. Mechanisms for resolving these disputes, which require immediate resolution, should be in place. Third-party mediators of such disputes may include the chief of staff or the involved service, the chief resident, a designated member of the institutional grievance committee, or, in large institutions, an institutional ombudsperson largely outside of the established hospital staff hierarchy.

Retaliatory or punitive actions against those who raise complaints are unethical and are a legitimate cause for filing a grievance with the appropriate institutional committee. (II, III, VII)

Issued June 1994 based on the report, "Disputes Between Medical Supervisors and Trainees," adopted December 1993 (JAMA. 1994; 272: 1861-1865).

Journal 1997 Discusses professionalism among attorneys. Emphasizes the need for individual accountability. Concludes that the rules of professional conduct should be modified to hold lawyers responsible for their actions. Quotes Opinion 9.055. Rice, *The Superior Orders Defense in Legal Ethics: Sending the Wrong Message to Young Lawyers*, 32 Wake Forest L. Rev. 887, 908-09 (1997).

Journal 1995 Examines the rights of health care professionals to refuse to participate in patient care on the basis of conscientious objection. Discusses rights and duties of health care facilities in this context. Suggests steps that facilities may take when dealing with health care professionals who object to participating in patient care. Quotes Principles I and VI and Opinions 1.02, 2.035, and 9.055. Dellinger & Vickery, *When Staff Object to Participating In Care*, 28 J. Health & Hospital Law 269, 272, 276 (1995).

9.06   Free Choice

Free choice of physicians is the right of every individual. One may select and change at will one's physicians, or one may choose a medical care plan such as that provided by a closed panel or group practice or health maintenance or service organization. The individual's freedom to select a preferred system of health care and free competition among physicians and alternative systems of care are prerequisites of ethical practice and optimal patient care.

In choosing to subscribe to a health maintenance or service organization or in choosing or accepting treatment in a particular hospital, the patient is thereby accepting limitations upon free choice of medical services.

The need of an individual for emergency treatment in cases of accident or sudden illness may, as a practical matter, preclude free choice of a physician, particularly where there is loss of consciousness.

Although the concept of free choice assures that an individual can generally choose a physician, likewise a physician may decline to accept that individual as a patient. In selecting the physician of choice, the patient may sometimes be obliged to pay for medical services which might otherwise be paid by a third party. (IV)

Issued prior to April 1977.

E.D. N.Y. 1975 Medical laboratories sought injunction against city's award of exclusive contracts for Medicaid services. The court granted a preliminary injunction and held that the laboratories had a substantial probability of success on the merits of the claim that Medicaid recipients would be deprived of statutory right of free choice of providers. In balancing the equities, the court also noted that the contracts would create an ethical dilemma for physicians who are required to provide patients with free choice of ancillary services under Opinions and Reports of the Judicial Council Sec. 1, Paras. 6 and 14 (1971) [now Opinions 8.03, 8.06, and 9.06]. Bay Ridge Diagnostic Laboratory, Inc. v. Dumpson, 400 F. Supp. 1104, 1109-10.

Ariz. 1965 Physician appealed denial of medical license which was based on alleged violations of local medical society rules and Principles 3, 5, and 10 (1957) [now Principles III, VII, and Opinions 3.01, 8.11, and 9.06]. Alleged violations included treating a patient without first obtaining a prior treating physician's permission, inadequate patient care, performing operations without hospital privileges, and signing the medical record of a deceased patient who had been treated by interns. The court held that the evidence failed to show any clear violation of the Principles and that a local medical society had no right to prescribe a code of ethics for state licensing purposes. *Arizona State Bd. of Medical Examiners v. Clark*, 97 Ariz. 205, 398 P.2d 908, 914-915, 915 n.3.

Cal. App. 1978 Surviving spouse sued physicians who were on emergency surgical call panel for malpractice where patient died during surgery. Although defendants claimed immunity under state Good Samaritan statute, the court held the statute inapplicable since the legislative purpose was to encourage physicians to render care on an irregular basis to unattended persons discovered by chance at the scene of an emergency. In so holding, the court noted that Principle 5 (1957) [now Principle VI and Opinions 8.11 and 9.06] imposed an ethical duty to render emergency medical care. *Colby v. Schwartz*, 78 Cal. App. 3d 885, 144 Cal. Rptr. 624, 627 n.2.

Ohio App. 1991 Medical corporation sought an injunction to enforce a covenant not to compete against defendant-physician. The lower court granted summary judgment based on a referee's report which concluded that, under Principle VI and Opinions 6.11, 9.02, and 9.06 (1989) restrictive covenants were *per se* unenforceable as a matter of public policy. While recognizing a strong public interest in allowing open access to health care, the appellate court in reversing held that Opinion 9.02, which applied specifically to restrictive covenants, only "discouraged" such covenants. *Ohio Urology, Inc. v. Poll*, 72 Ohio. App. 446, 450, 451, 594 N.E.2d 1027, 1030, 1031.

Wash. 1951 Plaintiff, a charitable, not for profit medical corporation, offered prepaid health care services to members and their families. Suit was filed against county medical society and others for damages and injunction for defendants' alleged efforts to monopolize prepaid medical care in area and unlawfully restrain competition by plaintiff and its physicians. Defendants alleged as affirmative defense that their efforts were designed to curb "unethical" prepaid contract practice by plaintiff. Court examined at length American Medical Association's position regarding "contract practice" including Principles Ch. III, Art. VI, Secs. 3 and 4 (1947) [now Principle VI and Opinions 8.05 and 9.06] concluding nothing in plaintiff's practice violated the Association's ethical guidelines. Further, quoting Principles Ch. III, Art. III, Sec.1 (1947) [now Opinion 8.04] dealing with consultations, court noted that defendants' efforts impeded plaintiff's physicians from obtaining consultations. Court concluded that defendants' actions constituted unlawful, monopolistic behavior and issued an injunction, although it declined to award damages. *Group Health Coop. v. King County Medical Soc'y*, 39 Wash. 2d 586, 237 P.2d 737, 744, 750-51, 759-60.

Journal 1997 Examines noncompetition clauses in the medical field. Reviews policy concerns and historical and common-law analyses of agreements not to compete. Posits that, the more commercialized the medical profession becomes, the more noncompetition clauses infringe upon the physician-patient relationship and patients' rights. Quotes Opinions 9.02 and 9.06. Cites Preamble and Opinion 6.11. Comment, *Noncompetition Clauses in Physician Employment Contracts in Oregon*, 76 Or. L. Rev. 195, 204-06 (1997).

Journal 1997 Examines the evolution of the Indiana health care system. Discusses developments in Indiana jurisprudence regarding the physician-patient relationship. Explores various challenges facing the relationship and recognizes the need for legal rules to help address these challenges. Quotes Opinion 8.08. Cites Opinions 2.20, 9.06, and 9.12. Kinney & Selby, *History and Jurisprudence of the Physician-Patient Relationship in Indiana*, 30 Ind. L. Rev. 263, 269, 272, 276 (1997).

Journal 1995 Analyzes South Carolina judicial treatment of covenants not to compete and liquidated damages provisions. Considers approaches in other jurisdictions and proposes guidelines for drafting contractual agreements. Quotes Opinion 9.06. Cites Opinion 9.01 (1982) [now Opinion 9.02]. Note, *Covenants Not to Compete and Liquidated Damages Clauses: Diagnosis and Treatment for Physicians*, 46 S.C. L. Rev. 505, 514 (1995).

Journal 1991 Considers the question of whether physicians should provide medical treatment to those who come to them for second opinions. Analyzes important ethical and legal guidelines. Concludes that each physician must individually decide whether to treat these patients. Quotes Opinions 6.11, 9.06, and 9.12. Cites Opinion 9.02. Ile, *Should Physicians Treat Patients Who Seek Second Opinions?*, 266 J.A.M.A. 273, 274 (1991).

Journal 1987 Considers arguments for and against active voluntary euthanasia, including arguments based on self-determination and various slippery-slope scenarios. Concludes that a policy or practice of active voluntary euthanasia is not desirable, linking a moral prohibition against active voluntary euthanasia to the moral prohibition against physicians actively participating in capital punishment. In place of any practice of active voluntary euthanasia, recommends increased use of hospices, greater emphasis on training physicians to care for the dying patient, and further research aimed at producing symptomatic relief in dying patients. Cites Opinions 2.06, 8.10 (1986) [now Opinion 8.11], and 9.06. Shewmon, *Active Voluntary Euthanasia: A Needless Pandora's Box*, 3 Issues in Law and Med. 219, 220, 222, 243 (1987).

9.065   Caring for the Poor

Each physician has an obligation to share in providing care to the indigent. The measure of what constitutes an appropriate contribution may vary with circumstances such as community characteristics, geographic location, the nature of the physician's practice and specialty, and other conditions. All physicians should work to ensure that the needs of the poor in their communities are met. Caring for the poor should be a regular part of the physician's practice schedule.

In the poorest communities, it may not be possible to meet the needs of the indigent for physicians' services by relying solely on local physicians. The local physicians should be able to turn for assistance to their colleagues in prosperous communities, particularly those in close proximity.

Physicians are meeting their obligation, and are encouraged to continue to do so, in a number of ways such as seeing indigent patients in their offices at no cost or at reduced cost, serving at freestanding or hospital clinics that treat the poor, and participating in government programs that provide health care to the poor. Physicians can also volunteer their services at weekend clinics for the poor and at shelters for battered women or the homeless.

In addition to meeting their obligation to care for the indigent, physicians can devote their energy, knowledge, and prestige to designing and lobbying at all levels for better programs to provide care for the poor. (I, VII)

Issued June 1994 based on the report, "Caring for the Poor," adopted December 1992 (JAMA. 1993; 269: 2533-2537).

Journal 1997 Considers the current approach to health care in the United States. Examines financing mechanisms, and suggests that reform could be effected through a decentralized, community-based approach. Proposes use of volunteer systems in which medical personnel would care for certain patients free of charge or at reduced rates. Quotes Fundamental Elements (6). References Opinion 9.065. Solomon & Asaro, *Community-Based Health Care: A Legal and Policy Analysis, 24 Fordham Urb. L. J. 235, 276-77 (1997).*

Journal 1996 Describes the problem of lack of access to medical care by the indigent. Recognizes the commitment of the medical profession to providing care for indigent patients. Observes that state initiatives that provide physicians tort immunity in exchange for volunteer service can improve access to care by the indigent. Quotes Fundamental Elements (6). References Opinion 9.065. Comment, *Statutory Immunity for Volunteer Physicians: A Vehicle for Reaffirmation of the Doctor's Beneficent Duties: Absent the Rights Talk, 1 Widener L. Symp. J. 425, 448, 449 (1996).*

9.07   Medical Testimony

As a citizen and as a professional with special training and experience, the physician has an ethical obligation to assist in the administration of justice. If a patient who has a legal claim requests a physician's assistance, the physician should furnish medical evidence, with the patient's consent, in order to secure the patient's legal rights.

Medical experts should have recent and substantive experience in the area in which they testify and should limit testimony to their sphere of medical expertise. Medical witnesses should be adequately prepared and should testify honestly and truthfully to the best of their medical knowledge.

The medical witness must not become an advocate or a partisan in the legal proceeding. The medical witness should be adequately prepared and should testify honestly and truthfully. The attorney for the party who calls the physician as a witness should be informed of all favorable and unfavorable information developed by the physician's evaluation of the case. It is unethical for a physician to accept compensation that is contingent upon the outcome of litigation. (II, IV, V, VII)

Issued June 1986.

Updated June 1996 based on the report, "Ethical Guidelines for Medical Experts," adopted December 1995.

M.D. Pa. 1947 Motion for new trial in malpractice action following verdict for defendant-physicians. Patient had been treated surgically for tube-ovarian abscess, had profuse post-operative bleeding, and died of infection secondary to ruptured ectopic pregnancy. Plaintiff moved for a new trial on grounds that an officer of a local medical society persuaded plaintiff's expert not to testify. Although it denied the motion on other grounds, the court criticized the officer's conduct, noting that it was contrary to Principles Ch. 1, Sec. 7 (1947) [now Opinion 9.07], but refused to impute the impropriety to the defendants. *McHugh v. Audet, 72 F. Supp. 394, 404.*

Cal. App. 1956 Physician-petitioner sought mandamus against local medical association whose bylaws provided for the expulsion of any member who violated the Principles. Petitioner had been expelled under the provision and the expulsion was affirmed by the American Medical Association's Judicial Council. The initial grounds for expulsion was alleged violation of Principles, Ch. III, Art. IV, Sec. 4 (1947) [now Opinions 9.04 and 9.07] for disparaging statements regarding another physician in a report used in judicial proceedings. In holding that application of the provision to petitioner was contrary to public policy, the court noted that the physician's statements had been made at the request of a civil litigant and enjoyed a statutory testimonial privilege. Further, the court found that the American Medical Association's right to formulate ethical principles did not extend to defining the duties of witnesses. Expulsion was also based on petitioner's critical comments about other physicians overheard by their patients in violation of Principles, Ch. III, Art. IV, Sec. 1 (1947) [now Principle II and Opinion 9.04]. The court found application of this Principle under the circumstances reasonable and not contrary to public policy. *Bernstein v. Alameda-Contra Costa Medical Ass'n, 139 Cal. App. 2d 241, 293 P.2d 862, 863, 863 nn.1, 2, 865 nn.4, 6, 866, 866 n.8, 867.*

N. J. 1995 Plaintiffs sued physician and manufacturer claiming that DPT shot administered to their daughter caused her to suffer seizures. Plaintiffs consulted pediatric neurologists, none of whom found a connection between the DPT vaccine and seizures. Court concluded that the videotaped depositions of two of the neurologists could be introduced by defendants because plaintiffs had waived all patient-physician privileges on this issue by bringing suit and because the neurologists did not examine the child in anticipation of litigation. The court cited Opinion 9.07 to support view that physicians have an obligation to assist in the administration of justice. *Stigliano v. Connaught Labs., Inc., 140 N.J. 305, 658 A.2d 715, 720-721.*

Wash. 1994 In a medical malpractice action against her former physician, plaintiff waived her physician-patient privilege with all physicians who had provided her care or treatment. In an ex parte interview, plaintiff's treating physician opined that defendant's conduct was not negligent. The defense listed the treating physician as an expert witness and plaintiff objected. The court concluded that waiver of the physician-patient privilege extends to all knowledge of the plaintiff's physicians. In holding that a patient cannot insist on physician confidentiality after bringing a civil proceeding, the court quoted Opinion 9.07. *Carson v. Fine, 123 Wash. 2d 206, 867 P.2d 610, 618.*

Journal 1997 Reports on a study of physician attitudes regarding expert witnesses. Notes that a majority of physicians believe that medical expert testimony should be subject to peer review and, when appropriate, medical licensing board discipline. Quotes Principles II and VI, and Opinion 9.07. Eitel, Hegeman, & Evans, *Medicine on Trial: Physicians' Attitudes about Expert Medical Witnesses, 18 J. Legal Med. 345, 355, 358 (1997).*

Journal 1994 Establishes guidelines for members of the American Academy of Pediatrics who are expert witnesses in medical liability cases. Emphasizes knowledge of the area of medicine involved, impartial testimony, evaluations based on generally accepted standards, and the duty to distinguish between malpractice and maloccurrence. Quotes Opinion 9.07. Cohn, Berger, Holzman, Lockhart, Reuben, Robertson, & Selbst, *Guidelines for Expert Witness Testimony in Medical Liability Cases*, 94 Pediatrics 755, 756 (1994).

Journal 1993 Discusses controversies surrounding how medical-legal consulting services and expert witnesses may be compensated. Examines relevant ethical guidelines in evaluating whether it is acceptable for a physician to be paid a flat fee for expert services rendered on behalf of a consulting business that receives a contingent fee. Quotes Opinion 9.07. Devlin, *Medical-Legal Consulting Services and Expert Witnesses: Payment Controversies*, 9 Medical Practice Management 141 (Nov./Dec. 1993).

Journal 1990 Considers the proper role of the expert witness in the realm of toxic tort litigation. Discusses problems with this type of testimony. Examines evidentiary rules regarding the admission of scientific evidence and considers various ways to solve testimonial problems. Concludes by discussing how the Supreme Court could respond to this issue. Quotes Opinion 9.07. Bernstein, *Out of the Frying Pan and Into the Fire: The Expert Witness Problem in Toxic Tort Litigation*, 10 Rev. Litigation 117, 143 (1990).

Journal 1990 Examines conflicting court decisions that have addressed the appropriateness of medical-legal consulting services and their use of contingent fee arrangements. Considers ethical opinions on this issue. Cautions against engaging the services of consulting groups charging contingent fees. Concludes by discussing the need for a less troublesome solution to the problems plaintiffs face in malpractice and personal injury cases. Quotes Opinion 6.01. Cites Opinions 6.12 (1989) [now Opinion 6.05] and 9.07. Dillon, *Contingent Fees and Medical-Legal Consulting Services: Economical or Unethical?*, 11 J. Legal Med. 93, 101, 111 (1990).

9.08 New Medical Procedures

In the ethical tradition expressed by Hippocrates and continuously affirmed thereafter, the role of the physician has been that of a healer who serves patients, a teacher who imparts knowledge of skills and techniques to colleagues, and a student who constantly seeks to keep abreast of new medical knowledge.

Physicians have an obligation to share their knowledge and skills and to report the results of clinical and laboratory research. Both positive and negative studies should be included even though they may not support the author's hypothesis. This tradition enhances patient care, leads to the early evaluation of new technologies, and permits the rapid dissemination of improved techniques.

The intentional withholding of new medical knowledge, skills, and techniques from colleagues for reasons of personal gain is detrimental to the medical profession and to society and is to be condemned.

Prompt presentation before scientific organizations and timely publication of clinical and laboratory research in scientific journals are essential elements in the foundation of good medical care. (I, II, V, VII)

Issued December 1984.

Updated June 1994.

Journal 1997 Explores the debate enveloping the patenting of medical procedures. Examines the beneficial and detrimental aspects of a ban on medical patents and pertinent ethical and economical factors. Suggests that allowing patents exacts too great a toll on society and science. Quotes Opinion 9.08. References Opinion 9.095. Judge, *Issues Surrounding the Patenting of Medical Procedures*, 13 Santa Clara Computer & High Tech. L. J. 181, 202-03 (1997).

Journal 1997 Examines the controversy surrounding the patenting of medical procedures. Concludes that patenting medical procedures has a negative effect on the physician-patient relationship and the medical profession. Quotes Opinion 9.095. References Opinions 9.08 and 9.09. Note, *Patenting Medical Procedures: A Search for a Compromise Between Ethics and Economics*, 18 *Cardozo L. Rev.* 1527, 1544, 1547, 1554 (1997).

Journal 1996 Examines the current status of medical procedure patents and discusses the statutory and case law requirements for obtaining a patent. Considers the ethical implications of patenting medical procedures. Argues against a legislative ban on such patents. Quotes Opinions 9.08, 9.09, and 9.095. Garris, *The Case for Patenting Medical Procedures*, XXII *Am. J. Law & Med.* 85, 93, 94-95 (1996).

Journal 1996 Explores the current rules for patenting medical procedures. Discusses the AMA's position that medical procedure patents are unethical. Concludes that a failure to grant patents will deter the development of new medical procedures. Quotes Opinion 9.08 (see also Opinion 9.095). Lafferty, *Statutory and Ethical Barriers in the Patenting of Medical and Surgical Procedures*, 29 *J. Marshall L. Rev.* 891, 912 (1996).

Journal 1995 Examines the conflict between medical ethics and patent laws. Explores the debates and commentaries regarding patenting medical instruments and processes. Concludes that current patent law fails to address the ethical concerns of physicians and their patients. Quotes Principles of Medical Ethics § 10 (1971) [now Principle VII] and Principle § 2 (1971) [now Opinion 9.095] and Opinions 9.08 and 9.09. Reisman, *Physicians and Surgeons as Inventors: Reconciling Medical Process Patents and Medical Ethics*, 10 *High Tech. L. J.* 355, 356, 368-70, 385 (1995).

9.09   Patent for Surgical or Diagnostic Instrument

A physician may patent a surgical or diagnostic instrument he or she has discovered or developed. The laws governing patents are based on the sound doctrine that one is entitled to protect one's discovery. (V, VII)

Issued prior to April 1977.

Journal 1997 Examines the controversy surrounding the patenting of medical procedures. Concludes that patenting medical procedures has a negative effect on the physician-patient relationship and the medical profession. Quotes Opinion 9.095. References Opinions 9.08 and 9.09. Note, *Patenting Medical Procedures: A Search for a Compromise Between Ethics and Economics*, 18 *Cardozo L. Rev.* 1527, 1544, 1547, 1554 (1997).

Journal 1996 Examines the current status of medical procedure patents and discusses the statutory and case law requirements for obtaining a patent. Considers the ethical implications of patenting medical procedures. Argues against a legislative ban on such patents. Quotes Opinions 9.08, 9.09, and 9.095. Garris, *The Case for Patenting Medical Procedures*, XXII *Am. J. Law & Med.* 85, 93, 94-95 (1996).

Journal 1995 Examines the conflict between medical ethics and patent laws. Explores the debates and commentaries regarding patenting medical instruments and processes. Concludes that current patent law fails to address the ethical concerns of physicians and their patients. Quotes Principles of Medical Ethics § 10 (1971) [now Principle VII] and Principle § 2 (1971) [now Opinion 9.095] and Opinions 9.08 and 9.09. Reisman, *Physicians and Surgeons as Inventors: Reconciling Medical Process Patents and Medical Ethics*, 10 *High Tech. L. J.* 355, 356, 368-70, 385 (1995).

Journal 1990 Discusses the relationship between patent law and medicine. Explains how medical patents have developed into widely accepted legal instruments that receive broad respect from the courts. Questions the lack of Congressional expansion of patent protection in the field of biotechnology and suggests that Congress should begin expanding protection in this area. References Opinion 9.09. Noonan, *Patenting Medical Technology*, 11 *J. Legal Med.* 263, 268 (1990).

9.095 Patenting of Medical Procedures

A physician has the ethical responsibility not only to learn from but also to contribute to the total store of scientific knowledge when possible. Physicians should strive to advance medical science and make their advances known to patients, colleagues and the public. This obligation provides not merely incentive but imperative to innovate and share the ensuing advances. The patenting of medical procedures poses substantial risks to the effective practice of medicine by limiting the availability of new procedures to patients and should be condemned on this basis. Accordingly, it is unethical for physicians to seek, secure or enforce patents on medical procedures.

Issued June 1996 based on the report, "Ethical Issues in the Patenting of Medical Procedures," adopted June 1995.

Journal 1997 Explores the debate enveloping the patenting of medical procedures. Examines the beneficial and detrimental aspects of a ban on medical patents and pertinent ethical and economical factors. Suggests that allowing patents exacts too great a toll on society and science. Quotes Opinion 9.08. References Opinion 9.095. Judge, *Issues Surrounding the Patenting of Medical Procedures, 13 Santa Clara Computer & High Tech. L. J. 181, 202-03 (1997).*

Journal 1997 Considers the issues surrounding medical procedure patents. Reviews the adoption of federal legislation granting patent infringement immunity to physicians while performing medical or surgical procedures. Discusses the medical community's position favoring immunity. Concludes that such a law sets a dangerous precedent. References Opinion 9.095. Lee, *35 U.S.C. § 287(C)—The Physician Immunity Statute, 79 J. Pat. & Trademark Off. Soc'y 701, 702-04 (1997).*

Journal 1997 Examines the controversy surrounding the patenting of medical procedures. Concludes that patenting medical procedures has a negative effect on the physician-patient relationship and the medical profession. Quotes Opinion 9.095. References Opinions 9.08 and 9.09. Note, *Patenting Medical Procedures: A Search for a Compromise Between Ethics and Economics, 18 Cardozo L. Rev. 1527, 1544, 1547, 1554 (1997).*

Journal 1997 Discusses federal patent legislation that protects physicians from liability for patent infringements. Describes legal and medical opinions on the matter. Notes that the legislation was passed in response to concerns regarding health care costs and patients' interests. Proposes that Congress reconsider the legislation. References Opinion 9.095. Note, *The New Patent Infringement Liability Exception for Medical Procedures, 23 J. Legis. 265, 268 (1997).*

Journal 1996 Examines the current status of medical procedure patents and discusses the statutory and case law requirements for obtaining a patent. Considers the ethical implications of patenting medical procedures. Argues against a legislative ban on such patents. Quotes Opinions 9.08, 9.09, and 9.095. Garris, *The Case for Patenting Medical Procedures, XXII Am. J. Law & Med. 85, 93, 94-95 (1996).*

Journal 1996 Discusses possible effects of a 1996 legislative enactment that was designed to limit the remedies for infringements on patented medical activities. Describes the legislative history of this enactment and notes the AMA's position against patenting of medical and surgical procedures. References Opinion 9.095. Mossinghoff, *Remedies Under Patents on Medical and Surgical Procedures, 78 J. Pat. & Trademark Off. Soc'y 789, 790 (1996).*

Journal 1995 Examines the conflict between medical ethics and patent laws. Explores the debates and commentaries regarding patenting medical instruments and processes. Concludes that current patent law fails to address the ethical concerns of physicians and their patients. Quotes Principles of Medical Ethics § 10 (1971) [now Principle VII] and Principle § 2 (1971) [now Opinion 9.095] and Opinions 9.08 and 9.09. Reisman, *Physicians and Surgeons as Inventors: Reconciling Medical Process Patents and Medical Ethics, 10 High Tech. L. J. 355, 356, 368-70, 385 (1995).*

Peer Review

Medical society ethics committees, hospital credentials and utilization committees, and other forms of peer review have been long established by organized medicine to scrutinize physicians' professional conduct. At least to some extent, each of these types of peer review can be said to impinge upon the absolute professional freedom of physicians. They are, nonetheless, recognized and accepted. They are necessary and committees performing such work act ethically as long as principles of due process (Opinion 9.05) are observed. They balance the physician's right to exercise medical judgment freely with the obligation to do so wisely and temperately. (II, III, VII)

Issued prior to April 1977.

Updated June 1994.

9.11 **Ethics Committees in Health Care Institutions**

The following guidelines have been developed to aid in the establishment and functioning of ethics committees in hospitals and other health care institutions that may choose to form such committees.

(1) Ethics committees in health care institutions should be educational and advisory in purpose. Generally, the function of the ethics committee should be to consider and assist in resolving unusual, complicated ethical problems involving issues that affect the care and treatment of patients within the health care institution. Recommendations of the ethics committee should impose no obligation for acceptance on the part of the institution, its governing board, medical staff, attending physician, or other persons. However, it should be expected that the recommendations of a dedicated ethics committee will receive serious consideration by decision makers.

(2) The size of the committee should be consistent with the needs of the institution but not so large as to be unwieldy. Committee members should be selected on the basis of their concern for the welfare of the sick and infirm, their interest in ethical matters, and their reputation in the community and among their peers for integrity and mature judgment. Experience as a member of hospital or medical society committees concerned with ethical conduct or quality assurance should be considered in selecting ethics committee members. Committee members should not have other responsibilities that are likely to prove incompatible with their duties as members of the ethics committee. Preferably, a majority of the committee should consist of physicians, nurses, and other health care providers. In hospitals, medical staff bylaws should delineate the functions of the committee, general qualifications for membership, and manner of selection of members, in accordance with these guidelines.

(3) The functions of the ethics committee should be confined exclusively to ethical matters. The Code of Medical Ethics of the American Medical Association is recommended for the guidance of ethics committees in making their own recommendations. The matters to be considered by the

committee should consist of ethical subjects that a majority of its members may choose to discuss on its own initiative, matters referred to it by the executive commitee of the organized medical staff or by the governing board of the institution, or appropriate requests from patients, families, or health care providers.

(4) In denominational health care institutions or those operated by religious orders, the recommendations of the ethics committee may be anticipated to be consistent with published religious tenets and principles. Where particular religious beliefs are to be taken into consideration in the committee's recommendations, this fact should be publicized to physicians, patients, and others concerned with the committee's recommendations.

(5) In its deliberations and communication of recommendations, the procedures followed by the ethics committee should comply with institutional and ethical policies for preserving the confidentiality of information regarding patients.

(6) Committee members should be prepared to meet on short notice and to render their recommendations in a timely and prompt fashion in accordance with the demands of the situation and the issues involved. (II, IV, VII)

Issued June 1994 based on the report, "Guidelines for Ethics Committees in Health Care Institutions," adopted December 1984 (JAMA. 1985; 253: 2698-2699).

9.11   **Opinion 9.11, Physician Impairment,** issued December 1986, was deleted in June 1994.

9.12   Patient-Physician Relationship: Respect for Law and Human Rights

The creation of the physician-patient relationship is contractual in nature. Generally, both the physician and the patient are free to enter into or decline the relationship. A physician may decline to undertake the care of a patient whose medical condition is not within the physician's current competence. However, physicians who offer their services to the public may not decline to accept patients because of race, color, religion, national origin, sexual orientation, or any other basis that would constitute invidious discrimination. Furthermore, physicians who are obligated under preexisting contractual arrangements may not decline to accept patients as provided by those arrangements. (I, III, V, VI)

Issued July 1986.

Updated June 1994 and June 1998.

N.Y. Sup. 1993 Plaintiff brought malpractice action against attending physician, resident, and hospital alleging that they caused premature birth and cerebral palsy of twin daughters. Plaintiff, pregnant and complaining of abdominal pains, was admitted to hospital by attending physician. She was also examined by resident. Despite indication of polyhydramnios, an increase of amniotic fluid creating a risk of premature delivery, attending physician released plaintiff from hospital. Resident and hospital moved for summary judgment on grounds that neither had provided independent treatment for plaintiff. They also relied on the principle that if a hospital properly follows attending physician's orders, it cannot be held responsible for the physician's actions in caring for patients. The court affirmed denial of motion for summary judgment stating that a question of fact existed as to whether plaintiff's release from hospital was so contrary to normal practice that resident physician should have inquired into situation. Quoting Opinion 9.12, the dissent argued that the motion for summary judgment should be granted because the attending physician makes medical decisions regarding the patient and neither hospital nor its residents should interfere. *Somoza v. St. Vincent's Hosp. & Med. Ctr. of New York*, 192 A.D.2d 429, 596 N.Y.S.2d 789, 793.

Journal 1997 Compares past ethical opinions to current opinions and notes the differences. Comments on the forces that have changed medical ethics through the years. Notes differing theories on the future course of medical ethics. Quotes Fundamental Elements (Preamble) and Opinions 5.05, 5.057, 7.01, 8.12, 9.12, and 9.131. Cites Fundamental Elements (5) and Opinions 8.115 and 8.13. Buchanan, *Medical Ethics at the Millennium: A Brief Retrospective*, 26 Colo. Law. 141, 142, 143, 144, 145 (1997).

Journal 1997 Examines the evolution of the Indiana health care system. Discusses developments in Indiana jurisprudence regarding the physician-patient relationship. Explores various challenges facing the relationship and recognizes the need for legal rules to help address these challenges. Quotes Opinion 8.08. Cites Opinions 2.20, 9.06, and 9.12. Kinney & Selby, *History and Jurisprudence of the Physician-Patient Relationship in Indiana*, 30 Ind. L. Rev. 263, 269, 272, 276 (1997).

Journal 1995 Provides legal and medical definitions of physician-assisted suicide and euthanasia. Offers relevant historical perspectives and provides comprehensive ethical and legal discussion of these compelling social issues. Highlights important legislative developments, including the Oregon Death with Dignity Act, and analyzes significant judicial opinions. Advocates legal tolerance of physician-assisted suicide and euthanasia. Quotes Principles III, IV, and VI and Opinions 2.21 and 9.12. Cites Opinions 2.20 and 8.11. Stone & Winslade, *Physician-Assisted Suicide and Euthanasia in the United States: Legal and Ethical Observations*, 16 J. Legal Med. 481, 483, 490, 497, 498, 499 (1995).

Journal 1994 Explores how the Americans with Disabilities Act has created, through federal civil rights mechanisms, a legal duty to treat HIV-infected patients. Discusses previous attempts to create a professional obligation to treat patients with AIDS. Quotes Principle VI and Opinion 9.131. Cites Opinion 9.12. Halevy & Brody, *Acquired Immunodeficiency Syndrome and the Americans with Disabilities Act: A Legal Duty to Treat*, 96 Am. J. Med. 282, 283, 284 (1994).

Journal 1993 Examines challenges in New York to a lawyer's right to discriminate in the context of selecting clients. Explores the traditional view that lawyers have unfettered discretion to select clients and New York's anti-discrimination disciplinary rule, statutes, and case law. Concludes that the legal profession should prohibit invidious or improper discrimination. Quotes Principle VI and Opinions 9.12 and 9.131. Begg, *Revoking the Lawyers' License to Discriminate in New York: The Demise of a Traditional Professional Prerogative*, 7 Geo. J. Legal Ethics 275, 298, 299 (1993).

Journal 1991 Considers the question of whether physicians should provide medical treatment to those who come to them for second opinions. Analyzes important ethical and legal guidelines. Concludes that each physician must individually decide whether to treat these patients. Quotes Opinions 6.11, 9.06, and 9.12. Cites Opinion 9.02. Ile, *Should Physicians Treat Patients Who Seek Second Opinions?*, 266 J.A.M.A. 273, 274 (1991).

Journal 1991 Discusses the problem of noncompliant patients and whether a physician may deny treatment to these individuals. Notes relevant legal and ethical considerations. Concludes that physicians are not relieved of their duty to treat noncompliant patients, especially because these patients may not be able to adequately control their behavior. Cites Principle VI and Opinion 9.12. Orentlicher, *Denying Treatment to the Noncompliant Patient*, 265 J.A.M.A. 1579, 1581 (1991).

Journal 1988 Observes that the view of medicine as a profession committed to the sick conflicts with the apparent position of the AMA, that a physician is free to choose his or her patients. (See Principle VI). The notion of the medical profession's commitment to the sick gives rise to two interpretations. The weak interpretation is that the profession as a whole has such a commitment, but not each physician. The stronger interpretation is that each physician must have such a commitment. This position is embodied in the 1987 Report of the Council on Ethical and Judicial Affairs, which addresses ethical issues involved in the AIDS crisis. Concludes that physicians have a duty to treat AIDS patients and must be ready to assume certain levels of risk in fulfilling the duty. References Opinion 9.12. Emanuel, *Do Physicians Have an Obligation to Treat Patients With AIDS?*, 318 New Eng. J. Med. 1686, 1687 (1988).

Journal 1988 Discusses the question of whether health professionals are obligated to subject themselves to the risks that attend treating patients with communicable diseases, particularly AIDS. Examines the ethical pronouncements and codes of the nursing and medical professions in this respect, noting that the most recent statements of professional values imply the existence of an obligation to treat HIV-infectious patients. Offers a discussion of the evolution of this viewpoint. Quotes Opinion 8.10 (1986) [now Opinion 8.11] and Principle VI. Cites Opinion 9.11 (1986) [now Opinion 9.12]. Freedman, *Health Professions, Codes, and the Right to Refuse to Treat HIV-Infectious Patients,* 18 Hastings Center Rep. 20 (Supp.), 23, 24 (April/May 1988).

9.121 Racial Disparities in Health Care

Disparities in medical care based on immutable characteristics such as race must be avoided. Whether such disparities in health care are caused by treatment decisions, differences in income and education, social and cultural factors, or failures by the medical profession, they are unjustifiable and must be eliminated. Physicians should examine their own practices to ensure that racial prejudice does not affect clinical judgment in medical care. (I, IV)

Issued March 1992 based on the report, "Black-White Disparities in Health Care," adopted December 1989 (JAMA. 1990; 263: 2344-2346).

Updated June 1994.

Journal 1997 Considers the use of race and gender to assess health care status and medical needs. Discusses the lack of consideration that Asian American women receive in the health care agenda. Proposes an examination of factors such as race, gender, and class status to provide a better understanding of the health needs of this group. References Opinions 9.121 and 9.122. Ikemoto, *The Fuzzy Logic of Race and Gender in the Mismeasure of Asian American Women's Health Needs,* 65 U. Cin. L. Rev. 799, 800, 804, 810 (1997).

Journal 1994 Observes that health care reform proposals present significant challenges to the role and ethics of attending physicians. Emphasizes that reform proposals must set forth the role envisioned for physicians and must articulate an acceptable ethical framework within which physicians may fulfill that role. Quotes Opinions 4.04, 9.121, and 9.122. Cites Opinions 2.03, 2.09, 5.01, and 8.03. Wolf, *Health Care Reform and the Future of Physician Ethics,* 24 Hastings Center Rep. 28, 32, 40 (March/April 1994).

Journal 1993 Presents findings by the Council on Graduate Medical Education regarding access to health care. Recommends that more emphasis be placed on primary care, the physician workforce be redistributed to increase the number of physicians in rural and inner city areas, and that there be more racial and ethnic diversity in the medical profession. Concludes that a national plan should be developed to respond to these needs. References Opinion 9.121. Rivo & Satcher, *Improving Access to Health Care Through Physician Workforce Reform,* 270 J.A.M.A. 1074, 1075 (1993).

Journal 1992 Discusses the impact of physicians' values on end-of-life decision making for patients. Examines how and why physician values may become dominant. Concludes that more research should be done regarding this important question. References Opinions 2.22 and 9.121. Orentlicher, *The Illusion of Patient Choice in End-Of-Life Decisions,* 267 J.A.M.A. 2101, 2102 (1992).

Journal 1991 Describes the attributes of women who self-report pelvic inflammatory disease (PID). Presents the results of a study that examined these attributes, noting that risk factors were consistent with prior studies. Concludes that PID is still widely prevalent in this country. References Opinion 9.121. Aral, Mosher, & Cates, *Self-Reported Pelvic Inflammatory Disease in the United States, 1988,* 266 J.A.M.A. 2570, 2573 (1991).

Journal 1991 Compares the health conditions of blacks in South Africa with those in the United States. Finds that American blacks suffer from increased risk of illness and lack of access to health care. Concludes that policy changes to address the health problems of South African blacks are also needed in this country. Proposes a community-oriented primary care system in both countries. References Opinion 9.121. Brooks, Smith, & Anderson, *Medical Apartheid: An American Perspective*, 266 J.A.M.A. 2746, 2748 (1991).

Journal 1991 Discusses the lack of health care among the poor and uninsured. Notes the traditional role of physician as advocate for the poor and prescribes a method by which physicians may act as spokespersons for underserved populations. References Opinion 9.121. Kleinman, *Health Care in Crisis: A Proposed Role for the Individual Physician as Advocate*, 265 J.A.M.A. 1991 (1991).

9.122 Gender Disparities in Health Care

A patient's gender plays an appropriate role in medical decision making when biological differences between the sexes are considered. However, some data suggest that gender bias may be playing a role in medical decision making. Social attitudes, including stereotypes, prejudices and other evaluations based on gender role expectations may play themselves out in a variety of subtle ways. Physicians must ensure that gender is not used inappropriately as a consideration in clinical decision making. Physicians should examine their practices and attitudes for influence of social or cultural biases which could be inadvertently affecting the delivery of medical care.

Research on health problems that affect both genders should include male and female subjects, and results of medical research done solely on males should not be generalized to females without evidence that results apply to both sexes. Medicine and society in general should ensure that resources for medical research should be distributed in a manner which promotes the health of both sexes to the greatest extent possible. (I, IV)

Issued March 1992 based on the report, "Gender Disparities in Clinical Decision Making," adopted December 1990 (JAMA. 1991; 266: 559-562).

Updated June 1994.

Journal 1997 Considers the use of race and gender to assess health care status and medical needs. Discusses the lack of consideration that Asian American women receive in the health care agenda. Proposes an examination of factors such as race, gender, and class status to provide a better understanding of the health needs of this group. References Opinions 9.121 and 9.122. Ikemoto, *The Fuzzy Logic of Race and Gender in the Mismeasure of Asian American Women's Health Needs*, 65 U. Cin. L. Rev. 799, 800, 804, 810 (1997).

Journal 1996 Considers the impact the doctrine of informed consent may have on the rate at which hysterectomy operations are performed. Discusses how stereotypes affect the quality of medical treatment women receive. Focuses on how informed consent may benefit the health and autonomy of women. References Opinion 9.122. Napoli, *The Doctrine of Informed Consent and Women: The Achievement of Equal Value and Equal Exercise of Autonomy*, 4 J. Gender & L. 335, 336 (1996).

Journal 1994 Observes that health care reform proposals present significant challenges to the role and ethics of attending physicians. Emphasizes that reform proposals must set forth the role envisioned for physicians and must articulate an acceptable ethical framework within which physicians may fulfill that role. Quotes Opinions 4.04, 9.121, and 9.122. Cites Opinions 2.03, 2.09, 5.01, and 8.03. Wolf, *Health Care Reform and the Future of Physician Ethics*, 24 Hastings Center Rep. 28, 32, 40 (March/April 1994).

Journal 1993 Discusses the underrepresentation of women in clinical trials and its medical relevance. Examines the extent to which women are underrepresented. Considers barriers to their participation and proposes ways to include women in clinical investigations. References Opinion 9.122. Bennett, *Inclusion of Women in Clinical Trials—Policies for Population Subgroups*, 329 New Eng. J. Med. 288, 289 (1993).

Journal 1993 Discusses the role of women in clinical trials. Explains how their role has evolved historically. Examines specific current concerns related to women's involvement in clinical studies and how these concerns might be resolved. References Opinion 9.122. Merkatz, *Women in Clinical Trials: An Introduction, 48 Food & Drug L. J. 161, 163 (1993).*

Journal 1992 Investigates the exclusion of women and minorities from medical research study groups. Considers justifications offered by the scientific community. Presents the argument against exclusion, as well as the dangers of possible remedies. Concludes that this problem illustrates the extent to which bias is still present in contemporary medicine and science. References Opinion 9.122. Dresser, *Wanted: Single, White Male for Medical Research, 22 Hastings Center Rep. 24, 28 (Jan./Feb. 1992).*

Journal 1992 Investigates gender disparities in the quality of medical care for the elderly. Presents the results of a study analyzing the differences in quality of care for patients hospitalized with one of four diseases. Finds very little evidence of gender bias in the hospital setting. Concludes that these results are positive, but notes that concerns regarding gender discrimination are not entirely eliminated. References Opinion 9.122. Pearson, Kahn, Harrison, Rubenstein, Rogers, Brook, & Keeler, *Differences in Quality of Care for Hospitalized Elderly Men and Women, 268 J.A.M.A. 1883 (1992).*

Journal 1992 Analyzes the impact of gender and age on hospital admissions for acute asthma attacks. Presents results of a study that looked at age and gender as factors affecting admissions and length of hospital stay. Concludes that biological distinctions between the sexes may play a role in the disease. References Opinion 9.122. Skobeloff, Spivey, St. Clair, & Schoffstall, *The Influence of Age and Sex on Asthma Admissions, 268 J.A.M.A. 3437, 3439, 3440 (1992).*

9.13   Physicians and Infectious Diseases

A physician who knows that he or she has an infectious disease, which if contracted by the patient would pose a significant risk to the patient, should not engage in any activity that creates an identified risk of transmission of that disease to the patient. The precautions taken to prevent the transmission of a contagious disease to a patient should be appropriate to the seriousness of the disease and must be particularly stringent in the case of a disease that is potentially fatal. (I, IV)

Issued August 1989.

Updated June 1996.

Md. 1993 Patients sued hospital and physician alleging that an operating surgeon has a duty to disclose his or her HIV-infected status. Quoting Opinions 9.13 and 9.131 (1992) for the proposition that a seropositive physician should not engage in activity that would create a risk of transmission of the disease to his or her patients, the court held that it could not say as a matter of law that an HIV-infected physician did not have a duty to warn patients of his condition or refrain from operating on them. *Faya v. Almaraz, 329 Md. 435, 449, 450, 620 A.2d 327, 334.*

Minn. App. 1993 Patients sued HIV-positive physician alleging negligent infliction of emotional distress. Trial court granted summary judgment holding that plaintiffs had failed to produce evidence sufficient to show "actual exposure" to the AIDS virus. The appellate court, in an unpublished opinion, held that the plaintiffs need only show that they were in the "zone of danger" of contracting HIV. The court referred to Faya v. Almaraz, 329 Md. 435, 449, 620 A.2d 327, 334 (1993) which had quoted Opinions 9.13 and 9.131 for the proposition that a physician who has an infectious disease should not engage in any activity that creates a risk of transmission of that disease to the patient. *K.A.C. v. Benson, 1993 Minn. App. LEXIS 1201.*

N.J. Super. 1991 Physician's estate sued hospital alleging that it violated state law against discrimination by restricting the physician's surgery privileges and requiring him to inform patients of his HIV-infected status before performing invasive procedures. The defendant hospital was also alleged to have breached its duty to maintain confidentiality of his seropositive diagnosis. The court held that the hospital had not discriminated against the physician since the hospital had relied on ethical and professional standards, including a report of the Council on Ethical and Judicial Affairs of the AMA dealing with the issue of AIDS [now Opinions 9.13 and 9.131]. However, the hospital was held to have breached its fiduciary duty to maintain the confidentiality of the physician's medical records. Referring to McIntosh v. Milano, 168 N.J. Super. 466, 403 A.2d 500 (1979) which had quoted AMA Principles of Medical Ethics sec. 9 (1957) [now Principle IV and Opinion 5.05] in applying the "duty to warn" exception, the court noted that the disclosure in this case went far beyond the medical personnel directly involved in the treatment of the physician and those patients entitled to informed consent. *Estate of Behringer v. Medical Ctr.*, 249 N.J. Super. 597, 614, 633, 592 A.2d 1251, 1259, 1268.

Journal 1997 Opines that physicians infected with HIV have an ethical and legal duty to disclose their status to patients before beginning invasive procedures. Suggests that the doctrine of informed consent and medical ethics guidelines require disclosure. Disagrees with public policy arguments favoring nondisclosure. References Opinions 9.13 and 9.131. Iheukwumere, *HIV-Positive Medical Practitioners: Legal and Ethical Obligations to Disclose*, 71 St. John's L. Rev. 715, 732-34 (1997).

Journal 1996 Discusses the doctrine of informed consent and its purpose. Posits that, due to patients' rights of self-determination, and the deadly nature of AIDS, physicians are morally and legally obligated to disclose their HIV status to patients where risk of transmission exists. Quotes Opinion 9.13. Note, *Torts: Defining the Duty Imposed on Physicians by the Doctrine of Informed Consent*, 22 Wm. Mitchell L. Rev. 149, 160 (1996).

Journal 1994 Examines the scope of a physician's duty to reveal HIV status to a patient before performing invasive procedures. Discusses applicable case law and advocates use of comprehensive and objective scientific data in evaluating potential liability in cases where physicians fail to disclose HIV status to patients. Quotes Opinions 9.13 and 9.131. Beane, *AIDS Crisis and the Health Care Community: Public Concerns Triggering Questionable Private Rights of Action for Emotional Harms and Legislative Response*, 45 Mercer L. Rev. 633, 669 (1994).

Journal 1994 Discusses the issue of whom physicians must serve first: themselves, their patients, insurers, or society. Explores attempts by the legal system to resolve this issue within the framework of risks that may arise in the physician-patient relationship. Focuses on risks arising out of provider economic arrangements and risks arising out of other individual physician characteristics. Quotes Opinions 8.03 and 9.13. Cites Opinion 8.15. Bobinski, *Autonomy and Privacy: Protecting Patients from Their Physicians*, 55 U. Pitt. L. Rev. 291, 302, 313 (1994).

Journal 1994 Discusses emotional distress claims based on the fear of contracting AIDS. Analyzes problems in proving these claims, such as proof of exposure and injury, reasonableness of fear, and proof of negligence. Proposes that courts follow evidentiary and public policy standards developed in other phobia cases. Quotes Opinions 9.13 and 9.131. Comment, *AIDS Phobia: Forcing Courts to Face New Areas of Compensation for Fear of a Deadly Disease*, 39 Vill. L. Rev. 241, 277 (1994).

Journal 1994 Examines the responsibilities of real estate brokers to disclose a seller's AIDS status in light of a potential buyer's right to know all material facts affecting property value. Discusses disclosure of AIDS status in other contexts, including the health care field. Concludes that a seller's AIDS status is a material fact that a real estate broker must disclose. Quotes Opinions 9.13 and 9.131. Hartog, *The Psychological Impact of AIDS on Real Property and a Real Estate Broker's Duty to Disclose*, 36 Ariz. L. Rev. 757, 772 (1994).

Journal 1993 Provides an overview of the doctrine of informed consent and evaluates the disclosure obligations of HIV-positive health care professionals. Concludes that in developing coherent guidelines for informed consent in this context, the best approach is to have a public determination of what level of risk is tolerable. Cites Opinion 9.13. Nodzenski, *HIV-Infected Health Care Professionals and Informed Consent*, 2 S. Cal. Interdisciplinary L. J. 299, 327 (1993).

9.131 HIV-Infected Patients and Physicians

A physician may not ethically refuse to treat a patient whose condition is within the physician's current realm of competence solely because the patient is seropositive for HIV. Persons who are seropositive should not be subjected to discrimination based on fear or prejudice.

When physicians are unable to provide the services required by an HIV-infected patient, they should make appropriate referrals to those physicians or facilities equipped to provide such services.

A physician who knows that he or she is seropositive should not engage in any activity that creates an identified risk of transmission of the disease to others. A physician who is seropositive should consult colleagues as to which activities the physician can pursue without creating a risk to patients. (I, II, IV)

Issued March 1992 based on the report, "Ethical Issues in the Growing AIDS Crisis," adopted December 1987 (*JAMA*. 1988; 259: 1360-1361).

Updated June 1996.

Md. 1993 Patients sued hospital and physician alleging that an operating surgeon has a duty to disclose his or her HIV-infected status. Quoting Opinions 9.13 and 9.131 (1992) for the proposition that a seropositive physician should not engage in activity that would create a risk of transmission of the disease to his or her patients, the court held that it could not say as a matter of law that an HIV-infected physician did not have a duty to warn patients of his condition or refrain from operating on them. *Faya v. Almaraz, 329 Md. 435, 449, 450, 620 A.2d 327, 334.*

Md. App. 1996 Members of patient's family sued physician, hospital, and laboratory for negligence in failing to inform the patient and his family of patient's human immunodeficiency virus (HIV) positive status. The patient was discharged from the hospital prior to receipt of test results. The patient's family provided home health care, and in so, doing came into contact with the patient's bodily secretions. The family all tested negative for HIV. The court noted that the common law duty of care owed by a health care provider to diagnose, evaluate, and treat a patient ordinarily flows only to the patient, not to third parties. However, courts have recognized a duty to third parties in limited circumstances, "mostly involving situations in which the patient has, or is thought to have, a communicable disease or otherwise presents a clear danger to a specific person." The court noted, with apparent reference to Opinion 9.131, that the AMA has urged that infected physicians should not engage in activity that creates a risk of transmission and therefore physicians have a duty to disclose their HIV positive status prior to invasive surgery. However, in the instant case, the court held that no duty to inform third parties of a patient's HIV status could exist because such a duty would constitute a wholly unwarranted invasion of the patient's privacy. *Lemon v. Stewart, 111 Md. App. 511, 523, 682 A.2d 1177, 1182.*

Minn. App. 1993 Patients sued HIV-positive physician alleging negligent infliction of emotional distress. Trial court granted summary judgment holding that plaintiffs had failed to produce evidence sufficient to show "actual exposure" to the AIDS virus. The appellate court, in an unpublished opinion, held that the plaintiffs need only show that they were in the "zone of danger" of contracting HIV. The court referred to Faya v. Almaraz, 329 Md. 435, 449, 620 A.2d 327, 334 (1993) which had quoted Opinions 9.13 and 9.131 for the proposition that a physician who has an infectious disease should not engage in any activity that creates a risk of transmission of that disease to the patient. *K.A.C. v. Benson, 1993 Minn. App. LEXIS 1201.*

N.J. Super. 1991 Physician's estate sued hospital alleging that it violated state law against discrimination by restricting the physician's surgery privileges and requiring him to inform patients of his HIV-infected status before performing invasive procedures. The defendant hospital was also alleged to have breached its duty to maintain confidentiality of his seropositive diagnosis. The court held that the hospital had not discriminated against the physician since the hospital had relied on ethical and professional standards, including a report of the Council on Ethical and Judicial Affairs of the AMA dealing with the issue of AIDS [now Opinions 9.13 and 9.131]. However, the hospital was held to have breached its fiduciary duty to maintain the confidentiality of the physician's medical records. Referring to McIntosh v. Milano, 168 N.J. Super. 466, 403 A.2d 500 (1979) which had quoted AMA Principles of Medical Ethics sec. 9 (1957) [now Principle IV and Opinion 5.05] in applying the "duty to warn" exception, the court noted that the disclosure in this case went far beyond the medical personnel directly involved in the treatment of the physician and those patients entitled to informed consent. *Estate of Behringer v. Medical Ctr., 249 N.J. Super. 597, 614, 633, 592 A.2d 1251, 1259, 1268.*

N.Y. 1996 Two dentists were found guilty of unlawful discriminatory practice, in violation of the state Human Rights Law, for refusing to treat patients who were known or suspected of having human immunodeficiency virus (HIV). On appeal the court affirmed the verdict and noted that both the American Dental Association and the American Medical Association, in Opinion 9.131, have adopted the position that it is unethical to refuse to treat an HIV positive patient solely because of that diagnosis. In clarifying its holding, the court noted that the decision does not interfere with the provider's ability to prescribe treatment or refer patients elsewhere, provided it is done for a legitimate nondiscriminatory reason. *Cahill v. Rosa, 89 N.Y.2d 14, 24, 674 N.E.2d 274, 278, 651 N.Y.S.2d 344, 348.*

Pa. Super. 1991 HIV-infected physician appealed order of lower court authorizing hospitals to disclose the physician's identity to the limited class of those patients whose contact with the physician involved intrusive procedures. Appellate court held that the hospitals met their burden of proving a compelling need under the state's confidentiality act. The court cited to AMA Council on Ethical and Judicial Affairs, Ethical Issues Involved in the Growing AIDS Crisis, 259 JAMA 1360, 1361 (March 4, 1988) [now Opinion 9.131] stating that medical professionals have an obligation to their patients to provide safe and adequate health care. *In re Milton S. Hershey Medical Ctr., 407 Pa. Super. 565, 575, 582 n.18, 595 A.2d 1290, 1295, 1300 n.18.*

Journal 1997 Compares past ethical opinions to current opinions and notes the differences. Comments on the forces that have changed medical ethics through the years. Notes differing theories on the future course of medical ethics. Quotes Fundamental Elements (Preamble) and Opinions 5.05, 5.057, 7.01, 8.12, 9.12, and 9.131. Cites Fundamental Elements (5) and Opinions 8.115 and 8.13. Buchanan, *Medical Ethics at the Millennium: A Brief Retrospective*, 26 Colo. Law. 141, 142, 143, 144, 145 (1997).

Journal 1997 Opines that physicians infected with HIV have an ethical and legal duty to disclose their status to patients before beginning invasive procedures. Suggests that the doctrine of informed consent and medical ethics guidelines require disclosure. Disagrees with public policy arguments favoring nondisclosure. References Opinions 9.13 and 9.131. Iheukwumere, *HIV-Positive Medical Practitioners: Legal and Ethical Obligations to Disclose*, 71 St. John's L. Rev. 715, 732-34 (1997).

Journal 1996 Considers the extent of discrimination against HIV-infected patients in the dental setting. Reviews approaches to solving the problem of discrimination in this context. Concludes that legal intervention may aid in ending non-treatment based on discrimination. Quotes Opinion 9.131. Burris, *Dental Discrimination Against the HIV-Infected: Empirical Data, Law and Public Policy*, 13 Yale J. On Reg. 1, 41 (1996).

Journal 1996 Considers the extreme risk to patients where physicians and surgeons infected with HIV perform invasive medical procedures. Advocates civil litigation and liability in situations where HIV-infected physicians refuse testing but perform invasive procedures on patients who are uninformed. References Opinion 9.131. Closen, *HIV-AIDS, Infected Surgeons and Dentists, and the Medical Profession's Betrayal of Its Responsibility to Patients*, 41 N.Y.L. Sch. L. Rev. 57, 65, 71-72, 129 (1996).

Journal 1996 Explores whether patients have a duty to disclose their HIV status to treating physicians. Suggests that recognizing such a duty may subject patients to a lower standard of care and provide a disincentive to be tested. Concludes that courts should not impose a duty to disclose on patients. Quotes Principle 9 (1957) [now Principle IV] and Opinion 9.131. DeNatale & Parrish, *Health Care Workers' Ability to Recover in Tort for Transmission or Fear of Transmission of HIV from a Patient*, 36 Santa Clara L. Rev. 751, 782-83, 787 (1996).

Journal 1995 Analyzes the secular approach to the duty to treat HIV-infected individuals and the duty to warn those who are sexual partners of, or who share needles with, people infected with HIV. Observes that the secular approach leaves these issues unresolved; but indicates that Jewish law compels physicians both to treat and to warn. Quotes Opinions 5.05 and 9.131. Shorr, *AIDS, Judaism, and the Limits of the Secular Society*, 20 Second Opinion 23, 24, 27 (1995).

Journal 1994 Examines the scope of a physician's duty to reveal HIV status to a patient before performing invasive procedures. Discusses applicable case law and advocates use of comprehensive and objective scientific data in evaluating potential liability in cases where physicians fail to disclose HIV status to patients. Quotes Opinions 9.13 and 9.131. Beane, *AIDS Crisis and the Health Care Community: Public Concerns Triggering Questionable Private Rights of Action for Emotional Harms and Legislative Response*, 45 Mercer L. Rev. 633, 669 (1994).

Journal 1994 Considers how the Americans with Disabilities Act (ADA) has affected health care providers. Illustrates various legal issues arising under the ADA by analyzing cases involving patients and health care providers with AIDS. Quotes Opinion 9.131. Benesch, *Disability Discrimination in the Health Care Workplace*, 9 Trends in Health Care, Law & Ethics 45, 46 (Summer 1994).

Journal 1994 Discusses emotional distress claims based on the fear of contracting AIDS. Analyzes problems in proving these claims, such as proof of exposure and injury, reasonableness of fear, and proof of negligence. Proposes that courts follow evidentiary and public policy standards developed in other phobia cases. Quotes Opinions 9.13 and 9.131. Comment, *AIDSphobia: Forcing Courts to Face New Areas of Compensation for Fear of a Deadly Disease*, 39 Vill. L. Rev. 241, 277 (1994).

Journal 1994 Explores how the Americans with Disabilities Act has created, through federal civil rights mechanisms, a legal duty to treat HIV-infected patients. Discusses previous attempts to create a professional obligation to treat patients with AIDS. Quotes Principle VI and Opinion 9.131. Cites Opinion 9.12. Halevy & Brody, *Acquired Immunodeficiency Syndrome and the Americans with Disabilities Act: A Legal Duty to Treat*, 96 Am. J. Med. 282, 283, 284 (1994).

Journal 1994 Examines the responsibilities of real estate brokers to disclose a seller's AIDS status in light of a potential buyer's right to know all material facts affecting property value. Discusses disclosure of AIDS status in other contexts, including the health care field. Concludes that a seller's AIDS status is a material fact that a real estate broker must disclose. Quotes Opinions 9.13 and 9.131. Hartog, *The Psychological Impact of AIDS on Real Property and a Real Estate Broker's Duty to Disclose*, 36 Ariz. L. Rev. 757, 772 (1994).

Journal 1994 Discusses obligation of HIV-infected health professionals to inform patients of their serological status. Discusses common law and regulatory developments that appear to favor patients' rights to know their health professional's serological status before consenting to treatment. Quotes Opinion 9.131. LeBlang, *Obligations of HIV-Infected Health Professionals to Inform Patients of Their Serological Status: Evolving Theories of Liability*, 27 J. Marshall L. Rev. 317, 318 (1994).

Journal 1994 Analyzes competing privacy and public health interests as they relate to HIV transmission in the dentist-patient relationship. Examines pertinent laws and dental association policies regarding HIV. Proposes a statute and possible dental association policies to minimize the risk of HIV transmission. Quotes Opinion 9.131. Note, *HIV and Dentistry*, 29 Val. U.L. Rev. 297, 317 (1994).

Journal 1994 Discusses the role of professional societies in establishing ethical guidelines for physicians in the context of using medical innovations and new technologies. Observes that these standards must be supplemented by additional external measures or incentives in order to be most effective. Concludes that professional societies are more successful at setting standards than ensuring acceptance and implementation of those standards by member professionals. Cites Opinions 1.01, 1.02, 8.061, 9.04, and 9.131. Orentlicher, *The Influence of a Professional Organization on Physician Behavior*, 57 Alb. L. Rev. 583, 592, 593, 594, 595, 596 (1994).

Journal 1993 Examines challenges in New York to a lawyer's right to discriminate in the context of selecting clients. Explores the traditional view that lawyers have unfettered discretion to select clients and New York's antidiscrimination disciplinary rule, statutes, and case law. Concludes that the legal profession should prohibit invidious or improper discrimination. Quotes Principle VI and Opinions 9.12 and 9.131. Begg, *Revoking the Lawyers' License to Discriminate in New York: The Demise of a Traditional Professional Prerogative*, 7 Geo. J. Legal Ethics 275, 298, 299 (1993).

Journal 1993 Addresses both patient rights under California consent and confidentiality laws relating to AIDS and prohibitions on unreasonable searches and seizures under the United States Constitution. Concludes that any health care worker who can document an exposure to blood or body fluids should have the option of compelling a nonconsenting patient to be tested for HIV. Quotes Principle VI and Opinion 9.131. Comment, *Nonconsensual HIV Testing in the Health Care Setting: The Case for Extending the Occupational Protections of California Proposition 96 to Health Care Workers*, 26 Loy. L.A. L. Rev. 1251, 1269 (1993).

Journal 1993 Discusses family privacy rights and a physician's ethical responsibility to report violence. Considers the meaning of justice, self respect, and the fundamental principles of physician ethics. Concludes that physicians have an ethical duty to intervene in domestic violence so long as such intervention does not breach confidentiality or violate patient autonomy. Quotes Principle IV and Opinion 5.05. References Opinions 8.14 and 9.131. Jecker, *Privacy Beliefs and the Violent Family: Extending the Ethical Argument for Physician Intervention*, 269 J.A.M.A. 776, 778, 779 (1993).

Journal 1993 Discusses Centers for Disease Control (CDC) guidelines governing HIV testing for health care workers. Examines the law in this area with particular emphasis on risk determination, mandatory testing, and duty to warn patients. Observes that common law and CDC guidelines are not synchronous. Proposes that CDC guidelines be reformed to more closely match evolving common law. References Opinion 9.131. Johnson, *HIV Testing of Health Care Workers: Conflict Between the Common Law and the Centers for Disease Control*, 42 Am. Univ. L. Rev. 479, 518 (1993).

Journal 1993 Explores the idea of reverse informed consent, which would impose a duty on patients to inform health care professionals of their infectious status. Concludes that such a duty is justified. Quotes Principles IV and VI and Opinions 8.11 and 9.131. Oddi, *Reverse Informed Consent: The Unreasonably Dangerous Patient*, 46 Vand. L. Rev. 1417, 1449, 1463, 1465, 1479 (1993).

Journal 1992 Discusses the problem of discrimination based on HIV status, particularly among women and children. Examines medical and public health issues involving HIV. Looks at types of HIV discrimination, the degree of prevalence, and causes. Focuses on federal, state, and local laws. Cites Principle VII. References Opinion 9.131. Gittler & Rennart, *HIV Infection Among Women and Children and Antidiscrimination Laws: An Overview*, 77 Iowa L. Rev. 1313, 1363 (1992).

Journal 1992 Considers the responsibility of HIV-infected health care workers to protect patients from infection. Examines several issues related to this subject including mandatory testing, disclosure to co-workers and supervisors, and the degree to which the practice of an HIV-infected health care worker should be modified. Focuses on whether there is a duty to disclose HIV-positive status to patients. Concludes that courts likely will impose such a requirement when there is a substantial risk of HIV transmission. Quotes Opinions 8.03 (1989) [now Opinion 8.032], and 8.07 (1989) [now Opinion 8.03]. References Opinion 9.131. Lieberman & Derse, *HIV-Positive Health Care Workers and the Obligation to Disclose: Do Patients Have a Right to Know?*, 13 J. Legal Med. 333, 353, 354 (1992).

Journal 1992 Discusses the lack of access to emergency medical care that many indigent patients face. Claims that a number of teaching hospitals deny emergency care to the impoverished. Argues that this sets a poor example for medical students and residents. Concludes that medical educators must instill more altruistic values in their students. References Opinion 9.131. Miles, *What Are We Teaching About Indigent Patients?*, 268 J.A.M.A. 2561, 2562 (1992).

Journal 1992 Discusses discrimination against HIV-infected patients and the resulting lack of access to health care. Argues that the ADA and other laws prohibiting discrimination will not alone solve this problem. Proposes additional steps to augment anti-discrimination laws including implementing protections for health care workers against accidental transmission and adequately funding health care needs of AIDS patients. References Opinion 9.131. Note, *The Americans With Disabilities Act: Magic Bullet or Band-Aid for Patients and Health Care Workers Infected With the Human Immunodeficiency Virus?*, 57 Brooklyn L. Rev. 1277, 1279, 1305 (1992).

Journal 1991 Discusses the risk of HIV transmission in the health care setting. Considers important issues in this context, including testing of patients and health care workers, prevention of HIV transmission, and costs that attend accidental transmission. Proposes that hospitals develop comprehensive policies to address these issues. Quotes Opinion 9.131. Brennan, *Transmission of the Human Immunodeficiency Virus in the Health Care Setting—Time for Action*, 324 New Eng. J. Med. 1504, 1505, 1506 (1991).

Journal 1991 Considers whether physicians have an obligation to provide medical care to HIV-infected patients. Examines various sources for such a duty, including a moral obligation not to discriminate and a social responsibility to provide access to health care. Concludes that physicians have a duty to treat. Quotes Opinion 9.131. Cites Principle VI. Daniels, *Duty to Treat or Right to Refuse?*, 21 Hastings Center Rep. 36, 37, 42 (March/April 1991).

Journal 1991 Considers the issue of mandatory AIDS testing. Examines several state statutes, both enacted and proposed, requiring HIV screening. Looks at two testing schemes and whether these schemes actually serve the public interest. Concludes that mandatory HIV testing does not further legitimate public health concerns, except in the area of sexual assault. Quotes Opinion 9.131. Eisenstat, *An Analysis of the Rationality of Mandatory Testing for the HIV Antibody: Balancing the Governmental Public Health Interests With the Individual's Privacy Interest*, 52 Univ. Pittsburgh L. Rev. 327, 347 (1991).

Journal 1991 Discusses CDC report indicating the possibility of dentist-to-patient HIV transmission. Finds that a majority of dentists do not believe the report and feel that transmission is unlikely. Also finds, however, that most dentists believe HIV-infected practitioners should modify their practice and that patients should be informed if their dentist is HIV-positive. References Opinion 9.131. Gerbert, Bleecker, Miyasaki, & Maguire, *Possible Health Care Professional-to-Patient HIV Transmission: Dentists' Reactions to a Centers for Disease Control Report*, 265 J.A.M.A. 1845, 1846, 1847 (1991).

Journal 1991 Examines the extent to which physicians provide primary care to AIDS patients and various barriers that stand in the way. Presents the results of a survey indicating that many physicians are responding professionally to the AIDS crisis but that attitudinal barriers block some physicians from providing care. References Opinion 9.131. Gerbert, Maguire, Bleecker, Coates, & McPhee, *Primary Care Physicians and AIDS: Attitudinal and Structural Barriers to Care*, 266 J.A.M.A. 2837, 2838 (1991).

Journal 1991 Examines why HIV-infected individuals have difficulty receiving medical care from private physicians. Presents a Virginia community's response to this problem, which is based on a voluntary rotating referral system using a pool of primary care physicians. References Opinion 9.131. Green, Haggerty, & Hale, *Community-Based Plan for Treating Human Immunodeficiency Virus-Infected Individuals Sponsored by Local Medical Societies and an Acquired Immunodeficiency Syndrome Service Organization*, 151 Arch. Intern. Med. 2061, 2064 (1991).

Journal 1991 Discusses the issue of HIV-infected surgeons in light of the New Jersey case decision in *Behringer v. Medical Center*. Summarizes the case and presents its implications. Considers future developments. References Opinions 8.032 and 9.131. Orentlicher, *HIV-Infected Surgeons: Behringer v. Medical Center*, 266 J.A.M.A. 1134, 1136 (1991).

Journal 1990 Examines concerns regarding the risk of HIV transmission by infected health care workers. Explains that the risk of transmission is highly remote. Suggests that hospitals should focus on infection control in general, rather than HIV transmission in particular. Concludes that HIV-infected health care workers should be allowed to continue working as long as they take prudent measures to avoid the risk of transmission. References Opinion 9.131. Barnes, Rango, Burke, & Chiarello, *The HIV-Infected Health Care Professional: Employment Policies and Public Health*, 18 Law, Med. & Health Care 311, 314, 315 (1990).

Journal 1990 Discusses ways in which physicians attempt to avoid malpractice liability, including use of written contracts and refusal to see certain types of patients. Examines the impact of these actions on patient rights, treatment, and the physician-patient relationship. Concludes that this behavior is undesirable and that more positive steps can be taken to eliminate much of the tension between physicians, patients, and lawyers. Quotes Opinion 9.131. Comment, *Physician Retaliation: Can the Physician-Patient Relationship Be Protected?*, 94 Dickinson L. Rev. 965, 986 (1990).

Journal 1990 Analyzes the major issues involved in mandatory AIDS testing. Considers whether forced testing should ever be required and, if so, who should be tested. Concludes that forced testing is inappropriate and that resources could be used better in other ways. References Opinion 9.131. Field, *Testing for AIDS: Uses and Abuses*, XVI Am. J. Law & Med. 34, 50 (1990).

Journal 1990 Examines patients' fears about AIDS, their knowledge about transmission of the disease, and their perceived risk of HIV transmission by health care workers. Finds that fear of AIDS is inversely proportional to knowledge. Recommends that physicians actively work to educate the public. References Opinion 9.131. Marshall, O'Keefe, Fisher, Caruso, & Surdukowski, *Patients' Fear of Contracting the Acquired Immune Deficiency Syndrome From Physicians*, 150 Arch. Intern. Med. 1501, 1505 (1990).

Journal 1990 Examines the risk of HIV transmission from surgeon to patient. Presents the results of a study which analyzed over 2000 patients of an HIV-positive surgeon and found that no patient became infected. Concludes that the risk of HIV transmission is extremely low. References Opinion 9.131. Mishu, Schaffner, Horan, Wood, Hutcheson, & McNabb, *A Surgeon With AIDS: Lack of Evidence of Transmission to Patients*, 264 J.A.M.A. 467 (1990).

Journal 1990 Considers the propriety of HIV testing for hospital patients prior to non-emergency surgery. Discusses the medical aspects of AIDS and the risk of HIV transmission. Looks at available HIV tests, including reliability and cost. Concludes that testing of patients should be permitted so long as it is not done with the intent, nor the effect, of discriminating against individual patients. Quotes Principle VI and Opinion 9.131. Naccasha, *The Permissibility of Routine AIDS Testing in the Health Care Context*, 5 Notre Dame J.L. Ethics & Pub. Pol'y, 223, 241 (1990).

Journal 1989 Explores factors contributing to the stigmatization of HIV-infected individuals. Discusses the legal and ethical challenges that AIDS poses for health care providers. Proposes that health care providers actively participate in preventing HIV infection, providing care for HIV-infected individuals, and fighting AIDS and its associated stigma. Quotes Principle VI and Opinion 9.131. Forrester, *AIDS: The Responsibility to Care*, 34 Vill. L. Rev. 799, 811 (1989).

American Medical Association
Constitution and Bylaws
Council on Ethical and Judicial Affairs

Authority

The Council on Ethical and Judicial Affairs is the judicial authority of the American Medical Association and its decision shall be final.

Functions

The functions of the Council on Ethical and Judicial Affairs are:
- To interpret the Principles of Medical Ethics of the American Medical Association.
- To interpret the Constitution, Bylaws and rules of the Association.
- To investigate general ethical conditions and all matters pertaining to the relations of physicians to one another or to the public, and make recommendations to the House of Delegates or the constituent associations.
- To receive appeals filed by applicants who allege that they, because of color, creed, race, religion, ethnic origin, national origin, or sex, have been unfairly denied membership in a component and/or constituent association, to determine the facts in the case, and to report the findings to the House of Delegates. If the Council determines that the allegations are indeed true, it shall admonish, censure, or in the event of repeated violations, recommend to the House of Delegates that the constituent association involved be declared to be no longer a constituent member of the American Medical Association.
- To request the President to appoint investigating juries to which it may refer complaints or evidences of unethical conduct which in its judgment are of greater than local concern. Such investigative juries, if probable cause for action be shown, shall submit formal charges to the President, who shall appoint a prosecutor to prosecute such charges against the accused before the Council on Ethical and Judicial Affairs in the name and on behalf of the American Medical Association. The Council may acquit, admonish, suspend or expel the accused.
- To approve applications and nominate candidates for affiliate membership as otherwise provided for in 1.141 of these Bylaws.

Original Jurisdiction

The Council on Ethical and Judicial Affairs shall have original jurisdiction in:
- All questions involving membership.

- All controversies arising under this Constitution and Bylaws and under the Principles of Medical Ethics to which the American Medical Association is a party.
- Controversies between two or more state associations or their members and between a constituent association and a component society or societies of another state association or associations or their members.

Appellate Jurisdiction

The Council on Ethical and Judicial Affairs shall have appellate jurisdiction in questions of law and procedure but not of fact in all cases which arise:

A. Between a constituent association and one or more of its component societies.
B. Between component societies of the same constituent association.
C. Between a member or members and the component society to which said member or members belong following an appeal to the member's constituent association.
D. Between members of different component societies of the same constituent association following a decision by the constituent association.

Appeal Mechanisms

Notice of appeal shall be filed with the Council on Ethical and Judicial Affairs within thirty (30) days of the date of the decision by the state association and the appeal shall be perfected within sixty (60) days thereof; provided, however, that the Council on Ethical and Judicial Affairs, for what it considers good and sufficient cause, may grant an additional thirty (30) days for perfecting the appeal.

Membership

The Council on Ethical and Judicial Affairs shall consist of nine Active members of the American Medical Association, including one Resident Physician member and one Medical Student member. Members elected to the Council on Ethical and Judicial Affairs shall resign all other positions held by them in the Association upon their election to the Council. No member, while serving on the Council on Ethical and Judicial Affairs, shall be a delegate or an alternate delegate to the House of Delegates, or a General Officer of the Association, or serve on any other council, committee or as Representative to or Governing Council Member of a Special Section of the American Medical Association.

Limit on Medical Student Participation

The Medical Student member of the Council shall have the right to participate fully in the work of the Council, except that in disciplinary matters and in matters relating to membership the Medical Student member shall participate only if a medical student is the subject of the disciplinary matter or is the applicant for membership.

Nomination and Election

The members of the Council shall be elected by the House of Delegates on nomination by the President. State Medical Associations, National Medical Specialty Societies, Special Sections of the AMA, and other organizations represented in the AMA House of Delegates, and members of the Board of Trustees may submit the names and qualifications of candidates for consideration by the President.

Term of Service

Members of the Council on Ethical and Judicial Affairs shall be elected by the House of Delegates for the following terms of office:

- The Medical Student member of the Council shall be elected for a term of two years, provided that if the Medical Student member ceases to be enrolled in an approved medical school or in an osteopathic medical school approved by an appropriate accrediting agency at any time prior to the expiration of the term for which the Medical Student member was elected, the service of such Medical Student member on the Council shall thereupon terminate, and the position shall be declared vacant. The Council shall determine the voting privileges of the Medical Student member for each term of service.

- The Resident Physician Member of the Council shall be elected for a term of three years provided that if the Resident member ceases to be in an approved training program at any time prior to the expiration of the term for which the Resident Physician member was elected, the service of such Resident member on the Council shall thereupon terminate, and the position shall be declared vacant. The Resident Physician member shall have the right to vote in all matters in which said member participates under the rules of the Council.

- All other members of the Council shall be elected by the House of Delegates for a term of seven years, so arranged that at each Annual Convention the term of one member shall expire.

Tenure

Members of the Council on Ethical and Judicial Affairs shall serve only one term, except that the Resident Physician member and the Medical Student member shall be eligible to serve for two terms. A member elected to serve an unexpired term shall not be regarded as having served a term unless such member has served at least half of said term.

Vacancies

Members Other Than the Resident Member. Any vacancy among the members of the Council on Ethical and Judicial Affairs other than the Resident member shall be filled at the next meeting of the House of Delegates. The new member shall be elected by the House of Delegates, on nomination by the President, for the remainder of the unexpired term.

Resident Member. If the Resident Physician member of the Council is unable, for any reason, to complete the term for which he or she was elected, the remainder of the term shall be deemed to have expired. The successor shall be elected by the House of Delegates at its next meeting, on nomination by the President, for a term to expire at the conclusion of the third Annual Meeting of the House of Delegates following the meeting at which said Resident was elected.

Rules of the Council on Ethical and Judicial Affairs

American Medical Association

Rule I. Administration

A. **Meetings.** The Council on Ethical and Judicial Affairs will meet during the Annual and Interim Meetings of the American Medical Association. Other meetings of the Council may be called, on reasonable notice, by the Chair of the Council; or they shall be called, on reasonable notice, by the Executive Vice President of the American Medical Association on the written request of at least five members of the Council.

B. **Chair and Vice-Chair.** At the reorganization meeting of the Council which shall be held during each Annual Meeting of the AMA after election of members to the Council, the Council on Ethical and Judicial Affairs shall elect a chair and a vice-chair from among its members except that the resident physician and medical student members of the Council shall not be eligible to serve as chair or vice-chair. The chair and the vice-chair shall retain the right to vote on all matters. No member of the Council shall serve more than two consecutive years as chair or two consecutive years as vice-chair.

The chair and vice-chair to be so elected shall be elected on separate, secret ballots. The balloting and voting for chair shall be completed and a chair elected before the balloting and voting for the vice-chair begins. A majority vote of the entire Council shall be required to so elect either a chair or a vice-chair, with balloting and voting to be repeated, if necessary, until a member is elected to each position.

In the event that the position of chair becomes permanently vacant for any reason during the term of the then currently serving chair, the then currently serving vice-chair shall immediately assume the position of chair for the remainder of the term. A new vice-chair shall then be elected by secret ballot at the ensuing meeting of the Council to serve the remainder of the immediately preceding vice-chair's term. A majority vote of the entire Council, as then constituted, shall be required to so elect a vice-chair, with balloting and voting to be repeated, if necessary, until a member is elected vice-chair. The serving of the balance of a term as chair or vice-chair due to such a vacancy shall not be counted in determining whether a member of the Council has served more than two consecutive years as chair or two consecutive years as vice-chair.

In the event that the position of vice-chair becomes permanently vacant for any reason during the term of the then currently serving vice-chair, a new vice-chair shall be elected by secret ballot at the ensuing meeting of the Council to serve the remainder of the immediately preceding vice-chair's term. A majority vote of the entire Council, as then constituted, shall be required to so elect a vice-chair, with balloting and voting to be repeated, if necessary, until a member is elected vice-chair. The serving of the balance of a term as vice-chair due to such a vacancy shall not be counted in determining whether a member of the Council has served more than two consecutive years as vice-chair.

C. **Student Members.** The medical student member of the Council shall participate as a regular member in the interpretation of the Principles of Medical Ethics of the American Medical Association, the interpretation of the Constitution, Bylaws and rules of the Association, and the investigation of general ethical conditions and all matters pertaining to the relations of physicians to one another or to the public. The medical student member of the Council shall have the right to participate in disciplinary matters and in matters relating to membership only if a medical student is the subject of the disciplinary matter or is the applicant for membership.

D. **Quorum.** A majority of the members of the Council on Ethical and Judicial Affairs eligible to vote on a matter shall constitute a quorum and shall be required to adopt any action.

E. **Confidentiality.** All matters under consideration for adoption by the Council shall be treated as confidential until adopted by the Council.

Rule II. Applications for Membership

A. **Active Membership.** Applications for membership in the American Medical Association will be considered by the Council on Ethical and Judicial Affairs at any meeting upon presentation of the applications by the Executive Vice President of the Association.

B. **Affiliate Membership.** Applications for affiliate membership submitted by (1) physicians in foreign countries who have attained distinction in medicine and who are members of the national medical society or such other organization as will verify their professional credentials, (2) American physicians located in foreign countries or possessions of the United States and engaged in medical missionary, educational or philanthropic endeavors, (3) dentists who hold the degree of D.D.S. or D.M.D., who are members of the American Dental Association and their state and local dental societies, (4) pharmacists who are active members of the American Pharmaceutical Association, (5) teachers of medicine or of the sciences allied to medicine who are citizens of the United States and are ineligible for active or associate membership, or (6) individuals engaged in scientific endeavors allied to medicine and others who have attained distinction in their fields of endeavor who are not otherwise eligible for membership, may be considered at any meeting of the Council on presentation of the applications by the Executive Vice President of the Association. The Council will consider and approve only those applications which are accompanied by a statement of a responsible and qualified individual attesting to the requirements set forth above. (Employees of the AMA or any AMA affiliate or subsidiary may be eligible affiliate members under subsection (6). They must have five yeares of employment at the AMA, affiliate, or subsidiary and their distinction in their field of endeavor must be certified by an AMA Senior Vice President or if the employee is a Senior Vice President, the Executive Vice President.)

C. **Refusal of Approval.** An applicant for membership in the American Medical Association whose application has not been approved by the Council on Ethical and Judicial Affairs will be promptly notified of such fact.

Rule III. Physicians Denied Membership in Component or Constituent Associations

Pursuant to 6.4024 of the Bylaws, any physician whose application for membership in a component and/or constituent association has allegedly been denied unfairly because of color, creed, race, religion, ethnic origin, national origin, or sex may appeal to the Council on Ethical and Judicial Affairs. The Council shall determine the facts in the case and report the findings to the House of Delegates. If the Council determines that the allegations are indeed true, it shall admonish, censure or, in the event of repeated violations, recommend to the House of Delegates that the state association involved be declared to be no longer a constituent member of the American Medical Association.

Proceedings for such determination shall be initiated by a written statement. Such statement shall: (1) identify the parties to the case, (2) show that the appellant has exhausted remedies made available by the constitution and bylaws of the component society and the state association, and (3) include a concise factual resume of the case in sufficient detail to enable the Council to ascertain the facts. The appellant should also furnish such other information as may be requested by or helpful to the Council in determining the facts.

Rule IV. Original Controversies

Original proceedings before the Council on Ethical and Judicial Affairs shall be initiated by a written statement. Such statement shall include information (1) identifying the parties to the controversy, including membership affiliations, if applicable, and (2) explaining the nature of the controversy, setting forth the provisions of the Constitution, Bylaws, Rules, or Principles of Medical Ethics concerned.

Rule V. Appeals

Appellate proceedings before the Council on Ethical and Judicial Affairs shall be perfected by a written statement of appeal. Such statement shall include information (1) identifying the parties to the case and indicating membership affiliations when appropriate, (2) showing that the appellant has exhausted remedies made available by the constitution and bylaws of the component society and the state association, and (3) describing the error of law or proce-dure which is believed to have occurred during the proceedings. The statement shall also include a concise, factual resume of the case. Appellant shall submit with the statement the charges, complaints, findings, opinions, and decisions previously entered in the case.

Rule VI. Interpretation of the Constitution, Bylaws, Rules, and Principles of Medical Ethics of the American Medical Association

A. **Requests for Interpretation.** Requests for interpretation of the Constitution, Bylaws, Rules, or Principles of Medical Ethics of the Association shall be in writing and shall describe the matter to be inter-preted in sufficient detail to enable the members of the Council on Ethical and Judicial Affairs to evaluate the request in all its aspects.

B. **Interpretations Initiated by the Council.** The Council on Ethical and Judicial Affairs on its own motion, may render an opinion concerning the interpretation or application of the Constitution, Bylaws, Rules, or Principles of Medical Ethics of the Association and may, on its own motion, consider and decide the constitutionality and validity of all rules and regulations adopted by Councils and Committees of the Association pursuant to the Bylaws of the Association.

C. **Discretionary Power.** The Council on Ethical and Judicial Affairs may, in its own discretion, refuse to consider requests for interpretation of the Principles of Medical Ethics which in the opinion of the Council should be resolved by a component society or a state association. Requests for interpretation of the Principles of Medical Ethics which are not of national interest and relate to the observance of local customs and ideals may be readdressed to the component society or constituent association primarily responsible for knowledge of the requirements of such local cus-toms and recognized ideals.

Rule VII. Jurisdiction

The Council on Ethical and Judicial Affairs may, on its own motion or on the motion of any party, determine the question of jurisdiction at any stage of the proceedings.

Rule VIII. Additional Statements and Record

After a statement has been submitted to the Council on Ethical and Judicial Affairs with the intention of initiating an action, all other parties in interest shall have the right to submit a statement on their behalf. Such statement shall be filed within thirty days after the filing of the initiating statement unless additional time is granted by the Council.

The Council on Ethical and Judicial Affairs may thereafter require the par-ties to submit such transcripts of testimony, records, written statements support-ing their contentions, or other material as the Council may deem necessary.

Rule IX. Hearings

A. **Notice of Hearings.** The Council may in its discretion determine whether a hearing is necessary or advisable. The Council will designate the time and place for all hearings, giving reasonable notice thereof to all parties.

B. **Attendance.** Attendance at hearings may be limited to the members of the Council on Ethical and Judicial Affairs, the staff, witnesses, if any, the parties, and counsel, who may speak in their behalf. Should any party to the controversy fail to appear, the Council may in its discretion continue, dismiss, or decide the matter.

C. **Evidence and Argument.** The Council on Ethical and Judicial Affairs will not be bound by technical rules of evidence usually employed in legal proceedings but may accept any evidence it deems appropriate and pertinent.

In any appeal case the review, if any, of the evidence will be limited to the evidence presented in the proceedings before the component society and constituent association or appropriate committee, board, or group thereof; provided, however, that in the event the Council is of the opinion such evidence is inadequate to determine the question of law or procedure presented, the Council, on its own motion or on the suggestion of any party, may require the production of additional evidence before the Council or refer the matter to the appropriate body for additional evidence.

In matters other than appeal cases, the Council will grant the parties the right to present evidence to the extent the Council believes appropriate to the particular matter in controversy.

In all hearings, the Council, within reasonable limitations, will allow oral argument.

D. **Record.** In hearings of original controversies, appeals, and in other proceedings, a transcript may be made at the discretion of the Council.

Rule X. Opinions

All opinions or decisions of the Council on Ethical and Judicial Affairs shall be in writing. Copies of the opinion or decision and the dissent, if any, will be filed as a part of the record and furnished to all the parties involved.

Rule XI. Filing and Copies

Ten (10) copies of all documents shall be submitted to the Secretary of the Council on Ethical and Judicial Affairs. One copy of each document shall be submitted at the same time to each of the other parties to the controversy.

Rule XII. AMA Membership Applications

A. Section 1.121 of the AMA Bylaws provides that Active Direct members shall be admitted to membership upon application to the Executive Vice President of the AMA, provided that there is no disapproval by the AMA Council on Ethical and Judicial Affairs. Section 1.1212 of the AMA

Bylaws provides that objections to applicants for Active Direct Membership will be referred to the Council for prompt disposition pursuant to the rules of the Council. Section 1.111 of the AMA Bylaws provides that Active Constituent members shall be admitted to membership upon certification by the secretary of the constituent association to the Executive Vice President of the AMA provided that there is no disapproval by the AMA Council on Ethical and Judicial Affairs.

B. In reviewing applications for AMA membership, the Council on Ethical and Judicial Affairs shall consider information contained in the application, information from other available sources and objections raised in response to notification of the state medical association or associations in the jurisdiction or jurisdictions in which the applicant practices. The Council may consider information pertaining to the character, ethics, professional status and professional activities of the applicant. Any significant misstatements or omissions from the application shall constitute cause for denial of AMA membership.

C. Following review of the application for AMA membership and related information, the applicant shall be notified of allegations, which if true, would justify denial of AMA membership. The applicant shall have thirty (30) days following receipt of the notice in which to file a written response. Failure of the applicant to respond within the thirty (30) day period waives any further consideration of the application. The Council on Ethical and Judicial Affairs shall consider any written response and determine whether additional information is needed to dispose of the matter in a fair and equitable manner.

D. If additional information is needed to resolve disputed issues of fact or the Council on Ethical and Judicial Affairs finds cause for disapproving an application, the applicant shall be notified in writing of the disputed issues of fact or reasons for disapproval and shall have thirty (30) days following receipt of the notice to request a hearing. Failure to request a hearing within the thirty (30) day period waives any further consideration of the application.

E. If the applicant submits a written request for a hearing, the Council on Ethical and Judicial Affairs shall notify the applicant of the date, place and time of the hearing and shall provide the applicant with a copy of these rules. Notice shall also be sent to anyone who submitted written objections to AMA membership by the applicant, informing them of the right, within seven (7) days after the date of the notice, to request to appear at their own expense to present evidence in support of the objections or refute evidence presented by the applicant. No objector shall have the right to cross-examine the applicant or any witnesses.

F. The Council on Ethical and Judicial Affairs shall not be bound by technical legal rules of evidence and may accept any evidence or information deemed reliable or relevant. The applicant shall not be required to, but may be accompanied by legal counsel and either the applicant or legal counsel may cross-examine any witnesses who appear in opposition to the applicant's application for AMA membership.

G. If a written transcript is made of the hearing, any party requesting a copy shall have it made available at his or her own expense.

H. The Council on Ethical and Judicial Affairs shall, within thirty (30) days after the hearing, notify the applicant and anyone who appeared at the hearing, of its decision.

I. If the decision is to deny membership, the applicant may reapply for membership after one year following the date of the decision.

Rule XIII. Discipline

Section 1.20 of the Bylaws provides that a member may retain membership only as long as the provisions of the Constitution and Bylaws and Principles of Medical Ethics of the American Medical Association are complied with. Section 1.621 of the Bylaws provides that the Council on Ethical and Judicial Affairs, after due notice and hearing, may censure, suspend or expel any active direct, associate, affiliate or honorary member of the AMA for an infraction of the Constitution and Bylaws or for a violation of the Principles of Medical Ethics of the AMA. Section 1.611 provides that the Council on Ethical and Judicial Affairs, after due notice and hearing, may censure, suspend or expel an active constituent association, for an infraction of the Constitution and Bylaws or for a violation of the Principles of Medical Ethics of the AMA. In addition, the AMA may take disciplinary action with respect to an active constituent member's AMA membership (1) when a state medical association to which a member belongs requests the AMA to take such action; or (2) when, at the request of the AMA, a state association to which the member belongs consents to such action. Section 6.4025 of the Bylaws provides that the Council on Ethical and Judicial Affairs may request the President of the Association to appoint investigating juries to which the Council may refer complaints or evidences of unethical conduct which, in its judgment, are of greater than local concern. The following Rules of Procedure, respecting notice of charges and the conduct of hearings before the Council, are based upon these Sections of the Bylaws.

A. **Statement of Charges**. The statement of charges shall allege in writing an infraction of the AMA's Constitution or Bylaws or a violation of the Principles of Medical Ethics of the AMA.

B. **Notice**. A copy of the statement of charges shall be sent to the member by registered or certified mail.

C. **Answer**. The member shall have sixty (60) days after receipt of the notice to file a written answer. The Council on Ethical and Judicial Affairs shall consider any written response and determine whether additional information is needed to dispose of the matter in a fair and equitable manner. Failure of the member to respond within the sixty (60) day period shall constitute an admission of the allegations.

D. **Hearings**. Where additional information is needed to resolve disputed issues of fact or in cases where the Council on Ethical and Judicial Affairs finds cause for censuring, suspending or expelling a member, the member shall be notified in writing of the disputed issues of fact or reasons for censure, suspension or expulsion and shall have thirty (30) days following receipt of the notice to request a hearing. Failure to request a hearing within the thirty (30) day period waives the right to a hearing on the matter.

If the member submits a written request for a hearing, the Council on Ethical and Judicial Affairs shall notify the applicant of the date, place and time of the hearing and shall provide the member with a copy of these rules. The member shall receive not less than thirty (30) days notice of the hearing. Notice shall also be sent to any state medical association to which an active constituent member belongs that has requested or consented to disciplinary action by the AMA; and such notice shall inform the state medical association of its right, within seven (7) days after the date of the notice, to request to appear at its own expense to present evidence in support of its allegation or refute evidence presented by the active constituent member, but the state medical association shall have no right to cross-examine the active constituent member or any witnesses.

The Council on Ethical and Judicial Affairs shall not be bound by technical legal rules of evidence and may accept any evidence or information deemed reliable or relevant. The General Counsel of the American Medical Association or her or his designee shall present the evidence against the member and may question the parties or their witnesses. The member shall not be required to, but may be accompanied by legal counsel and either the member or the member's legal counsel may cross-examine any witnesses who appear.

A written transcript shall be made of the hearing; any person requesting a copy shall have it made at his or her own expense.

E. **Decision**. The Council on Ethical and Judicial Affairs shall, within thirty (30) days after the hearing, notify the member of its decision and the reasons for any adverse decision. If the decision is to expel a member, he or she may reapply for membership after one year has elapsed from the date of the decision.

Rules of the Council on Ethical and Judicial Affairs in Original Jurisdiction Cases

Preamble

6.4025 of the Bylaws provides that the Council on Ethical and Judicial Affairs may request the President of the Association to appoint investigating juries to which the Council may refer complaints or evidences of unethical conduct which, in its judgment, are of greater than local concern.

The following Rules of Procedure, respecting notice of charges and the conduct of hearings before the Council on Ethical and Judicial Affairs are based upon this section of the Bylaws.

Investigating Jury

At the request of the Council on Ethical and Judicial Affairs, the President has appointed an investigating jury. Complaints or evidence of unethical conduct of greater than local concern will be submitted to this jury by the Council.

Institution of Proceedings

If after investigation a probable cause for action is shown, the investigating jury shall submit a statement of charges to the President. The President shall submit to the Council on Ethical and Judicial Affairs the statement of charges presented to him or her by the investigating jury for prosecution in the name and on behalf of the American Medical Association.

Statement of Charges

The statement of charges shall allege in writing an infraction of the AMA's Constitution or Bylaws or a violation of the Principles of Medical Ethics of the AMA. Exhibits may be attached.

Notice

A copy of the statement of charges shall be sent to the respondent physician by personal delivery or by registered or certified mail.

Answer

The respondent physician shall have thirty (30) days after personal delivery or mailing of the notice of statement of charges to file a written answer. If the respondent physician fails to file a written answer, the allegations shall be considered to be admitted.

Proceedings

The Chairman of the Council on Ethical and Judicial Affairs shall designate one or more members of the Council to conduct a hearing on the statement of charges. This member or these members shall be known as the Hearing Officer.

Hearings shall be held at such reasonable time and place, designated by the Hearing Officer, as may be consistent with the nature of the proceedings and the convenience of the parties. The parties shall receive not less than fifteen (15) days of notice of the hearing.

The General Counsel of the American Medical Association or his or her designee shall prosecute the charges against the respondent physician.

Attendance at hearings may be limited to the members of the Council on Ethical and Judicial Affairs, the staff, witnesses, if any, the parties and counsel who may speak in their behalf.

The Hearing Officer or his counsel may question the parties and their witnesses. The Hearing Officer shall not be bound by technical rules of evidence usually employed in legal proceedings but may accept any evidence deemed appropriate and pertinent.

Should any party to the controversy fail to appear at the hearing, the Hearing Officer may, in his or her discretion, continue, dismiss or proceed with the hearing.

Findings and Conclusions

At the conclusion of the hearing, the Hearing Officer shall render a report in writing containing findings and conclusions and recommendations, if any. This report, together with a transcript of the proceedings, shall be submitted to the Council on Ethical and Judicial Affairs. A copy of the report shall be mailed to all parties of record.

Written Objections

Any party to the proceedings may submit written objections to the report to the Council on Ethical and Judicial Affairs. These objections must be submitted within twenty-one (21) days after the report has been submitted by the Hearing Officer to the Council on Ethical and Judicial Affairs.

Oral Argument

In addition to written objections, any party may request an opportunity to present oral arguments on its objections to the report of the Hearing Officer before the Council on Ethical and Judicial Affairs. This request must be made within twenty-one (21) days after the report has been submitted to the Council. The granting of oral arguments shall be discretionary with the Council. If granted, the parties shall be notified by the Council of the place and date for such oral argument; all parties shall be given opportunity to be heard and the time allotted to argument may be limited by the Council with due regard to the magnitude and complexities of the issues involved.

If any party fails to appear, the Council may continue or proceed with the oral argument.

Final Decision

The Council on Ethical and Judicial Affairs, including the member or members who serve as the Hearing Officer, shall render a final decision. A copy of that decision shall be mailed or otherwise served upon all parties.

Disciplinary Action

The Council on Ethical and Judicial Affairs shall have the authority to acquit, admonish, or censure the accused physician or suspend or expel him or her from AMA membership as the facts may justify. This action shall be in accordance with the authority vested in the Council by 1.60 and 6.4024 of the Bylaws.

Transcript

A written transcript shall be made of the proceedings and of the oral argument before the Council on Ethical and Judicial Affairs.

If any party to the controversy requests a copy of the transcript, it shall be made available to the party at the party's expense.

Filing of Copies

Ten (10) copies of all pleadings and exhibits shall be submitted to AMA Headquarters to the Chairman of the Council on Ethical and Judicial Affairs. One copy of each document shall be submitted at the same time to each of the other parties to the controversy.

Index to Opinions

Table of Cases

Corbett v. D'Alessandro, 487 So. 2d 368 (Fla. App. 1986) [IV; 2.20].

Couture v. Couture, 48 Ohio App. 3d 208, 549 N.E.2d 571 (1989) [2.20].

Crist v. Moffatt, 326 N.C. 326, 333, 389 S.E.2d 41 (1990) [IV; 5.05].

Cruzan v. Director, Missouri Department of Health, 497 U.S. 261 (1990) [2.20].

Cruzan v. Harmon, 760 S.W.2d 408 (1988), aff'd, 497 U.S. 261 (1990) [2.20].

D.A.B v. Brown, 570 N.W. 2d 168 (Minn. App. 1997) [8.06].

Dade County Medical Ass'n v. Samartino, 213 So. 2d 627 (Fla. App. 1968) [5.02].

DeGrella v. Elston, 858 S.W.2d 698 (Ky. 1993) [2.20].

Delio v. Westchester County Medical Center, 134 Misc. 2d 206, 510 N.Y.S.2d 415 (Sup. Ct. 1986), rev'd, 129 A.D.2d 1, 516 N.Y.S.2d 677 (1987) [2.20].

Doe v. Roe, 93 Misc. 2d 201, 400 N.Y.S.2d 668 (Sup. Ct. 1977) [IV; 5.05].

Downey v. Weston, 451 Pa. 259, 301 A.2d 635 (1973) [IV; 5.05].

Dr. K. v. State Bd. of Physician Quality Assur., 98 Md. App. 103, 632 A.2d 453 (1993), cert. denied, 334 Md. 18, 637 A.2d 1191 (1994), and cert. denied, 115 S. Ct. 75, 130 L. Ed. 29 (1994) [II].

Dupree v. Malpractice Research, Inc., 179 Mich. App. 254, 445 N.W.2d 498 (1989) [6.01].

Duquette v. Superior Court, 161 Ariz. 269, 778 P.2d 634 (Ariz. Ct. App. 1989) [IV; 5.05].

Eli Lilly & Co. v. Marshall, 850 S.W.2d 155 (Tex. 1993) [V].

Estate of Behringer v. Medical Ctr., 249 N.J. Super. 597, 592 A.2d 1251, 1268 (1991) [IV; 5.05, 9.13, 9.131].

Estate of Finkle, 90 Misc. 2d 550, 395 N.Y.S.2d 343 (Sur. Ct. 1977) [IV; 5.05, 7.04].

Estates of Morgan v. Fairfield Family Counseling Center, 77 Ohio St. 3d 284, 303, 673 N.E.2d 1311 (1997) [IV; 5.05].

Falcon v. Alaska Pub. Offices Comm'n, 570 P.2d 469 (Alaska 1977) [IV; 5.05].

Falcone v. Middlesex County Medical Soc'y, 62 N.J. Super. 184, 162 A.2d 324 (1960), aff'd, 34 N.J. 582, 170 A.2d 791 (1961) [VI; 3.01].

Faya v. Almaraz, 329 Md. 435, 620 A.2d 327 (1993) [9.13, 9.131].

Fineman v. New Jersey Dept. of Human Servs., 272 N.J. Super. 606, 640 A.2d 1161 (App. Div. 1994), cert. denied, 138 N.J. 267, 649 A.2d 1287 (1994) [VI].

Forziati v. Board of Registration in Medicine, 333 Mass. 125, 128 N.E.2d 789 (1955) [II; 6.02].

Fosmire v. Nicoleau, 75 N.Y.2d 218, 551 N.E.2d 77, 551 N.Y.S.2d 876 (1990) [2.20].

Freeman v. Duluth Clinic, 334 N.W.2d 626 (Minn. 1983) [9.02].

Gadson v. Newman, 807 F. Supp. 1412 (C.D. Ill. 1992) [8.032].

Geisberger v. Willuhn, 72 Ill. App. 3d 435, 390 N.E.2d 945 (2d Dist. 1979) [IV; 5.05].

Gomez v. Chua Medical Corp., 510 N.E.2d 191 (Ind. Ct. App. 1987) [9.02].

Grabowski v. Quigley, 454 Pa. Super. 27, 684 A.2d 610 (1996) [8.16].

Greisman v. Newcomb Hosp., 40 N.J. 389, 192 A.2d 817 (1963) [3.01].

Gromis v. Medical Board, 8 Cal. App. 4th 589, 10 Cal. Rptr. 2d 452 (1st Dist. 1992), reh'g denied, 1992 Cal. App. LEXIS 1047, and review denied, 1992 Cal. LEXIS 5101 [8.14].

Group Health Coop. v. King County Medical Soc'y, 39 Wash. 2d 586, 237 P.2d 737 (1951) [VI; 8.04, 8.05, 9.06].

Hague v. Williams, 37 N.J. 328, 181 A.2d 345 (1962) [IV; 5.05].

Hammonds v. Aetna Casualty & Sur. Co., 243 F. Supp. 793 (N.D. Ohio 1965) [IV; 5.08].

Harlan v. Lewis, 141 F.R.D. 107 (E.D. Ark. 1992) [5.05].

Health Sys. Agency v. Virginia State Bd. of Medicine, 424 F.Supp. 267 (E.D. Va. 1976) [5.02].

Heller v. Norcal Mutual Ins. Co., 8 Cal. 4th 30, 876 P.2d 999, 32 Cal. Rptr. 2d 200 (1994), cert. denied, 115 S. Ct. 669, 130 L. Ed. 2d 602 (1994) [5.05].

Loudon v. Mhyre, 110 Wash. 2d 675, 756 P.2d 138 (1988) [IV; 5.05].

Loui v. Board of Medical Examiners, 78 Haw. 21, 889 P.2d 705 (1995) [Preamble].

Lurch v. United States, 719 F.2d 333 (10th Cir. 1983), cert. denied, 466 U.S. 927 (1984) [8.03, 8.05].

Magan Medical Clinic v. California State Bd. of Medical Examiners, 249 Cal. App. 2d 124, 57 Cal. Rptr. 256 (2d Dist. 1967) [8.03, 8.032, 8.06].

Manion v. N.P.W. Medical Center of N.E. Pa., Inc., 676 F.Supp. 585 (M.D. Pa. 1987) [IV; 5.05, 5.06, 5.07].

Martin v. Baehler, 1993 Del. Super. LEXIS 199 (1993) [IV].

Maryland Att'y Gen. Op., 62 Op. Att'y Gen. 157 (1977) [IV; 2.02, 5.05].

Maryland Att'y Gen. Op. No. 89-022 (1989) [IV].

Maryland Att'y Gen. Op. No. 86-030, 71 Op. Att'y. Gen. 407 (1986) [IV].

Maryland Att'y Gen. Op. No. 88-046, 73 Op. Att'y Gen. 162 (1988) [2.20].

Maxey v. United States, 1989 U.S. Dist. LEXIS 5827 (W.D. Ark. 1989) [VI].

McConnell v. Beverly Enterprises-Connecticut, Inc., 209 Conn. 692, 553 A.2d 596 (1989) [2.20].

McCormick v. England, 328 S.C. 627, 494 S.E. 2d 431 (S.C. App. 1997) [IV].

McHugh v. Audet, 72 F.Supp. 394 (M.D. Pa. 1947) [9.07].

McIntosh v. Milano, 168 N.J. Super. 466, 403 A.2d 500 (1979) [Preamble; I, IV; 5.05].

McMurray v. Johnson, 481 So. 2d 887 (Ala. 1985) [8.16].

Mich. Att'y Gen. Opinion No. 5229, 1977-78 Att'y. Gen. Op. 234 (1977) [8.03, 8.032].

Mich. Att'y Gen. Opinion No. 5024, 1977-78 Att'y. Gen. Op. 299 (1978) [5.02].

Missouri Att'y Gen. Op. N. 6 (July 8, 1982) (LEXIS, States Library, Mo. file) [8.06].

Modi v. West Virginia Board of Medicine, 465 S.E.2d 230 (W. Va. 1995) [8.08].

Montefiore Hosp. & Medical Center v. NLRB, 621 F.2d 510 (2d Cir. 1980) [VI].

Monturi v. Englewood Hosp., 246 N.J. Super. 547, 588 A.2d 408 (1991) [8.16].

Morrison v. Abramovice, 206 Cal. App. 3d 304, 309, 253 Cal. Rptr. 530, 533 (1988) [2.20].

Moses v. McWilliams, 379 Pa. Super. 150, 549 A.2d 950 (1988), appeal denied, 521 Pa. 630, 558 A.2d 532 (1989) [IV; 5.05, 5.07].

Ms. B. v. Montgomery County Emergency Service, Inc., 799 F. Supp. 534 (E.D. Pa. 1992) cert. denied, 114 S.Ct. 174 (1993) [5.05].

Nash v. Wennar, 645 F.Supp. 238 (D. Vt. 1986) [I, IV; 8.05].

Noble v. Sartori, 1989 Ky. App. LEXIS 67 (1989) [VI; 8.11].

Ohio Urology, Inc. v. Poll, 72 Ohio. App. 446, 594 N.E.2d 1027 (1991) [VI; 6.11, 9.02, 9.06].

Ojeda v. Sharp Cabrillo Hosp., 8 Cal. App. 4th 1, 10 Cal. Rptr. 2d 230 (1992) [6.01].

People v. Anyakora, 162 Misc. 2d 47, 616 N.Y.S.2d 149 (N.Y. Sup. Ct. 1993) [VI].

People v. Stritzinger, 137 Cal. App. 3d 126, 186 Cal. Rptr. 750 (2d Dist. 1982), rev'd 34 Cal. 3d 505, 668 P.2d 738, 194 Cal. Rptr. 431 (1983) [IV; 2.02, 5.05].

Perna v. Pirozzi, 182 N.J. Super 510, 442 A.2d 1016 (1982), revd, 92 N.J. 446, 457 A.2d 431 (1983) [8.16].

Perna v. Pirozzi, 92 N.J. 446, 457 A.2d 431 (1983) [8.16].

Perreira v. State, 768 P.2d 1198 (Colo. 1989) [IV; 5.05].

Petrillo v. Syntex Laboratories, Inc., 148 Ill. App. 3d 581, 499 N.E.2d 952 (1st Dist. 1986), cert. denied, 483 U.S. 1007 (1987) [II, IV; 5.05, 5.06, 5.07, 5.08].

Phoenix Orthopaedic Surgeons, Ltd. v. Peairs, 164 Ariz. 54, 790 P.2d 752 (App. 1989) [9.02].

Pierce v. Ortho Pharmaceutical Corp., 84 N.J. 58, 417 A.2d 505 (1980) [2.07].

Planned Parenthood League of Massachusetts, Inc. v. Attorney General, 424 Mass. 586, 677 N.E.2d 101, 107 (1997) [2.015].

Planned Parenthood v. Miller, 63 F.3d 1452 (8th Cir. 1995) [2.015].

Plastic Surgical Servs. of New England, P.C. v. Hall, 1993 WL 818637 (Mass. Super. 1993) [8.115].

Polo v. Gotchel, 225 N.J. Super. 429, 542 A.2d 947 (1987) [6.01].

Pons v. Ohio State Medical Bd., 66 Ohio St. 3d 619, 614 N.E.2d 748 (1993) [I, II, IV; 8.14].

Quilico v. Kaplan, 749 F.2d 480 (7th Cir. 1984) [8.03, 8.05].

Rasmussen v. Fleming, 154 Ariz. 200, 741 P.2d 667 (Ct. App. 1986), aff'd in part and rev'd in part, 154 Ariz. 207, 741 P.2d 674 (1987) [2.20].

Rasmussen v. Fleming, 154 Ariz. 207, 741 P.2d 674 (1987) [2.20].

Ritt v. Ritt, 98 N.J. Super. 590, 238 A.2d 196 (1967), rev'd, 52 N.J. 177, 244 A.2d 497 (1968) [IV; 5.05].

Rocca v. Southern Hills Counseling Center, Inc., 671 N.E. 2d 913 (Ind. App. 1996) [IV; 5.05].

Roe v. Wade, 410 U.S. 113 (1973) [2.01].

Salt River Project v. Industrial Comm'n, 1992 Ariz. App. LEXIS 323, 129 Ariz. Adv. Rep. 39 (1992) [IV].

Shankman v. Coastal Psychiatric Assoc., 258 Ga. 294, 368 S.E.2d 753 (1988) [9.02].

Singleton v. State, 437 S.E.2d 53 (S.C. 1993) [2.06].

Somoza v. St. Vincent's Hosp. & Medical Ctr. of New York, 192 A.D.2d 429, 596 N.Y.S.2d 789 (N.Y. App. Div. 1993) [9.12].

South Carolina Att'y Gen. Op. 1978 S.C. AG LEXIS 806 [7.01, 7.02, 7.03].

Sperry Rand Corp. v. Hill, 356 F.2d 181 (1st Cir.), cert. denied, 384 U.S. 973 (1966) [5.02].

Spock v. Pocket Books, Inc., 48 Misc. 2d 812, 266 N.Y.S.2d 77 (Sup. Ct. 1965) [II; 5.02].

State ex rel. Woytus v. Ryan, 776 S.W.2d 389 (Mo. 1989) [IV; 5.05].

State ex. rel. Kitzmiller v. Henning, 437 S.E.2d 452 (W.Va. 1993) [IV; 5.05].

State ex. rel. Stufflebam v. Appelquist, 694 S.W.2d 882 (Mo. App. 1985) overuled by State ex. rel. Woytus v. Ryan, 776 S.W.2d 389 (Mo. 1989) [IV; 5.05].

State v. AMA, 1981-2 Trade Cas. (CCH) ¶ 64,195 (1981) [V, VI; 3.04, 3.07].

State v. Perry, 610 So. 2d 746 (La. 1992) [2.06].

Steeves v. United States, 294 F. Supp. 446 (D.S.C. 1968) [V; 8.04].

Steinberg v. Jensen, 186 Wis. 2d 237, 519 N.W.2d 753 (Wis. Ct. App. 1994), rev'd, 194 Wis. 2d 440, 534 N.W.2d 361 (1995) [IV; 5.05].

Steinberg v. Jensen, 194 Wis. 2d 440, 534 N.W.2d 361 (1995) [IV; 5.05].

Stempler v. Speidell, 100 N.J. 368, 495 A.2d 857 (1985), cert. denied, 483 U.S. 1007 (1987) [IV; 5.05].

Stewart v. Midani, 525 F. Supp. 843 (N.D. Ga. 1981) [VI].

Stigliano v. Connaught Labs., Inc., 140 N.J. 305, 658 A.2d 715 (1995) [9.07].

Tarasoff v. Regents of Univ. of Cal., 17 Cal.3d 425, 551 P.2d 334, 131 Cal. Rptr. 14 (1976) [IV; 5.05].

Thompson v. Sun City Community Hosp., Inc., 141 Ariz. 597, 688 P.2d 605 (1984) [VI].

Treister v. American Academy of Orthopaedic Surgeons, 78 Ill. App. 3d 746, 396 N.E.2d 1225 (1st Dist. 1979) [9.05].

United States v. Neufeld, 908 F. Supp. 491 (S.D. Ohio 1995) [3.04].

Utah Att'y Gen. Op. No. 77-294 (Feb. 15, 1978) [IV; 5.05].

Va. Att'y Gen. Op., 1994 Va. AG LEXIS 12 (1994) [2.06].

Va. Att'y Gen. Op., 1990 Va. AG LEXIS 63 (1990) [2.20].

Vacco v. Quill, 117 S. Ct. 2293, 138 L. Ed. 2d 834 (U.S. 1997) [2.20, 2.211].

Vassiliades v. Garfinckel's, Brooks Bros., 492 A.2d 580 (D.C. App. 1985) [IV; 5.05].

Washington v. Glucksberg, 117 S. Ct. 2258, 138 L. Ed. 2d 772 (U.S. 1997) [2.211].

Webb v. Jarvis, 575 N.E.2d 992 (Ind. 1991) [Preamble].

Weiss v. Cigna Healthcare, Inc., 972 F. Supp. 748 (S.D.N.Y. 1997) [8.13].

Weiss v. York Hosp., 745 F.2d 786 (3d Cir. 1984), *cert. denied*, 470 U.S. 1060 (1985) [3.01].

Wenninger v. Muesing, 307 Minn. 405, 240 N.W.2d 333 (1976) [IV; 5.05].

Wilk v. American Medical Association, 895 F.2d 352 (7th Cir. 1990) [3.01].

Wilk v. American Medical Association, 671 F.Supp. 1465 (N.D. Ill. 1987), *aff'd*, 895 F.2d 352 (7th Cir. 1990) [3.01].

Wilk v. American Medical Association, 735 F.2d 217 (7th Cir. 1983), *cert. denied*, 467 U.S. 1210 (1984) [3.01].

Wilk v. American Medical Association, 719 F.2d 207 (7th Cir. 1983), *Cert. denied*, 467 U.S. 1210 (1984) [3.01].

Wisconsin Att'y Gen. Op. 10-87 (Mar. 16, 1987), (LEXIS, States library, Wis. file) [IV; 2.02, 5.05].

Wood v. Upjohn Co., No. 6093-1-II (Wash. Ct. App. Sept. 4, 1984) (LEXIS, States library, Wash. file) [VI].

Wright v. Wasudev, 1994 Tenn. App. LEXIS 657 (1994) [IV; 5.05].

Yates v. El-Deiry, 160 Ill. App. 3d 198, 513 N.E.2d 519 (3d Dist. 1987) [IV; 5.05].

Table of Articles

Bernstein, *Out of the Frying Pan and Into the Fire: The Expert Witness Problem in Toxic Tort Litigation*, 10 Rev. Litigation 117, 143 (1990) [9.07].

Berrol, *Considerations for Management of the Persistent Vegetative State*, 67 Arch. Phys. Med. Rehabil. 283 (1986) [2.20].

Blair, *Lifting the Genealogical Veil: The Blueprint for Legislative Reform of the Disclosure of Health-Related Information in Adoption*, 70 No. Carolina L. Rev. 681, 692 (1992) [IV].

Bobinski, *Autonomy and Privacy: Protecting Patients from Their Physicians*, 55 U. Pitt. L. Rev. 291, 302, 313 (1994) [8.03, 8.15, 9.13].

Bodenheimer & Grumbach, *Capitation or Decapitation: Keeping Your Head in Changing Times*, 276 J.A.M.A. 1025, 1031 (1996) [8.13].

Bond, *Diverse and Perverse Incentives In Managed Care: Where Will the Pendulum Stop?*, 1 Widener L. Symp. J. 141, 151, 154 (1996) [8.13].

Boozang, *Death Wish: Resuscitating Self-Determination for the Critically Ill*, 35 Ariz. L. Rev. 23, 24, 28, 52 (1993) [2.22, 8.08].

Bopp & Coleson, *The Constitutional Case Against Permitting Physician-Assisted Suicide for Competent Adults With "Terminal Conditions,"* 11 Issues in Law & Med. 239, 250 (1995) [2.211].

Boyle, *Managed Care in Mental Health: A Cure, or a Cure Worse Than the Disease?*, 40 St. Louis U. L. J. 437, 448 (1996) [8.13].

Brennan, *Ensuring Adequate Health Care for the Sick: The Challenge of the Acquired Immunodeficiency Syndrome as an Occupational Disease*, 1988 Duke L. J. 29 (1988) [VI].

Brennan, *Transmission of the Human Immunodeficiency Virus in the Health Care Setting—Time for Action*, 324 New Eng. J. Med. 1504, 1505, 1506 (1991) [9.131].

Brock, *Voluntary Active Euthanasia*, 22 Hastings Center Rep. 10 (March/April 1992) [2.20, 2.21].

Brody, *Ethical Questions Raised by the Persistent Vegetative Patient*, 18 Hastings Center Rep. 33 (Feb./March 1988) [2.20].

Brody, *New Perspectives on Emergency Room Research*, 27 Hastings Center Rep. 7, 9 (Jan./Feb. 1997) [2.07].

Brody, *Special Ethical Issues in the Management of PVS Patients*, 20 Law, Med. & Health Care 104, 109 (1992) [2.20, 2.22].

Brody, *The Physician as Professional and the Physician as Honest Businessman*, 119 Arch. Otolaryngol. Head Neck Surg. 495, 496 (1993) [6.11].

Brooks, Smith, & Anderson, *Medical Apartheid: An American Perspective*, 266 J.A.M.A. 2746, 2748 (1991) [9.121].

Bruening, Andrew, & Smith, *Concurrent Care: An Ethical Issue for Family Physicians*, 36 J. Fam. Practice 606, 607 (1993) [Preamble].

Brunetti, Weiss, Studenski, & Clipp, *Cardiopulmonary Resuscitation Policies and Practices: A Statewide Nursing Home Study*, 150 Arch. Intern. Med. 121, 122 (1990) [2.20, 2.22].

Buchanan, *Medical Ethics at the Millennium: A Brief Retrospective*, 26 Colo. Law. 141, 142, 143, 144, 145 (1997) [FE (Preamble), (5); 5.05, 5.057, 7.01, 8.115, 8.12, 8.13, 9.12, 9.131].

Burris, *Dental Discrimination Against the HIV-Infected: Empirical Data, Law and Public Policy*, 13 Yale J. On Reg. 1, 41 (1996) [9.131].

Cantor, *Discarding Substituted Judgment and Best Interests: Toward a Constructive Preference Standard for Dying, Previously Competent Patients Without Advance Instructions*, 48 Rutgers L. Rev. 1193, 1234, 1247 (1996) [2.17].

Cantor, *My Annotated Living Will*, 18 Law, Med. & Health Care 114 (1990) [2.20].

Cantor, *The Permanently Unconscious Patient, Non-Feeding and Euthanasia*, XV Am. J. Law & Med. 381 (1989) [2.20].

Caplan, Cooper, Garcia-Prats, & Brody, *Diffusion of Innovative Approaches to Managing Hypoplastic Left Heart Syndrome*, 150 Arch. Pediatr. Adolesc. Med. 487, 490 (1996) [2.162].

Capron, *Ethics: Public and Private*, 24 Hastings Center Rep. 26, 27 (November/December 1994) [2.162].

Childress, *Ethics, Public Policy, and Human Fetal Tissue Transplantation Research*, Kennedy Inst. Ethics J. 93, 116 (June 1991) [2.10].

Clark, *Autonomy and Death*, 71 Tul. L. Rev. 45, 89 (1996) [2.21, 2.211].

Closen, *HIV-AIDS, Infected Surgeons and Dentists, and the Medical Profession's Betrayal of Its Responsibility to Patients*, 41 N.Y.L. Sch. L. Rev. 57, 65, 71-72, 129 (1996) [9.131].

Cohen & Cohen, *Required Reconsideration of "Do-Not-Resuscitate" Orders in the Operating Room and Certain Other Treatment Settings*, 20 Law, Med. & Health Care 354, 356 (1992) [2.22].

Cohen, *Holistic Health Care: Including Alternative and Complementary Medicine in Insurance and Regulatory Schemes*, 38 Ariz. L. Rev. 83, 92 (1996) [3.01].

Cohen, *Toward a Bioethics of Compassion*, 28 Ind. L. Rev. 667, 673, 681-82, 683 (1995) [2.01, 2.211, 8.18].

Cohn, Berger, Holzman, Lockhart, Reuben, Robertson, & Selbst, *Guidelines for Expert Witness Testimony in Medical Liability Cases*, 94 Pediatrics 755, 756 (1994) [9.07].

Cole, *Beyond Unconstitutional Conditions: Charting Spheres of Neutrality in Government-Funded Speech*, 67 N.Y.U. L. Rev. 675, 744 (1992) [8.08].

Coleman, *"Brother, Can You Spare a Liver?" Five Ways to Increase Organ Donation*, 31 Val. U.L. Rev. 1, 30, 31 (1996) [2.06].

Coleson, *The Glucksberg & Quill Amicus Curiae Briefs: Verbatim Arguments Opposing Assisted Suicide*, 13 Issues in Law & Med. 3, 67 (1997) [2.211].

Comment, *A Right to Die: Can a Massachusetts Physician Withdraw Artificial Nutrition and Hydration From a Persistently Vegetative Patient Following Cruzan v. Director, Missouri Department of Health?*, 26 New Eng. L. Rev. 199, 216, 220 (1991) [2.20].

Comment, *AIDSphobia: Forcing Courts to Face New Areas of Compensation for Fear of a Deadly Disease*, 39 Vill. L. Rev. 241, 277 (1994) [9.13, 9.131].

Comment, *Alliances for the Future: Cultivating a Cooperative Environment for Biotech Success*, 11 Berkeley Tech. L. J. 311, 344 (1996) [8.031].

Comment, *An Illinois Physician-Assisted Suicide Act: A Merciful End to a Terminally Ill Criminal Tradition*, 28 Loy. U. Chi. L. J. 763, 775 (1997) [2.20].

Comment, *Artificial Nutrition and the Terminally Ill: How Should Washington Decide?*, 61 Wash. L. Rev. 419 (1986) [2.20].

Comment, *Beyond Autonomy: Judicial Restraint and the Legal Limits Necessary to Uphold the Hippocratic Tradition and Preserve the Ethical Integrity of the Medical Profession*, 9 J. Contemp. Health L. & Pol'y 451, 467, 468 (1993) [FE(5); 2.20].

Comment, *Curing the Health Care Industry: Government Response to Medicare Fraud and Abuse*, 5 J. Contemp. Health L. & Pol'y 175 (1989) [8.03].

Comment, *Dangerous Relations: Doctors and Extracorporeal Embryos, The Need For New Limits To Medical Inquiry*, 7 J. Contemp. Health L. & Pol'y 307, 309 (1991) [2.10, 2.14].

Comment, *Ethical Considerations in Resuscitation*, 268 J.A.M.A. 2282, 2283, 2287 (1992) [2.20, 2.22].

Comment, *From the Land of Lincoln a Healing Rule: Proposed Texas Rule of Civil Procedure Prohibiting Ex Parte Contact Between Defense Counsel and a Plaintiff's Treating Physician*, 25 Tex. Tech L. Rev. 1081, 1081, 1082 (1994) [II, IV; 5.05].

Comment, *Hold On Courts: May a Comatose Patient Be Denied Food and Water*, 31 St. Louis Univ. L. J. 749 (1987) [2.20].

Comment, *Medical Use of Marijuana: Legal and Ethical Conflicts in the Patient-Physician Relationship*, 30 U. Rich. L. Rev. 249, 268-69 (1996) [2.17].

Comment, *Noncompetition Clauses in Physician Employment Contracts in Oregon*, 76 Or. L. Rev. 195, 204-06 (1997) [Preamble; 6.11, 9.02, 9.06].

Comment, *Nonconsensual HIV Testing in the Health Care Setting: The Case for Extending the Occupational Protections of California Proposition 96 to Health Care Workers*, 26 Loy. L.A. L. Rev. 1251, 1269 (1993) [VI; 9.131].

Comment, *One Step Forward, Two Steps Back: A Constitutional and Critical Look at Ohio's New Living Will Statute*, 54 Ohio St. L. J. 445, 447, 460, 470 (1993) [2.20].

Comment, *Physician Assisted Suicide and the Right to Die With Assistance*, 105 Harvard L. Rev. 2021, 2027, 2035 (1992) [2.20].

Comment, *Physician Gag Clauses—The Hypocrisy of the Hippocratic Oath*, 21 So. Ill. U. L. J. 313, 318, 320 (1997) [8.13].

Comment, *Physician Retaliation: Can the Physician-Patient Relationship Be Protected?*, 94 Dickinson L. Rev. 965, 986 (1990) [9.131].

Comment, *Physician-Assisted Suicide: Should Texas Be Different?*, 33 Hous. L. Rev. 1475, 1480, 1488 (1997) [2.21, 2.211].

Comment, *Protecting Children Exposed to Domestic Violence in Contested Custody and Visitation Litigation*, 6 B.U. Pub. Int. L. J. 501, 502, 505 (1997) [2.02].

Comment, *Regulating Physician Investment and Referral Behavior in the Competitive Health Care Marketplace of the '90s—An Argument for Decentralization*, 65 Wash. L. Rev. 657, 658 (1990) [8.03].

Comment, *Right to Die: Oklahoma's Position on Nutrition and Hydration: Confusing or Unconstitutional?*, 43 Okla. L. Rev. 143, 151 (1990) [2.20].

Comment, *Shielding the Plaintiff and Physician: The Prohibition of Ex Parte Contacts With a Plaintiff's Treating Physician*, 13 Campbell L. Rev. 233, 243, 248 (1991) [IV; 5.06].

Comment, *Statutory Immunity for Volunteer Physicians: A Vehicle for Reaffirmation of the Doctor's Beneficent Duties—Absent the Rights Talk*, 1 Widener L. Symp. J. 425, 448, 449 (1996) [FE(6); 9.065].

Comment, *Surrogate Health Care Decision Making: The Pennsylvania Supreme Court Recognizes the Right of an Individual in a Permanent Vegetative State to Refuse Life-Sustaining Measures through a Surrogate Decision Maker*, 35 Duq. L. Rev. 849, 859-60 (1997) [2.20].

Comment, *Taking Tarasoff Where No One Has Gone Before: Looking at "Duty to Warn" Under the AIDS Crisis*, 15 St. Louis U. Pub. L. Rev. 471, 499 (1996) [2.23, 5.057].

Comment, *The Hospice Movement: A Renewed View of the Death Process*, 4 J. Contemp. Health L. & Pol'y 295 (1988) [2.20].

Comment, *The Living Will: Preservation of the Right-To-Die Demands Clarity and Consistency*, 95 Dickinson L. Rev. 209, 217 (1990) [2.20].

Comment, *The Right to Refuse Life Sustaining Medical Treatment and the Nonterminally Ill Patient: An Analysis of Abridgment and Anarchy*, 17 Pepperdine L. Rev. 461, 462 (1990) [2.20].

Comment, *The Role of the Family in Medical Decisionmaking for Incompetent Adult Patients: A Historical Perspective and Case Analysis*, 48 Univ. Pittsburgh L. Rev. 539 (1987) [2.20].

Comment, *Tort Reform to Ensure the Inclusion of Fertile Women in Early Phases of Commercial Drug Research*, 3 U. Chi. L. Sch. Roundtable 355, 359 (1996) [9.035].

Comment, *Who's in Charge: The Doctor or the Dollar?, Assessing the Relative Liability of Third Party Payors and Doctors After Wickline and Wilson*, 18 J. Contemp. L. 285, 301, 302 (1992) [2.03].

Comment, *Withholding Lifesaving Treatment From Defective Newborns: An Equal Protection Analysis*, 29 St. Louis Univ. L. J. 853 (1985) [2.17].

Cooper, *Restrictive Covenants*, 248 J.A.M.A. 3091 (1982) [9.02].

Crane, *The Problem of Physician Self-Referral Under the Medicare and Medicaid Antikickback Statute: The Hanlester Network Case and the Safe Harbor Regulation*, 268 J.A.M.A. 85, 89, 90 (1992) [8.032].

Cranford, *Neurologic Syndromes and Prolonged Survival: When Can Artificial Nutrition and Hydration Be Foregone?*, 19 Law, Med. & Health Care 13, 14, 16, 17 (1991) [2.20].

Crespi, *Overcoming the Legal Obstacles to the Creation of a Futures Market in Bodily Organs*, 55 Ohio St. L. J. 1, 74 (1994) [2.15].

Crossley, *Infants with Anencephaly, the ADA, and the Child Abuse Amendments*, 11 Issues in Law & Med. 379, 385, 409 (1996) [2.162, 2.17].

Crossley, *Of Diagnoses and Discrimination: Discriminatory Nontreatment of Infants With HIV Infection*, 93 Columbia L. Rev. 1581, 1620, 1621 (1993) [2.09, 2.17, 2.20, 2.22, 4.04, 8.03].

Cultice, *Medical Futility: When Is Enough, Enough?*, 27 J. Health & Hosp. Law 225, 230, 256 (1994) [2.03, 2.035, 2.095, 2.17, 2.19, 2.20, 2.22].

Cuzmanes & Orlando, *Automation of Medical Records: The Electronic Superhighway and Its Ramifications for Health Care Providers*, 6 J. Pharmacy & L. 19, 27 (1997) [IV].

Daar, *A Clash at the Bedside: Patient Autonomy v. A Physician's Professional Conscience*, 44 Hastings L. J. 1241, 1257, 1268, 1286 (1993) [2.20, 2.22].

Daar, *Medical Futility and Implications for Physician Autonomy*, XXI Am. J. Law & Med. 221, 234 (1995) [2.035].

Dahm, *Using DNA Profile as the Unique Patient Identifier in the Community Health Information Network: Legal Implications*, 15 J. Marshall J. Computer & Info. L. 227, 266, 275 (1997) [5.05].

Dalton, *Domestic Violence, Domestic Torts and Divorce: Constraints and Possibilities*, 31 New. Eng. L. Rev. 319, 354 (1997) [2.02].

Daniels, *Duty to Treat or Right to Refuse?*, 21 Hastings Center Rep. 36, 37, 42 (March/April 1991) [VI; 9.131].

Davis & Grimaldi, *Sexual Confusion: Attorney-Client Sex and the Need for a Clear Ethical Rule*, 7 Notre Dame J. Law, Ethics, & Pub. Pol. 57, 61 (1993) [8.14].

Deftos, *Genomic Torts: The Law of the Future—The Duty of Physicians to Disclose the Presence of a Genetic Disease to the Relatives of Their Patients with the Disease*, 32 U.S.F. L. Rev. 105, 130 (1997) [FE(4)].

Dellinger & Vickery, *When Staff Object to Participating In Care*, 28 J. Health & Hospital Law 269, 272, 276 (1995) [I, VI; 1.02, 2.035, 9.055].

DeNatale & Parrish, *Health Care Workers' Ability to Recover in Tort for Transmission or Fear of Transmission of HIV from a Patient*, 36 Santa Clara L. Rev. 751, 782-83, 787 (1996) [IV; 9.131].

Dennis, *Promotion of Devices: An Extension of FDA Drug Regulation or a New Frontier?*, 48 Food & Drug L. J. 87 (1993) [8.061].

Denno, *Getting to Death: Are Executions Constitutional?*, 82 Iowa L. Rev. 319, 385-86 (1997) [2.06].

Devettere, *The Imprecise Language of Euthanasia and Causing Death*, 1 J. Clinical Ethics 268, 268 (1990) [2.20].

Dickey, *Euthanasia: A Concept Whose Time Has Come?*, 8 Issues in Law & Med. 521, 523, 524 (1993) [2.17, 2.20].

Dillon, *Contingent Fees and Medical-Legal Consulting Services: Economical or Unethical?*, 11 J. Legal Med. 93, 101, 111 (1990) [6.01, 6.05, 9.07].

Dowell, *The Corporate Practice of Medicine Prohibition: A Dinosaur Awaiting Extinction*, 27 J. Health & Hospital Law 369, 370 (1994) [VI].

Doyal, *Human Need and the Right of Patients to Privacy*, 14 J. Contemp. Health L. & Pol'y 1, 3 (1997) [IV].

Dresser, *Relitigating Life and Death*, 51 Ohio St. L. J. 425, 436 (1990) [2.20].

Dresser, *Wanted: Single, White Male for Medical Research*, 22 Hastings Center Rep. 24, 28 (Jan./Feb. 1992) [9.122].

Duncan & Lubin, *The Use and Abuse of History in Compassion in Dying*, 20 Harv. J.L. & Pub. Pol'y 175, 183 (1996) [2.211].

Eisenstat, *An Analysis of the Rationality of Mandatory Testing for the HIV Antibody: Balancing the Governmental Public Health Interests With the Individual's Privacy Interest*, 52 Univ. Pittsburgh L. Rev. 327, 347 (1991) [9.131].

Eitel, Hegeman, & Evans, *Medicine on Trial: Physicians' Attitudes about Expert Medical Witnesses*, 18 J. Legal Med. 345, 355, 358 (1997) [II, VI; 9.07].

Elsas, *A Clinical Approach to Legal and Ethical Problems in Human Genetics*, 39 Emory L. J. 811, 816, 820 (1990) [5.05].

Emanuel, Barry, Stoeckle, Ettelson, & Emanuel, *Advance Directives for Medical Care—A Case for Greater Use*, 324 New Eng. J. Med. 889 (1991) [2.20].

Emanuel, *Do Physicians Have an Obligation to Treat Patients With AIDS?*, 318 New Eng. J. Med. 1686 (1988) [9.12].

Emanuel, Emanuel, Stoeckle, Hummel, & Barry, *Advance Directives: Stability of Patients' Treatment Choices*, 154 Arch. Intern. Med. 209, 217 (1994) [2.20].

Falk & Cary, *Death-Defying Feats: State Constitutional Challenges to New York's Death Penalty*, 4 J. L. & Pol'y 161, 233, 234 (1995) [2.06].

Farber, Novack, & O'Brien, *Love, Boundaries, and the Physician-Patient Relationship*, 157 Arch. Intern. Med. 2291, 2292, 2293, 2294 (1997) [8.14].

Farley, *The Medicare Antifraud Statute and Safe Harbor Regulations: Suggestions for Change*, 81 Georgetown L. J. 167, 184 (1992) [8.032].

Field, *Overview: Computerized Medical Records Create New Legal and Business Confidentiality Problems*, 11 HealthSpan 3, 4 (1994) [5.05].

Field, *Testing for AIDS: Uses and Abuses*, XVI Am. J. Law & Med. 34, 50 (1990) [9.131].

Finks, *Lethal Injection: An Uneasy Alliance of Law and Medicine*, 4 J. Legal Med. 383 (1983) [2.06].

Fischer, Alpert, Stoeckle, & Emanuel, *Can Goals of Care Be Used to Predict Intervention Preferences in an Advance Directive?*, 157 Arch. Intern. Med. 801, 807 (1997) [2.20, 2.21].

FitzGibbon & Lai, *The Model Physician-Assisted Suicide Act and the Jurisprudence of Death*, 13 Issues in Law & Med. 173, 203-04 (1997) [2.211].

Flick, *The Due Process of Dying*, 79 Cal. L. Rev. 1121, 1152 (1991) [2.22].

Forrester, *AIDS: The Responsibility to Care*, 34 Vill. L. Rev. 799, 811 (1989) [VI; 9.131].

Freedman & Halpern, *The Erosion of Ethics and Morality in Medicine: Physician Participation in Legal Executions in the United States*, 41 N.Y.L. Sch. L. Rev. 169, 174 (1996) [2.06].

Freedman, *Health Professions, Codes, and the Right to Refuse to Treat HIV-Infectious Patients*, 18 Hastings Center Rep. 20 (Supp.) (April/May 1988) [VI; 8.11, 9.12].

Friedland, *HIV Confidentiality and the Right to Warn—The Health Care Provider's Dilemma*, 80 Mass. L. Rev. 3, 4 (March 1995) [IV; 5.05].

Friedland, *Physician-Patient Confidentiality: Time to Re-Examine a Venerable Concept in Light of Contemporary Society and Advances in Medicine*, 15 J. Legal Med. 249, 257, 264, 276 (1994) [I, IV; 5.05].

Furrow, *Incentivizing Medical Practice: What (If Anything) Happens to Professionalism?*, 1 Widener L. Symp. J. 1, 9 (1996) [2.03].

Garris, *The Case for Patenting Medical Procedures*, XXII Am. J. Law & Med. 85, 93, 94-95 (1996) [9.08, 9.09, 9.095].

Gellman, *Prescribing Privacy: The Uncertain Role of the Physician in the Protection of Patient Privacy*, 62 No. Carolina L. Rev. 255 (1984) [5.03, 5.04, 5.06, 5.07, 5.08, 5.09].

Gerbert, Bleecker, Miyasaki, & Maguire, *Possible Health Care Professional-to-Patient HIV Transmission: Dentists' Reactions to a Centers for Disease Control Report*, 265 J.A.M.A. 1845, 1846, 1847 (1991) [9.131].

Gerbert, Maguire, Bleecker, Coates, & McPhee, *Primary Care Physicians and AIDS: Attitudinal and Structural Barriers to Care*, 266 J.A.M.A. 2837, 2838 (1991) [9.131].

Gilmore, *Employment Protection for Lesbians and Gay Men*, 6 L. & Sex. 83, 95 (1996) [9.03].

Gittler & Rennart, *HIV Infection Among Women and Children and Antidiscrimination Laws: An Overview*, 77 Iowa L. Rev. 1313, 1363 (1992) [VII; 9.131].

Glynn, *Multidisciplinary Representation of Children: Conflicts Over Disclosures of Client Communications*, 27 J. Marshall L. Rev. 617, 625, 626, 630-32, 637, 639, 643 (1994) [III, IV; FE(4);1.02, 2.02, 5.05].

Goldberg, *Sex and the Attorney-Client Relationship: An Argument for a Prophylactic Rule*, 26 Akron L. Rev. 45 (1992) [8.14].

Goldman, *Revising Iowa's Life-Sustaining Procedures Act: Creating a Practical Guide to Living Wills in Iowa*, 76 Iowa L. Rev. 1137, 1149 (1992) [2.20].

Gostin, *Deciding Life and Death in the Courtroom: From Quinlan to Cruzan, Glucksberg, and Vacco—A Brief History and Analysis of Constitutional Protection of the 'Right to Die,'* 278 J.A.M.A. 1523, 1525, 1528 (1997) [2.211].

Gostin, *Drawing a Line Between Killing and Letting Die: The Law, and Law Reform, on Medically Assisted Dying*, 21 J. Law, Med. & Ethics 94, 98 (1993) [2.20].

Gray, *Trust and Trustworthy Care in the Managed Care Era*, 16 Health Affairs 34, 38, 47-48 (1997) [8.03].

Greely, *Direct Financial Incentives in Managed Care: Unanswered Questions*, 6 Health Matrix 53, 81 (1996) [8.13].

Green, Haggerty, & Hale, *Community-Based Plan for Treating Human Immunodeficiency Virus-Infected Individuals Sponsored by Local Medical Societies and an Acquired Immunodeficiency Syndrome Service Organization*, 151 Arch. Intern. Med. 2061, 2064 (1991) [9.131].

Green, *NHGRI's Intramural Ethics Experiment*, 7 Kennedy Inst. of Ethics J. 181, 185, 188 (1997) [2.138].

Guise, *Expansion of the Scope of Disclosure Required Under the Informed Consent Doctrine: Moore v. The Regents of the University of California*, 28 San Diego L. Rev. 455, 462 (1991) [Preamble].

Gutheil, Jorgenson, & Sutherland, *Prohibiting Lawyer-Client Sex*, 20 Bull. Am. Acad. Psychiatry Law 365 (1992) [8.14].

Hackler & Hiller, *Family Consent to Orders Not To Resuscitate: Reconsidering Hospital Policy*, 264 J.A.M.A. 1281, 1282 (1990) [2.17].

Haddon, *Baby Doe Cases: Compromise and Moral Dilemma*, 34 Emory L. J. 545 (1985) [2.20].

Halevy & Brody, *Acquired Immunodeficiency Syndrome and the Americans with Disabilities Act: A Legal Duty to Treat*, 96 Am. J. Med. 282, 283, 284 (1994) [VI; 9.12, 9.131].

Hall, *A Theory of Economic Informed Consent*, 31 Ga. L. Rev. 511, 521, 524-25 (1997) [8.13].

Hall, *Rationing Health Care at the Bedside, 69 N.Y.U. L. Rev. 693, 704 (1994)* [2.03].

Hammes & Webster, *Professional Ethics and Managed Care in Dermatology, 132 Arch. Dermatol. 1070, 1072, 1073 (1996)* [8.13].

Hartog, *The Psychological Impact of AIDS on Real Property and a Real Estate Broker's Duty to Disclose, 36 Ariz. L. Rev. 757, 772 (1994)* [9.13, 9.131].

Harvey, *Confidentiality: A Measured Response to the Failure of Privacy, 140 Univ. Pa. L. Rev. 2385, 2454 (1992)* [8.08].

Hashimoto, *The Future Role of Managed Care and Capitation in Workers' Compensation, XXII Am. J. Law & Med. 233, 258, 259 (1996)* [8.13].

Healey & Dowling, *Controlling Conflicts of Interest in the Doctor-Patient Relationship: Lessons From Moore v. Regents of the University of California, 42 Mercer L. Rev. 989, 997, 998 (1991)* [2.19, 8.032, 8.06].

Hillerich, Ellerin, & Frieder, *Selecting and Presenting a Failure to Diagnose Breast Cancer Case, 20 Am. J. Trial Advoc. 253, 271 (1996-97)* [5.05, 5.06].

Hirshfeld & Thomason, *Medical Necessity Determinations: The Need for a New Legal Structure, 6 Health Matrix 3, 8-9 (1996)* [I, II, III, IV, V, VI, VII; 2.03].

Hirshfeld, *Defining Full and Fair Disclosure in Managed Care Contracts, 60 The Citation 67 (1990)* [8.03, 8.032, 8.13].

Hirshfeld, *Economic Considerations in Treatment Decisions and the Standard of Care in Medical Malpractice Litigation, 264 J.A.M.A. 2004, 2007 (1990)* [2.03, 2.09].

Hirshfeld, *Should Ethical and Legal Standards for Physicians Be Changed to Accommodate New Models for Rationing Health Care?, 140 Univ. Pa. L. Rev. 1809, 1816 (1992)* [2.03, 2.09, 4.04].

Hirshfeld, *Should Third Party Payors of Health Care Services Disclose Cost Control Mechanisms to Potential Beneficiaries?, 14 Seton Hall Legis. J. 115 (1990)* [2.03, 2.09, 2.19, 4.04, 4.06, 8.03, 8.032].

Hodges, Tolle, Stocking, & Cassel, *Tube Feeding: Internists' Attitudes Regarding Ethical Obligations, 154 Arch. Intern. Med. 1013, 1020 (1994)* [2.20].

Hoge, *APA Resource Document: I. The Professional Responsibilities of Psychiatrists in Evolving Health Care Systems, 24 Bull. Am. Acad. Psychiatry Law 393, 405 (1996)* [2.095, 8.13, 8.132].

Hoge, *APA Resource Document: II. Regulatory Guidelines for Protecting the Interests of Psychiatric Patients in Emerging Health Care Systems, 24 Bull. Am. Acad. Psychiatry Law 407, 412, 418 (1996)* [8.13].

Hoge, *Proposed Federal Legislation Jeopardizes Patient Privacy, 23 Bull. Am. Acad. Psychiatry Law 495, 498, 500 (1995)* [IV; 5.07].

Holland, *Should Parents Be Permitted to Authorize Genetic Testing for Their Children?, 31 Fam. L. Q. 321, 346-47 (1997)* [2.132].

Horan & Grant, *The Legal Aspects of Withdrawing Nourishment, 5 J. Legal Med. 595 (1984)* [2.20].

Hyams, *Expert Psychiatric Evidence in Sexual Misconduct Cases Before State Medical Boards, XVIII Am. J. Law & Med. 171, 173, 174 (1992)* [8.14].

Hyams, Shapiro, & Brennan, *Medical Practice Guidelines in Malpractice Litigation: An Early Retrospective, 21 J. Health Pol. Pol'y & L. 289, 298 (1996)* [8.16].

Iheukwumere, *HIV-Positive Medical Practitioners: Legal and Ethical Obligations to Disclose, 71 St. John's L. Rev. 715, 732-34 (1997)* [9.13, 9.131].

Ikemoto, *The Fuzzy Logic of Race and Gender in the Mismeasure of Asian American Women's Health Needs, 65 U. Cin. L. Rev. 799, 800, 804, 810 (1997)* [9.121, 9.122].

Ile, *Should Physicians Treat Patients Who Seek Second Opinions?, 266 J.A.M.A. 273, 274 (1991)* [6.11, 9.02, 9.06, 9.12].

Isaacman & Miller, *Neonatal HIV Seroprevalence Studies, 14 J. Legal Med. 413, 428 (1993)* [2.07].

Jacobi, *Patients at a Loss: Protecting Health Care Consumers through Data Driven Quality Assurance, 45 U. Kan. L. Rev. 705, 720, 721, 759 (1997)* [2.03, 2.09, 8.13].

Jecker & Schneiderman, *An Ethical Analysis of the Use of "Futility" in the 1992 American Heart Association Guidelines for Cardiopulmonary Resuscitation and Emergency Cardiac Care, 153 Arch. Intern. Med. 2195, 2197 (1993)* [2.22].

Jecker, *Genetic Testing and the Social Responsibility of Private Health Insurance Companies, 21 J. Law, Med. & Ethics 109, 112 (1993)* [2.132].

Jecker, *Privacy Beliefs and the Violent Family: Extending the Ethical Argument for Physician Intervention, 269 J.A.M.A. 776, 778, 779 (1993)* [IV; 5.05, 8.14, 9.131].

Johnson, Gibbons, Goldner, Wiener, & Eton, *Legal and Institutional Policy Responses to Medical Futility*, 30 J. Health & Hosp. L. 21, 26, 31, 35, 36 (1997) [2.035, 2.22].

Johnson, *HIV Testing of Health Care Workers: Conflict Between the Common Law and the Centers for Disease Control*, 42 Am. Univ. L. Rev. 479, 518 (1993) [9.131].

Johnson, *Judicial Review of Disciplinary Action for Sexual Misconduct in the Practice of Medicine*, 270 J.A.M.A. 1596 (1993) [8.14].

Johnson, *Minnesota's "Crack Baby" Law: Weapon of War or Link in a Chain?*, 8 Law & Ineq. 485, 494, 495, 496 (1990) [8.08].

Johnson, *The Death-Prolonging Procedures Act and Refusal of Treatment in Missouri*, 30 St. Louis Univ. L. J. 805 (1986) [2.19].

Jones, *Battered Spouses' Damage Actions Against Non-Reporting Physicians*, 45 DePaul L. Rev. 191 (1996) [2.02].

Joynt, *Neurology*, 263 J.A.M.A. 2660 (1990) [2.161].

Jozefowicz, *The Case Against Having "Professional Privilege" in the Physician-Patient Relationship*, 16 Med. & L. 385, 386-87, 391 (1997) [Preamble; IV; 5.05].

Judge, *Issues Surrounding the Patenting of Medical Procedures*, 13 Santa Clara Computer & High Tech. L. J. 181, 202-03 (1997) [9.08, 9.095].

Jurevic, *Disparate Impact Under Title VI: Discrimination, By Any Other Name, Will Still Have the Same Impact*, 15 St. Louis U. Pub. L. Rev. 237, 253 (1996) [2.03].

Kamisar, *When is There A Constitutional "Right to Die"? When is There No Constitutional "Right to Live"?*, 25 Georgia L. Rev. 1203, 1207, 1208, 1222 (1991) [2.20].

Kapp, *Placebo Therapy and the Law: Prescribe With Care*, 8 Am. J. Law & Med. 371 (1983) [8.08, 8.12].

Kass & Lund, *Physician-Assisted Suicide, Medical Ethics and the Future of the Medical Profession*, 35 Duq. L. Rev. 395, 404 (1996) [2.211].

Kassel, *Counterpoint . . . Defense Counsel's Ex Parte Communication with Plaintiff's Doctors: A Bad One-Sided Deal*, 9 S.C. Law. 42, 43 (Sept./Oct. 1997) [IV; 5.05].

Katner, *The Ethical Dilemma Awaiting Counsel Who Represent Adolescents with HIV/AIDS: Criminal Law and Tort Suits Pressure Counsel to Breach the Confidentiality of the Clients' Medical Status*, 70 Tul. L. Rev. 2311, 2341 (1996) [5.05].

Katz, *Informed Consent—Must It Remain a Fairy Tale?*, 10 J. Contemp. Health L. & Pol'y 69, 80 (1994) [8.08].

Kelly, *The "Right to Die" in America: The Ninth Circuit's Decision in Compassion in Dying v. The State of Washington*, 29 J. Health & Hosp. L. 246, 255 (1996) [2.211].

Kerr, Hays, Mittman, Siu, Leake, & Brook, *Primary Care Physicians' Satisfaction with Quality of Care in California Capitated Medical Groups*, 278 J.A.M.A. 308, 312 (1997) [8.13].

Kinney & Selby, *History and Jurisprudence of the Physician-Patient Relationship in Indiana*, 30 Ind. L. Rev. 263, 269, 272, 276 (1997) [2.20, 8.08, 9.06, 9.12].

Kinney, *Procedural Protections for Patients in Capitated Health Plans*, XXII Am. J. Law & Med. 301, 319-20 (1996) [8.13].

Kirschenbaum & Kuhlik, *Federal and State Laws Affecting Discounts, Rebates, and Other Marketing Practices for Drugs and Devices*, 47 Food & Drug L. J. 533, 560 (1992) [6.04, 8.061].

Kleinman, *Health Care in Crisis: A Proposed Role for the Individual Physician as Advocate*, 265 J.A.M.A. 1991 (1991) [9.121].

Koniak, *The Law Between the Bar and the State*, 70 No. Carolina L. Rev. 1389, 1396 (1992) [1.02].

Kumar & Kinney, *Indiana Lawmakers Face National Health Policy Issues*, 25 Indiana L. Rev. 1271, 1275, 1276 (1992) [2.20].

Labowitz, *Beyond Tarasoff: AIDS and the Obligation to Breach Confidentiality*, 9 St. Louis Univ. Pub. L. Rev. 495, 514 (1990) [2.23].

Lafferty, *Statutory and Ethical Barriers in the Patenting of Medical and Surgical Procedures*, 29 J. Marshall L. Rev. 891, 912 (1996) [9.08].

Larson, *Prescription For Death: A Second Opinion*, 44 DePaul L. Rev. 461, 472 (1995) [2.21, 2.211].

Law, *Silent No More: Physicians' Legal and Ethical Obligations to Patients Seeking Abortions*, 21 N.Y.U. Rev. L. & Soc. Change 279, 289, 290, 300 (1994) [3.04, 8.04].

LeBlang, *Obligations of HIV-Infected Health Professionals to Inform Patients of Their Serological Status: Evolving Theories of Liability*, 27 J. Marshall L. Rev. 317, 318 (1994) [9.131].

Lee, *35 U.S.C. § 287(C)—The Physician Immunity Statute*, 79 J. Pat. & Trademark Off. Soc'y 701, 702-04 (1997) [9.095].

Leflar, *Advance Health Care Directives Under Arkansas Law*, 1994 Ark. L. Notes 37, 42. [2.20].

Levine, *Medicalization of Psychoactive Substance Use and the Doctor-Patient Relationship*, 69 Milbank Quarterly 623, 624 (1991) [III].

Levy, *Because Judges Went to Law School, Not Medical School: Restrictive Covenants in the Practices of Law and Medicine*, 30 J. Health & Hosp. L. 89, 92, 101 (1997) [9.02].

Lieberman & Derse, *HIV-Positive Health Care Workers and the Obligation to Disclose: Do Patients Have a Right to Know?*, 13 J. Legal Med. 333, 353, 354, (1992) [8.03, 8.032, 9.131].

Livingston, *When Libido Subverts Credo: Regulation of Attorney-Client Sexual Relations*, 62 Fordham L. Rev. 5, 55 (1993) [8.14].

Loftus, Paddock, & Guernsey, *Patient-Psychotherapist Privilege: Access to Clinical Records in the Tangled Web of Repressed Memory Litigation*, 30 U. Rich L. Rev. 109, 127 (1996) [IV; 5.05].

Lonchyna, *To Resuscitate or Not . . . In the Operating Room: The Need for Hospital Policies for Surgeons Regarding DNR Orders*, 6 Annals Health L. 209, 215, 217 (1997) [2.22, 8.08].

Loue, *Access to Health Care and the Undocumented Alien*, 13 J. Legal Med. 271, 291 (1992) [VI, VII].

Lundmark, *Surgery by an Unauthorized Surgeon as a Battery*, 10 J. L. & Health 287, 293 (1996) [8.16].

MacDonald, *Organ Donation: The Time Has Come to Refocus the Ethical Spotlight*, 8 Stan. L. & Pol'y Rev. 177, 179, 185 (1997) [2.155].

Madow, *Forbidden Spectacle: Executions, the Public and the Press in Nineteenth Century New York*, 43 Buff. L. Rev. 461, 475 (1995) [2.06].

Malinowski, *Capitation, Advances in Medical Technology, and the Advent of a New Era in Medical Ethics*, XXII Am. J. Law & Med. 331, 337 (1996) [2.09].

Malone, *Medical Authority and Infanticide*, 1 J. Law & Health 77 (1985-86) [2.17].

Mancino, *New GCM Suggests Rules for Ventures Between Nonprofit Hospitals and Doctors*, 76 J. Taxation 164, 167 (1992) [8.032].

Mars, *The Corporate Practice of Medicine: A Call for Action*, 7 Heath Matrix 241, 267 (1997) [VI].

Marshall, O'Keefe, Fisher, Caruso, & Surdukowski, *Patients' Fear of Contracting the Acquired Immune Deficiency Syndrome From Physicians*, 150 Arch. Intern. Med. 1501, 1505 (1990) [9.131].

Martin & Bjerknes, *The Legal and Ethical Implications of Gag Clauses in Physician Contracts*, XXII Am. J. Law & Med. 433, 465-66 (1996) [Preamble; II, V, VI, FE(1)].

Martin & Lagod, *The Human Preembryo, the Progenitors, and the State: Toward a Dynamic Theory of Status, Rights, and Research Policy*, 5 High Tech. L. J. 257, 304 (1990) [2.141].

Marzen, *"Out, Out Brief Candle": Constitutionally Prescribed Suicide for the Terminally Ill*, 21 Hastings Const. L.Q. 799, 821 (1994) [2.06, 2.211].

McConnell, *Confidentiality and the Law*, 20 J. Med. Ethics 47, 47 (1994) [IV; FE(4)].

McGonnigal, *This is Who Will Die When Doctors Are Allowed To Kill Their Patients*, 31 J. Marshall L. Rev. 95, 103 (1997) [2.211].

McGuire, *AIDS and the Sexual Offender: The Epidemic Now Poses New Threats to the Victim and the Criminal Justice System*, 96 Dickinson L. Rev. 95, 109, 110 (1991) [5.05].

McIntyre, *Loosening Criteria for Withholding Prehospital Cardiopulmonary Resuscitation*, 153 Arch. Intern. Med. 2189, 2190 (1993) [2.22].

McKnight & Bollis, *Foregoing Life-Sustaining Treatment for Adult Developmentally Disabled, Public Wards: A Proposed Statute*, XVIII Am. J. Law & Med. 203, 206, 220, 227 (1992) [2.20].

McNoble, *The Cruzan Decision—A Surgeon's Perspective*, 20 Memphis State Univ. L. Rev. 569, 581, 600, 601 (1990) [2.20].

Mehlman & Massey, *The Patient-Physician Relationship and the Allocation of Scarce Resources: A Law and Economics Approach*, 4 Kennedy Inst. Ethics J. 291, 292 (1994) [2.09, 2.095].

Mehlman, *Medical Advocates: A Call for a New Profession*, 1 Widener L. Symp. J. 299, 314 (1996) [2.03].

Mehlman, *Rationing Expensive Lifesaving Medical Treatments,* 1985 Wisconsin L. Rev. 239, 250, 260 (1985) [2.03].

Mehlman, *The Patient-Physician Relationship in an Era of Scarce Resources: Is There a Duty to Treat?,* 25 Conn. L. Rev. 349 (1993) [2.09].

Meisel, *A Retrospective on* Cruzan, 20 Law, Med. & Health Care 340, 345 (1992) [2.20].

Meisel, *Barriers to Forgoing Nutrition and Hydration in Nursing Homes,* XXI Am. J. Law & Med. 335, 353-54 (1995) [2.20].

Meisel, *Legal Myths About Terminating Life Support,* 151 Arch. Intern. Med. 1497, 1499 (1991) [2.20].

Meisel, *Lessons from* Cruzan, 1 J. Clinical Ethics 245, 248 (1990) [2.20].

Meisel, *The Legal Consensus About Forgoing Life-Sustaining Treatment: Its Status and Its Prospects,* 2 Kennedy Inst. Ethics J. 309, 325 (1992) [2.20].

Merkatz, *Women in Clinical Trials: An Introduction,* 48 Food & Drug L. J. 161, 163 (1993) [9.122].

Merz, *Psychosocial Risks of Storing and Using Human Tissues in Research,* 8 Risk: Health Safety & Env't 235, 236 (1997) [2.132].

Michalos, *Medical Ethics and the Executing Process in the United States of America,* 16 Med. & Law 125, 131, 133 (1997) [2.06].

Milani, *Better Off Dead Than Disabled?: Should Courts Recognize A "Wrongful Living" Cause of Action When Doctors Fail to Honor Patients' Advance Directives?,* 54 Wash. & Lee L. Rev. 149, 151-52 (1997) [2.22].

Miles, *Medical Futility,* 20 Law, Med. & Health Care 310, 311, 313 (1992) [2.20, 2.21, 2.22].

Miles, *What Are We Teaching About Indigent Patients?,* 268 J.A.M.A. 2561, 2562 (1992) [9.131].

Miller, *Managed Care Regulation: In the Laboratory of the States,* 278 J.A.M.A. 1102, 1104, 1108-09 (1997) [8.13].

Minor, *Identity Cards and Databases in Health Care: The Need for Federal Privacy Protections,* 28 Colum. J.L. & Soc. Probs. 253, 279 (1995) [5.05].

Mishu, Schaffner, Horan, Wood, Hutcheson, & McNabb, *A Surgeon With AIDS: Lack of Evidence of Transmission to Patients,* 264 J.A.M.A. 467 (1990) [9.131].

Mitchell & Scott, *Evidence on Complex Structures of Physician Joint Ventures,* 9 Yale J. Regulation 489, 503 (1992) [8.032].

Mitchell & Scott, *New Evidence of the Prevalence and Scope of Physician Joint Ventures,* 268 J.A.M.A. 80, 84 (1992) [8.032].

Mitchell & Scott, *Physician Ownership of Physical Therapy Services: Effects on Charges, Utilization, Profits, and Service Characteristics,* 268 J.A.M.A. 2055, 2058 (1992) [8.032].

Mitchell & Sunshine, *Consequences of Physicians' Ownership of Health Care Facilities—Joint Ventures in Radiation Therapy,* 327 New Eng. J. Med. 1497, 1500 (1992) [8.032].

Mitten, *Team Physicians and Competitive Athletes: Allocating Legal Responsibility for Athletic Injuries,* 55 U. Pitt. L. Rev. 129, 140 (1993) [3.06].

Modlin, *Forensic Psychiatry and Malpractice,* 18 Bull. Am. Acad. Psychiatry Law 153, 161 (1990) [II, IV].

Morgan & Sutherland, *Last Rights? Confronting Physician-Assisted Suicide in Law and Society: Legal Liturgies on Physician-Assisted Suicide,* 26 Stetson L. Rev. 481, 484 (1996) [2.20, 2.21, 2.211].

Morgan, Marks, & Harty-Golder, *The Issue of Personal Choice: The Competent Incurable Patient and the Right to Commit Suicide?,* 57 Mo. L. Rev. 1, 44, 45 (1992) [2.21, 2.211].

Morreim, *Am I My Brother's Warden? Responding to the Unethical or Incompetent Colleague,* 23 Hastings Center Rep. 19, 23 (May/June 1993) [II; 8.14, 9.031].

Morreim, *Blessed Be the Tie That Binds? Antitrust Perils of Physician Investment and Self-Referral,* 14 J. Legal Med. 359, 367, 374, 377, 394, 409 (1993) [8.032].

Morreim, *Diverse and Perverse Incentives of Managed Care: Bringing Patients into Alignment,* 1 Widener L. Symp. J. 89, 129 (1996) [8.13].

Morreim, *Economic Disclosure and Economic Advocacy: New Duties in the Medical Standard of Care,* 12 J. Legal Med. 275, 306 (1991) [8.08, 8.12].

Morreim, *Patient-Funded Research: Paying the Piper or Protecting the Patient?,* 13 IRB 1, 2 (May/June 1991) [8.031].

Morreim, *Physician Investment and Self-Referral: Philosophical Analysis of a Contentious Debate,* 15 J. Med. & Phil. 425, 428, 429, 430, 431 (1990) [8.032].

Morreim, *Redefining Quality by Reassigning Responsibility,* 20 Am. J. Law & Med. 79, 103 (1994) [Patient Responsibilities (1), (4), (5)].

Mossinghoff, *Remedies Under Patents on Medical and Surgical Procedures*, 78 J. Pat. & Trademark Off. Soc'y 789, 790 (1996) [9.095].

Mullins, *The Need for Guidance in Decisionmaking for Terminally Ill Incompetents: Is the Ohio Legislature in a "Persistent Vegetative State"?*, 17 Ohio No. Univ. L. Rev. 827, 844 (1991) [2.20].

Myers, Sonenshein, & Hofstein, *To Regulate or Not To Regulate Attorney-Client Sex? The Ethical Question in Pennsylvania*, 69 Temp. L. Rev. 741, 780 (1996) [II].

Naccasha, *The Permissibility of Routine AIDS Testing in the Health Care Context*, 5 Notre Dame J.L. Ethics & Pub. Pol'y, 223, 241 (1990) [VI; 9.131].

Napoli, *The Doctrine of Informed Consent and Women: The Achievement of Equal Value and Equal Exercise of Autonomy*, 4 J. Gender & L. 335, 336 (1996) [9.122].

Nelson & Cranford, *Legal Advice, Moral Paralysis and the Death of Samuel Linares*, 17 Law, Med. & Health Care 316 (1989) [2.20].

Newman, *Baby Doe, Congress and the States: Challenging the Federal Treatment Standard for Impaired Infants*, XV Am. J. Law and Med. 1 (1989) [2.17].

Noah, *Death of a Salesman: To What Extent Can the FDA Regulate the Promotional Statements of Pharmaceutical Sales Representatives?*, 47 Food & Drug L. J. 309, 316 (1992) [8.061].

Nodzenski, *HIV-Infected Health Care Professionals and Informed Consent*, 2 S. Cal. Interdisciplinary L. J. 299, 327 (1993) [9.13].

Noonan, *Patenting Medical Technology*, 11 J. Legal Med. 263, 268 (1990) [9.09].

Note, *A Case Study of New Textualism in State Courts: Doe v. Marselle and the Confidentiality of HIV-Related Information*, 30 Conn. L. Rev. 295, 297 (1997) [5.05].

Note, *Administrative Agencies Get Their Way Over Constitutional Rights in Rust v. Sullivan*, 28 Willamette L. Rev. 173, 193 (1991) [8.08].

Note, *Aid-in-Dying: Should We Decriminalize Physician-Assisted Suicide and Physician-Committed Euthanasia?*, XVIII Am. J. Law & Med. 369, 370 (1992) [2.211].

Note, *AIDS: Establishing a Physician's Duty to Warn*, 21 Rutgers L. J. 645, 652 (1990) [5.05].

Note, *Constitutional Aspects of Physician-Assisted Suicide After Lee v. Oregon*, XXIII Am. J. Law & Med. 69 (1997) [2.211].

Note, *Constitutional Law—Judicial Deference—Supreme Court Will Defer to "Reasonable" Abortion Restrictions*, 14 Univ. Ark. Little Rock 557, 573 (1992) [8.08].

Note, *Contingent Expert Witness Fees: Access and Legitimacy*, 64 So. Cal. L. Rev. 1363, 1374, 1382 (1991) [8.04].

Note, *Covenants Not to Compete and Liquidated Damages Clauses: Diagnosis and Treatment for Physicians*, 46 S.C. L. Rev. 505, 514 (1995) [9.02, 9.06].

Note, *Cruzan v. Director, Missouri Department of Health: To Die or Not to Die: That is the Question—But Who Decides?*, 51 Louisiana L. Rev. 1307, 1327, 1333 (1991) [2.20].

Note, *Denial of Coverage for "Experimental" Medical Procedures: The Problem of De Novo Review Under ERISA*, 79 Kentucky L. J. 801, 824 (1990-91) [2.03, 2.09].

Note, *Ethics and AIDS: A Summary of the Law and a Critical Analysis of the Individual Physician's Ethical Duty to Treat*, XVI Am. J. Law & Med. 249, 262 (1990) [VI].

Note, *Exercising the Right to Die: North Carolina's Amended Natural Death Act and the 1991 Health Care Power of Attorney Act*, 70 No. Carolina L. Rev. 2108, 2116 (1992) [2.20].

Note, *Healer-Patient Privilege: Extending the Physician-Patient Privilege to Alternative Health Practitioners in California*, 48 Hastings L. J. 633, 657 (1997) [5.05].

Note, *Health Care Proxies: New York's Attempt to Resolve the Right to Die Dilemma*, 57 Brooklyn L. Rev. 145, 168 (1991) [2.20].

Note, *HIV and Dentistry*, 29 Val. U.L. Rev. 297, 317 (1994) [9.131].

Note, *HMO Exclusion of Chiropractors*, 66 So. Cal. L. Rev. 807, 823 (1993) [3.04].

Note, *I Have A Conscience, Too: The Plight of Medical Personnel Confronting the Right to Die*, 65 Notre Dame L. Rev. 699, 706 (1990) [2.20].

Note, *Informed Choice: Physicians' Duty to Disclose Nonreadily Available Alternatives*, 43 Case W. Res. L. Rev. 491, 491, 498-499, 508, 509 (1993) [I, II, III, IV, V; 8.08].

Note, *Patenting Medical Procedures: A Search for a Compromise Between Ethics and Economics*, 18 Cardozo L. Rev. 1527, 1544, 1547, 1554 (1997) [9.08, 9.09, 9.095].

Note, *Perry v. Louisiana: Medical Ethics on Death Row—Is Judicial Intervention Warranted?*, 4 Georgetown J. Legal Ethics 707, 714 (1991) [2.06].

Note, *Physician-Patient Sexual Contact: The Battle Between the State and the Medical Profession*, 50 Wash. & Lee L. Rev. 1725, 1725-1726, 1734, 1752 (1993) [8.14].

Note, *Physicians, Bound and Gagged: Federal Attempts to Combat Managed Care's Use of Gag Clauses*, 21 Seton Hall Legis. J. 567, 601-02 (1997) [II, V; FE(1); 8.13].

Note, *Preventing Patient Dumping: Sharpening the COBRA's Fangs*, 61 N. Y. U. L. Rev. 1186 (1986) [VI; 8.11].

Note, *Professional Ethics Codes in Court: Redefining the Social Contract Between the Public and the Professions*, 25 Georgia L. Rev. 1327, 1335, 1351 (1991) [II; 2.19].

Note, *Redefining the Right to Die in Illinois*, 15 So. Ill. Univ. L. J. 1261, 1273 (1991) [2.20].

Note, *Restricting Ex Parte Interviews With Nonparty Treating Physicians: Crist v. Moffatt*, 69 No. Carolina L. Rev. 1381, 1391, 1392 (1991) [5.50].

Note, *Rust on the Constitution: Politics and Gag Rules*, 37 How. L. J. 83, 96 (1993) [8.08].

Note, *Sexual Conduct Within the Physician-Patient Relationship: A Statutory Framework for Disciplining this Breach of Fiduciary Duty*, 1 Widener L. Symp. J. 501, 507 (1996) [II; 8.14].

Note, *Something Worth Writing Home About: Clear and Convincing Evidence, Living Wills, and Cruzan v. Director, Missouri Department of Health*, 22 Univ. Toledo L. Rev. 871, 879 (1991) [2.20].

Note, *State Natural Death Acts: Illusory Protection of Individuals' Life-Sustaining Treatment Decisions*, 29 Harvard J. Legis. 175, 186, 194, 195, 201 (1992) [2.20, 2.22].

Note, *Stop Gagging Physicians!*, 7 Health Matrix 187, 193, 200, 208-09 (1997) [8.13].

Note, *The Americans With Disabilities Act: Magic Bullet or Band-Aid for Patients and Health Care Workers Infected With the Human Immunodeficiency Virus?*, 57 Brooklyn L. Rev. 1277, 1279, 1305 (1992) [9.131].

Note, *The Economic Wisdom of Regulating Pharmaceutical "Freebies,"* 1991 Duke L. J. 206, 216, 233, 234 (1991) [8.061, 8.08].

Note, *The Informed-Consent Policy of the International Conference on Harmonization of Technical Requirements for Registrations of Pharmaceuticals for Human Use: Knowledge is the Best Medicine*, 30 Cornell Int'l L. J. 203, 209 (1997) [2.07].

Note, *The New Patent Infringement Liability Exception for Medical Procedures*, 23 J. Legis. 265, 268 (1997) [9.095].

Note, *The Ohio Physician-Patient Privilege: Modified, Revised, and Defined*, 49 Ohio St. L. J. 1147 (1989) [II, IV; 5.05].

Note, *The Policy Against Federal Funding for Abortions Extends Into the Realm of Free Speech After Rust v. Sullivan*, 19 Pepperdine L. Rev. 637, 681 (1992) [8.08].

Note, *Torts: Defining the Duty Imposed on Physicians by the Doctrine of Informed Consent*, 22 Wm. Mitchell L. Rev. 149, 160 (1996) [9.13].

Note, *Toward a More Perfect Union: A Federal Cause of Action for Physician Aid-In-Dying*, 27 U. Mich. J.L. Ref. 521, 538 (1994) [I, III; 2.06].

Note, *Who Decides if There is "Triumph in the Ultimate Agony?" Constitutional Theory and the Emerging Right to Die With Dignity*, 37 Wm. & Mary L. Rev. 827, 829 (1996) [2.20, 2.211].

Obade, *Whisper Down the Lane: AIDS, Privacy, and the Hospital "Grapevine,"* 2 J. Clinical Ethics 133, 133 (1991) [5.05].

Oddi, *Reverse Informed Consent: The Unreasonably Dangerous Patient*, 46 Vand. L. Rev. 1417, 1449, 1463, 1465, 1479 (1993) [IV, VI; 8.11, 9.131].

Olson, *Physician Specialty Advertising: The Tendency to Deceive?*, 11 J. Legal Med. 351, 354 (1990) [5.02].

Oppenheim, *Physicians as Experts Against Their Own Patients? What Happened to the Privilege?*, 63 Def. Couns. J. 254, 257, 261 (1996) [IV; 5.05].

Orentlicher, *Advance Medical Directives*, 263 J.A.M.A. 2365 (1990) [2.20].

Orentlicher, *Denying Treatment to the Noncompliant Patient*, 265 J.A.M.A. 1579, 1581 (1991) [VI; 9.12].

Orentlicher, *Health Care Reform and the Patient-Physician Relationship*, 5 Health Matrix 141, 143, 148 (1995) [FE(5); 5.05].

Orentlicher, *HIV-Infected Surgeons: Behringer v. Medical Center*, 266 J.A.M.A. 1134, 1136 (1991) [8.032, 9.131].

Orentlicher, *Paying Physicians More to Do Less: Financial Incentives to Limit Care*, 30 U. Rich. L. Rev. 155, 167 (1996) [8.13].

Orentlicher, *The Illusion of Patient Choice in End-Of-Life Decisions*, 267 J.A.M.A. 2101, 2102 (1992) [9.121].

Orentlicher, *The Influence of a Professional Organization on Physician Behavior*, 57 Alb. L. Rev. 583, 592, 593, 594, 595, 596 (1994) [1.01, 1.02, 8.061, 9.04, 9.131].

Orentlicher, *The Legalization of Physician Assisted Suicide: A Very Modest Revolution*, 38 B.C.L. Rev. 443, 459-60 (1997) [2.211].

Ornish, Mills, & Ornish, *Prearraignment Forensic Evaluations: Toward a New Policy*, 24 Bull. Am. Acad. Psychiatry Law 453, 454, 469 (1996) [Preamble; IV; 5.05].

O'Shaughnessy, *The Worst of Both Worlds?: Parental Involvement Requirements and the Privacy Rights of Mature Minors*, 57 Ohio St. L. J. 1731, 1764-65 (1996) [2.015].

O'Toole, *HIV-Specific Crime Legislation: Targeting an Epidemic for Criminal Prosecution*, 10 J.L. & Health 183, 195, 199 (1995) [2.23].

Parker, *Corporate Practice of Medicine: Last Stand or Final Downfall?*, 29 J. Health & Hosp. L. 160, 167, 173 (1996) [VI].

Patterson, *Planning for Health Care Using Living Wills and Durable Powers of Attorney: A Guide for the South Carolina Attorney*, 42 So. Carolina L. Rev. 525, 535, 541, 547, 548 (1991) [2.20].

Patton, *A Call for Common Sense: Organ Donation and the Executed Prisoner*, 3 Va. J. Soc. Pol'y & L. 387, 404, 405, 407-10 (1996) [VII; 2.06, 2.162].

Pearlman, Cain, Patrick, Appelbaum-Maizel, Starks, Jecker, & Uhlmann, *Insights Pertaining to Patient Assessments of States Worse than Death*, 4 J. Clinical Ethics 33, 40 (1993) [2.20, 2.21].

Pearson, Kahn, Harrison, Rubenstein, Rogers, Brook, & Keeler, *Differences in Quality of Care for Hospitalized Elderly Men and Women*, 268 J.A.M.A. 1883 (1992) [9.122].

Peccarelli, *A Moral Dilemma: The Role of Judicial Intervention in Withholding or Withdrawing Nutrition and Hydration*, 23 John Marshall L. Rev. 537, 539, 540, 541 (1990) [Preamble; I, II, III, IV, V, VI, VII; 2.20].

Persels, *Forcing the Issue of Physician-Assisted Suicide: Impact of the Kevorkian Case on the Euthanasia Debate*, 14 J. Legal Med. 93, 115 (1993) [2.06, 2.20].

Petrila, *Ethics, Money, and the Problem of Coercion in Managed Behavioral Health Care*, 40 St. Louis U. L. J. 359, 377 (1996) [2.03, 4.04].

Pittman, *"Any Willing Provider" Laws and ERISA's Saving Clause: A New Solution for an Old Problem*, 64 Tenn. L. Rev. 409, 416 (1997) [8.13].

Porter, *Physician Advertising – What is Legal? What is Ethical? What is Acceptable?*, 80 Ohio State Med. J. 437 (1984) [5.02].

Post, Blustein, Gordon, & Dubler, *Pain: Ethics, Culture, and Informed Consent to Relief*, 24 J. Law, Med. & Ethics 348, 349, 356 (1996) [2.20].

Post, *Subsidized Speech*, 106 Yale L. J. 151, 173 (1996) [8.08].

Price, *Between Scylla and Charybdis: Charting a Course to Reconcile the Duty of Confidentiality and the Duty to Warn in the AIDS Context*, 94 Dickinson L. Rev. 435, 477 (1990) [2.23].

Pugno, *Hospital Privileges for Family Physicians: Rights, Rationale, and Resources*, 17 J. Fam. Practice 77 (1983) [9.05].

Quill & Cassel, *Nonabandonment: A Central Obligation for Physicians*, 10 Trends in Health Care, Law & Ethics 25, 27 (Winter/Spring 1995) [8.11].

Quill, Cassel, & Meier, *Care of the Hopelessly Ill: Proposed Clinical Criteria for Physician-Assisted Suicide*, 327 New Eng. J. Med. 1380, 1381 (1992) [2.20].

Quinn, *The Best Interests of Incompetent Patients: The Capacity for Interpersonal Relationships as a Standard for Decisionmaking*, 76 Cal. L. Rev. 897 (1988) [2.20].

Rabeneck, McCullough, & Wray, *Ethically Justified, Clinically Comprehensive Guidelines for Percutaneous Endoscopic Gastrostomy Tube Placement*, 349 Lancet 496, 497, 498 (1997) [2.17].

Regan, *Regulating the Business of Medicine: Models for Integrating Ethics and Managed Care*, 30 Colum. J.L. & Soc. Probs. 635, 651, 656, 657 (1997) [Preamble; I, II, III, IV, V; 8.13].

Reisman, *Physicians and Surgeons as Inventors: Reconciling Medical Process Patents and Medical Ethics*, 10 High Tech. L. J. 355, 356, 368-70, 385 (1995) [VII; 9.08, 9.09, 9.095].

Reiss, *Commentary on Payment and Reimbursement Issues Affecting the Marketing of Drugs, Medical Devices, and Biologics, with Emphasis on the Anti-Kickback Statute and Stark II*, 52 Food & Drug L. J. 99,107 (1997) [8.061].

Relman, *"Self-Referral"—What's at Stake?*, 327 New Eng. J. Med. 1522, 1524 (1992) [8.032].

Rheinstein, *MedWatch: The FDA Medical Products Reporting Program*, 48 Am. Fam. Physician 636, 636 (1993) [9.032].

Rice, *The Superior Orders Defense in Legal Ethics: Sending the Wrong Message to Young Lawyers*, 32 Wake Forest L. Rev. 887, 908-09 (1997) [9.055].

Rich, *The Assault on Privacy on Healthcare Decisionmaking*, 68 Denver L. Rev. 1, 10 (1991) [2.20].

Rie, *The Limits of a Wish*, 21 Hastings Center Rep. 24 (July/August 1991) [2.20].

Risley, *Ethical and Legal Issues in the Individual's Right to Die*, 20 Ohio N.U.L. Rev. 597, 605 (1993) [2.20].

Rivo & Satcher, *Improving Access to Health Care Through Physician Workforce Reform*, 270 J.A.M.A. 1074, 1075 (1993) [9.121].

Roach, *Paradox and Pandora's Box: The Tragedy of Current Right-to-Die Jurisprudence*, 25 Univ. Mich. J. Law Reform 133, 137, 158 (1991) [2.20].

Roberts, Roberts, Warner, Solomon, Hardee, & McCarty, *Internal Medicine, Psychiatry, and Emergency Medicine Residents' Views of Assisted Death Practices*, 157 Arch. Intern. Med. 1603, 1609 (1997) [2.211].

Roberts, *Rust v. Sullivan and the Control of Knowledge*, 61 Geo. Wash. L. Rev. 587, 641 (1993) [8.08].

Robertson, *Dilemma in Danville*, 11 Hastings Center Rep. 5 (Oct. 1981) [2.17].

Robertson, *Prior Agreements for Disposition of Frozen Embryos*, 51 Ohio St. L. J. 407, 419 (1990) [2.141].

Rodwin, *Strains in the Fiduciary Metaphor: Divided Physician Loyalties and Obligations in a Changing Health Care System*, XXI Am. J. Law & Med. 241, 246, 250 (1995) [Preamble; 8.032].

Rosato, *The Ultimate Test of Autonomy: Should Minors Have a Right to Make Decisions Regarding Life-Sustaining Treatment?*, 49 Rutgers L. Rev. 1, 80-81, 82 (1996) [2.20].

Rosner, Cassell, Friedland, Landolt, Loeb, Numann, Ora, Risemberg, & Sordillo, *Ethical Considerations of Reproductive Technologies*, 87 N.Y. State J. Med. 398 (1987) [2.04, 2.05, 2.14, 2.18].

Roth & Levin, *Dilemma of Tarasoff: Must Physicians Protect the Public or Their Patients?*, 11 Law, Med. & Health Care 104 (1983) [IV].

Rothenberg, *Gestational Surrogacy and the Health Care Provider: Put Part of the "IVF Genie" Back Into the Bottle*, 18 Law, Med. & Health Care 345, 346 (1990) [2.18].

Rothenberg, *Who Cares? The Evolution of the Legal Duty to Provide Emergency Care*, 26 Houston L. Rev. 21 (1989) [VI].

Sadoff, *Ethical Obligations for the Psychiatrist: Confidentiality, Privilege, and Privacy in Psychiatric Treatment*, 29 Loy. L.A. L. Rev. 1709, 1710, 1711 (1996) [IV; 5.05].

Sangree, *Control of Childbearing by HIV-Positive Women: Some Responses to Emerging Legal Policies*, 41 Buff. L. Rev. 309, 362 (1993) [8.08].

Sargent, *Treating the Condemned to Death*, 16 Hastings Center Rep. 5 (Dec. 1986) [I; 2.06].

Schiff, *The Lawyer's Role in Restoring Adolescents' Abortion Rights*, 44 Fed. Law. 60, 62 (May 1997) [2.015].

Schlesinger, Gray, & Perreira, *Medical Professionalism under Managed Care: The Pros and Cons of Utilization Review*, 16 Health Affairs 106, 119, 120, 124 (1997) [8.13, 9.031].

Schmid, *Protecting the Physician in HIV Misdiagnosis Cases*, 46 Duke L. J. 431, 458 (1996) [IV].

Schneiderman, Teetzel, & Kalmanson, *Who Decides Who Decides? When Disagreement Occurs Between the Physician and the Patient's Appointed Proxy About the Patient's Decision-Making Capacity*, 155 Arch. Intern. Med. 793, 796 (1995) [2.20].

Schnibbe, *Recent Legislative Developments in Utah Law: Family Law*, 1996 Utah L. Rev. 1335, 1394 (1996) [8.08].

Schoenholtz, Freedman, & Halpern, *The "Legal" Abuse of Physicians in Deaths in the United States: The Erosion of Ethics and Morality in Medicine*, 42 Wayne L. Rev. 1505, 1542 (1996) [2.06].

Schwartz & Gibson, *Defining the Role of the Physician: Medical Education, Tradition, and the Legal Process*, 18 Houston L. Rev. 779 (1981) [IV].

Schwartz, *Privacy and the Economics of Personal Health Care Information*, 76 Tex. L. Rev. 1, 59 (1997) [5.07].

Severyn, *Jacobson v. Massachusetts: Impact on Informed Consent and Vaccine Policy*, 5 J. Pharmacy & L. 249, 253, 274 (1996) [FE(2); 8.08].

Shepherd, *Sophie's Choices: Medical and Legal Responses to Suffering*, 72 Notre Dame L. Rev. 103, 106, 133 (1996) [VI; 2.162].

Shewmon, *Active Voluntary Euthanasia: A Needless Pandora's Box*, 3 Issues in Law and Med. 219 (1987) [2.06, 8.11, 9.06].

Shimm & Spece, *Conflict of Interest and Informed Consent in Industry—Sponsored Clinical Trials*, 12 J. Legal Med. 477, 481, 507, 510 (1991) [8.031].

Shiner, *Medical Futility: A Futile Concept?*, 53 Wash. & Lee L. Rev. 803, 834 (1996) [FE(5)].

Shorr, *AIDS, Judaism, and the Limits of the Secular Society*, 20 Second Opinion 23, 24, 27 (1995) [5.05, 9.131].

Shultz, *From Informed Consent to Patient Choice: A New Protected Interest*, 95 Yale L. J. 219 (1985) [II, IV; 6.02, 8.08].

Sigman, Kraut, & La Puma, *Disclosure of a Diagnosis to Children and Adolescents When Parents Object*, 147 Am. J. Diseases Children 764, 766 (1993) [II].

Silver, *From Baby Doe to Grandpa Doe: The Impact of the Federal Age Discrimination Act on the "Hidden" Rationing of Medical Care*, 37 Catholic Univ. L. Rev. 993 (1988) [2.03].

Simon, *Treatment Boundary Violations: Clinical, Ethical, and Legal Considerations*, 20 Bull. Am. Acad. Psychiatry Law 269, 282 (1992) [6.07].

Sirmon & Kreisberg, *The Invisible Patient*, 334 New Eng. J. Med. 908, 910, 911 (1996) [8.12].

Skiver & Hickey, *AIDS: Legal Issues 1992*, 19 Ohio No. Univ. L. Rev. 839, 860 (1993) [5.05].

Skobeloff, Spivey, St. Clair, & Schoffstall, *The Influence of Age and Sex on Asthma Admissions*, 268 J.A.M.A. 3437, 3439, 3440 (1992) [9.122].

Smith, *Legal Recognition of Neocortical Death*, 71 Cornell L. Rev. 850 (1986) [2.20].

Smith, *Murder, She Wrote or Was It Merely Selective Nontreatment?*, 8 J. Contemp. Health L. & Pol'y 49, 53 (1992) [2.17, 2.20].

Smith, *Our Hearts Were Once Young and Gay: Health Care Rationing and the Elderly*, 8 U. Fla. J.L. & Pub. Pol'y 1, 21 (1996) [2.09].

Snyder, *Artificial Feeding and the Right to Die: The Legal Issues*, 9 J. Legal Med. 349 (1988) [2.20].

Solomon & Asaro, *Community-Based Health Care: A Legal and Policy Analysis*, 24 Fordham Urb. L. J. 235, 276-77 (1997) [FE(6); 9.065].

Sprung, *Changing Attitudes and Practices in Forgoing Life-Sustaining Treatments*, 263 J.A.M.A. 2211, 2213 (1990) [2.20].

Steinbrook & Lo, *Artificial Feeding—Solid Ground, Not a Slippery Slope*, 318 New Eng. J. Med. 286 (1988) [2.20].

Stone & Winslade, *Physician-Assisted Suicide and Euthanasia in the United States: Legal and Ethical Observations*, 16 J. Legal Med. 481, 483, 490, 497, 498, 499 (1995) [III, IV, VI; 2.20, 2.21, 8.11, 9.12].

Sulmasy, Geller, Faden, & Levine, *The Quality of Mercy: Caring for Patients With "Do Not Resuscitate" Orders*, 267 J.A.M.A. 682 (1992) [2.22].

Swedlow, Johnson, Smithline, & Milstein, *Increased Costs and Rates of Use in the California Workers' Compensation System as a Result of Self-Referral By Physicians*, 327 New Eng. J. Med. 1502 (1992) [8.032].

Szczygiel, *Beyond Informed Consent*, 21 Ohio N.U.L. Rev. 171, 217, 218, 220, 225, 226, 256 (1994) [Preamble; I, II, III, IV, V, VI; FE(1), (2); 1.01, 1.02, 8.08].

Tabor, *The Battle for Hospital Privileges*, 251 J.A.M.A. 1602 (1984) [9.05].

Tarantino, *Withdrawal of Life Support: Conflict Among Patient Wishes, Family, Physicians, Courts and Statutes, and the Law*, 42 Buff. L. Rev. 623, 638, 639, 646 (1994) [2.20].

Taub, *Withholding Treatment From Defective Newborns*, 10 Law, Med. & Health Care 4 (Feb. 1982) [2.17].

Thomasma, *When Physicians Choose to Participate in the Death of Their Patients: Ethics and Physician-Assisted Suicide*, 24 J. Law, Med. & Ethics 183, 184, 195 (1996) [2.211].

Thompson, *Understanding Financial Conflicts of Interest*, 329 New Eng. J. Med. 573 (1993) [8.032].

Truog & Brennan, *Participation of Physicians in Capital Punishment*, 329 New Eng. J. Med. 1346 (1993) [2.06].

Turkington, *Medical Record Confidentiality Law, Scientific Research, and Data Collection in the Information Age,* 25 J. Law, Med. & Ethics 113, 126 (1997) [IV].

Underwood & Cadle, *Genetics, Genetic Testing, and the Specter of Discrimination: A Discussion Using Hypothetical Cases,* 85 Ky. L. J. 665, 684 (1996-97) [2.12].

Veatch, *Abandoning Informed Consent,* 25 Hastings Center Rep. 5, 6 (March/April 1995) [8.08].

Virmani, Schneiderman, & Kaplan, *Relationship of Advance Directives to Physician-Patient Communication,* 154 Arch. Intern. Med. 909, 913 (1994) [2.20].

Wallace, *Incompetency for Execution: The Supreme Court Challenges the Ethical Standards of the Mental Health Professions,* 8 J. Legal Med. 265 (1987) [2.06].

Waller & Fulton, *The Electronic Chart; Keeping it Confidential and Secure,* 26 J. Health & Hosp. L. 104, 105 (April 1993) [IV; 5.07].

Walters & Ashwal, *Organ Prolongation in Anencephalic Infants: Ethical and Medical Issues,* 18 Hastings Center Rep. 19 (Oct./Nov. 1988) [2.20].

Walzer, *Impaired Physicians: An Overview and Update of the Legal Issues,* 11 J. Legal Med. 131, 174, 192 (1990) [IV; 4.07].

Wanzer, Federman, Adelstein, Cassel, Cassem, Cranford, Hook, Lo, Moertel, Safar, Stone, & Van Eys, *The Physician's Responsibility Toward Hopelessly Ill Patients: A Second Look,* 320 New Eng. J. Med. 844 (1989) [2.20].

Watson, *Medicaid Physician Participation: Patients, Poverty, and Physician Self-Interest,* XXI Am. J. Law & Med. 191, 218 (1995) [VI].

Weiner & Wettstein, *Confidentiality of Patient-Related Information,* 112 Arch. Ophthalmology 1032, 1033 (1994) [IV; FE(4)].

Weinstock, Leong, & Silva, *Opinions by AAPL Forensic Psychiatrists on Controversial Ethical Guidelines: A Survey,* 19 Bull. Am. Acad. Psychiatry Law 237, 238 (1991) [1.02, 5.09].

Weir & Gostin, *Decisions to Abate Life-Sustaining Treatment for Nonautonomous Patients: Ethical Standards and Legal Liability for Physicians After Cruzan,* 264 J.A.M.A. 1846, 1849, 1850 (1990) [2.20].

Wentz, Osteen, & Gannon, *Continuing Medical Education: Unabated Debate,* 268 J.A.M.A. 1118 (1992) [8.061, 9.011].

Wentz, Osteen, & Gannon, *Refocusing Support and Direction,* 266 J.A.M.A. 953 (1991) [8.061, 9.011].

Westfall, McCabe, & Nicholas, *Personal Use of Drug Samples by Physicians and Office Staff,* 278 J.A.M.A. 141, 142 (1997) [8.061].

Wolf, *Health Care Reform and the Future of Physician Ethics,* 24 Hastings Center Rep. 28, 32, 40 (March/April 1994) [2.03, 2.09, 4.04, 5.01, 8.03, 9.121, 9.122].

Woodward, *Medical Record Confidentiality and Data Collection: Current Dilemmas,* 25 J. Law, Med. & Ethics 88, 90, 95 (1997) [5.07].

Zwirn, *Professionalism, Mental Disability, and the Death Penalty,* 41 N.Y.L Sch. L. Rev. 163, 165 (1996) [2.06].